Exotic Animal Clinical Pathology

Editors

J. JILL HEATLEY
KAREN E. RUSSELL

VETERINARY CLINICS OF NORTH AMERICA: EXOTIC ANIMAL PRACTICE

www.vetexotic.theclinics.com

Consulting Editor
JÖRG MAYER

September 2022 • Volume 25 • Number 3

ELSEVIER

1600 John F. Kennedy Boulevard • Suite 1800 • Philadelphia, Pennsylvania, 19103-2899
http://www.vetexotic.theclinics.com

VETERINARY CLINICS OF NORTH AMERICA: EXOTIC ANIMAL PRACTICE Volume 25, Number 3
September 2022 ISSN 1094-9194, ISBN-13: 978-0-323-84985-2

Editor: Stacy Eastman
Developmental Editor: Axell Ivan Jade M. Purificacion

Photocopying

Single photocopies of single articles may be made for personal use as allowed by national copyright laws. Permission of the Publisher and payment of a fee is required for all other photocopying, including multiple or systematic copying, copying for advertising or promotional purposes, resale, and all forms of document delivery. Special rates are available for educational institutions that wish to make photocopies for non-profit educational classroom use. For information on how to seek permission visit www.elsevier.com/permissions or call: (+44) 1865 843830 (UK)/(+1) 215 239 3804 (USA).

Derivative Works

Subscribers may reproduce tables of contents or prepare lists of articles including abstracts for internal circulation within their institutions. Permission of the Publisher is required for resale or distribution outside the institution. Permission of the Publisher is required for all other derivative works, including compilations and translations (please consult www.elsevier.com/permissions).

Electronic Storage or Usage

Permission of the Publisher is required to store or use electronically any material contained in this periodical, including any article or part of an article (please consult www.elsevier.com/permissions). Except as outlined above, no part of this publication may be reproduced, stored in a retrieval system or transmitted in any form or by any means, electronic, mechanical, photocopying, recording or otherwise, without prior written permission of the Publisher.

Notice

No responsibility is assumed by the Publisher for any injury and/or damage to persons or property as a matter of products liability, negligence or otherwise, or from any use or operation of any methods, products, instructions or ideas contained in the material herein. Because of rapid advances in the medical sciences, in particular, independent verification of diagnoses and drug dosages should be made.

Although all advertising material is expected to conform to ethical (medical) standards, inclusion in this publication does not constitute a guarantee or endorsement of the quality or value of such product or of the claims made of it by its manufacturer.

Veterinary Clinics of North America: Exotic Animal Practice (ISSN 1094-9194) is published in January, May, and September by Elsevier, Inc., 360 Park Avenue South, New York, NY 10010-1710. Subscription prices are $296.00 per year for US individuals, $697.00 per year for US institutions, $100.00 per year for US students and residents, $345.00 per year for Canadian individuals, $707.00 per year for Canadian institutions, $359.00 per year for international individuals, $707.00 per year for international institutions, $100.00 per year Canadian students/residents, and $165.00 per year for international students/residents. To receive student/resident rate, orders must be accompanied by name of affiliated institution, date of term, and the *signature* of program/residency coordinator on institution letterhead. Orders will be billed at individual rate until proof of status is received. Foreign air speed delivery is included in all *Clinics* subscription prices. All prices are subject to change without notice. **POSTMASTER:** Send address changes to *Veterinary Clinics of North America: Exotic Animal Practice*, Elsevier Health Sciences Division, Subscription Customer Service, 3251 Riverport Lane, Maryland Heights, MO 63043. **Customer Service: Telephone: 1-800-654-2452** (U.S. and Canada); **1-314-447-8871** (outside U.S. and Canada). **Fax: 1-314-447-8029. E-mail: journalscustomerservice-usa@ elsevier.com (for print support); journalsonlinesupport-usa@elsevier.com (for online support).**

Reprints. For copies of 100 or more of articles in this publication, please contact the Commercial Reprints Department, Elsevier Inc., 360 Park Avenue South, New York, New York 10010-1710. Tel.: 212-633-3874; Fax: 212-633-3820; E-mail: reprints@elsevier.com.

Veterinary Clinics of North America: Exotic Animal Practice is covered in *MEDLINE/PubMed (Index Medicus).*

Contributors

CONSULTING EDITOR

JÖRG MAYER, Dr med vet, Msc
Diplomate, American Board of Veterinary Practitioners (Exotic Companion Mammals); Diplomate, European College of Zoological Medicine (Small Mammals); Diplomate, American College of Zoological Medicine; Associate Professor of Zoological Medicine, Department of Small Animal Medicine and Surgery, University of Georgia College of Veterinary Medicine, Athens, Georgia

EDITORS

J. JILL HEATLEY, DVM, MS
Diplomate, American Board of Veterinary Practitioners (Avian, Reptilian, Amphibian); Diplomate, American College of Zoological Medicine; Associate Professor, Zoological Medicine, Department of Small Animal Clinical Sciences, College of Veterinary Medicine and Biomedical Sciences, Texas A&M University, College Station, Texas

KAREN E. RUSSELL, DVM, PhD
American College of Veterinary Pathologists (Clinical Pathology), Professor and Associate Department Head for Clinical Services and Residency Programs, Department of Veterinary Pathobiology, College of Veterinary Medicine and Biomedical Sciences, Texas A&M University, College Station, Texas

AUTHORS

LAURA ADAMOVICZ, DVM, PhD
Wildlife Epidemiology Laboratory, University of Illinois, College of Veterinary Medicine, Urbana, Illinois

MATTHEW C. ALLENDER, DVM, MS, PhD
Diplomate, American College of Zoological Medicine; Wildlife Epidemiology Laboratory, University of Illinois, College of Veterinary Medicine, Urbana, Illinois

HUGUES BEAUFRÈRE, DVM, PhD
Diplomate, American College of Zoological Medicine; Diplomate, American Board of Veterinary Practitioners (Avian); Diplomate, European College of Zoological Medicine (Avian); Associate Professor, Department of Veterinary Epidemiology and Medicine, School of Veterinary Medicine, University of California, Davis, Davis, California

JOÃO BRANDÃO, LMV, MS
Diplomate, European College of Zoological Medicine (Avian); Department of Veterinary Clinical Sciences, College of Veterinary Medicine, Oklahoma State University, Stillwater, Oklahoma

CLARK BROUGHTON, DVM
Clinical Pathology Resident, Department of Veterinary Pathobiology, Texas A&M College of Veterinary Medicine & Biomedical Sciences, College Station, Texas

SATHYA K. CHINNADURAI, DVM, MS
Diplomate, American College of Zoological Medicine; Diplomate, American College of Veterinary Anesthesia and Analgesia; Diplomate, American College of Animal Welfare; Director of Animal Health, Department of Animal Health, Saint Louis Zoo, St Louis, Missouri; Senior Vice President of Animal Health and Welfare, Chicago Zoological Society, Brookfield, Illinois

LINN CLARIZIO, DVM
Kansas State University, College of Veterinary Medicine, Manhattan, Kansas State

SABRINA D. CLARK, DVM, PhD, MRCVS
Diplomate, American College of Veterinary Pathologists (Clinical Pathology); Global Dx Digital Cytopathology, Zoetis, Inc, Parsippany, New Jersey

CHARLES O. CUMMINGS, DVM, Postdoctoral Fellow
Tufts Clinical and Translational Science Institute, Tufts Medical Center, Boston, Massachusetts

ARMELLE DELAFORCADE, DVM
Diplomate, American College of Veterinary Emergency Critical Care; Associate Professor, Department of Clinical Sciences, Cummings School of Veterinary Medicine at Tufts University, North Grafton, Massachusetts

RICHARD DULLI, DVM
Clinical Pathology Resident, Department of Veterinary Pathobiology, College of Veterinary Medicine and Biomedical Sciences, Texas A&M University, College Station, Texas

JESSICA EISENBARTH, DVM
Department of Clinical Sciences, Cummings School of Veterinary Medicine at Tufts University, North Grafton, Massachusetts

SUSAN FIELDER, DVM, MS
Diplomate, American College of Veterinary Pathologist (Clinical Pathology); Department of Pathobiology, College of Veterinary Medicine, Oklahoma State University, Stillwater, Oklahoma

J. JILL HEATLEY, DVM, MS
Diplomate, American Board of Veterinary Practitioners (Avian, Reptilian, Amphibian); Diplomate, American College of Zoological Medicine; Associate Professor, Zoological Medicine, Department of Small Animal Clinical Sciences, College of Veterinary Medicine and Biomedical Sciences, Texas A&M University, College Station, Texas

SARRAH KAYE, DVM
Diplomate, American College of Zoological Medicine; Staten Island Zoo, Staten Island, New York

JANE MERKEL, RVT, MS, VTS (Zoo)
Zoological Manager, Department of Animal Health, Saint Louis Zoo, St Louis, Missouri

CHERYL MOLLER, BSc, BVMS, MS
Diplomate, American College of Veterinary Pathologists (Clinical); ANTECH Diagnostics, Fountain Valley, California

MICHAEL F. ROSSER, DVM, MS
Diplomate, American College of Veterinary Pathologists (Clinical Pathology); Department of Veterinary Clinical Medicine and Veterinary Diagnostic Laboratory, College of Veterinary Medicine, University of Illinois at Urbana-Champaign, Urbana, Illinois

AMY N. SCHNELLE, DVM, MS
Diplomate, American College of Veterinary Pathologists; Clinical Assistant Professor, Veterinary Diagnostic Laboratory, University of Illinois, College of Veterinary Medicine, Urbana, Illinois

ANDREA SIEGEL, DVM
Diplomate, American College of Veterinary Pathologists (Clinical Pathology); Veterinary Clinical Pathologist, IDEXX Laboratories, Inc, New York, New York

NORA L. SPRINGER, DVM, PhD
Diplomate, American College of Veterinary Pathologists; University of Tennessee College of Veterinary Medicine, Knoxville, Tennessee

TRACY STOKOL, BVSc, PhD
Diplomate, American College of Veterinary Pathologists; Cornell University, Ithaca, New York

RAQUEL M. WALTON, VMD, MS, PhD
Diplomate, American College of Veterinary Pathologists (Clinical Pathology); Veterinary Clinical Pathologist, IDEXX Laboratories, Inc, Philadelphia, Pennsylvania

KYLE LAUREN WEBB, DVM
Diplomate, American College of Veterinary Pathologists (Clinical Pathology); Antech Diagnostics, Orlando, Florida

TREVOR T. ZACHARIAH, DVM, MS
Diplomate, American College of Zoological Medicine; Brevard Zoo, Melbourne, Florida

Contents

Comparative Utility of Select Diagnostics for Exotic Animals

The synthesis of bile acids occurs during the degradation of cholesterol in hepatocytes. Thus, this analyte is expected to be a sensitive indicator of hepatocellular dysfunction or alterations in portal circulation. Bile acids can be quantified via an enzymatic reaction to a highly conserved moiety across species. The evidence for the clinical utility of bile acids for the diagnosis of liver disease is strongest in birds and ferrets with equivocal evidence in rodents, rabbits, and reptiles. Current limitations to the interpretation of bile acids in exotic animal species include a paucity of species-specific reference intervals and incomplete understanding of bile acid metabolism in nonmammalian species and the diversity of bile acids synthesized by vertebrates.

Monitoring blood lactate concentrations with a handheld, point-of-care (POC) meter is an efficient and inexpensive method of monitoring critically ill or anesthetized exotic patients. Serial monitoring of lactate allows early recognition of hypoperfusion, allowing for prompt implementation of resuscitative efforts. Reference ranges for exotic animals are currently sparse and often gathered from field studies of wild animals. In the absence of reference ranges, extrapolations can be made regarding mammals and birds, but may be more difficult in reptiles and amphibians.

Whole blood viscoelastic coagulation testing (VCT) allows global assessment of hemostasis and fibrinolysis. Although not widely used in exotic animal practice, VCT has been used in exotic animal research settings. Differences in patient demographics and analytical variables can result in dramatically different results with the same analyzer. To improve the utility of VCT in exotic animal medicine, standardization of protocols is necessary to facilitate the establishment of reference intervals. Despite these challenges, the quantitative/qualitative nature of VCT has already proved its real-world value to some clinicians.

The mammalian hemostatic system is highly conserved, and companion exotic mammals are commonly used as biomedical models for normal and disordered hemostasis. Challenges associated with sample collection, test validation, and test interpretation have limited the use of these tests in clinical exotic animal practice. However, evaluation of platelet counts, coagulation screening times, and fibrin(ogen) degradation products can be valuable for monitoring exotic patients with a range of disease presentations including intoxications, anemia, systemic viral disease, hepatopathy, and endocrinopathy.

Endocrine disease in exotic species is less common than in small animals. Nevertheless, the diagnostic principles used in small animals can be adapted to evaluate endocrine disease in many of the exotic species although species-specific aspects need to be considered. This article covers important diseases such as thyroid dysfunction in reptiles and birds, hyperthyroidism in guinea pigs, and hyperadrenocorticism in ferrets. Glucose metabolism in neoplasms affecting normal physiology, such as insulinoma in ferrets and gastric neuroendocrine carcinoma in bearded dragons, is discussed. Calcium abnormalities, including metabolic bone disease in reptiles and hypocalcemia in birds, are also covered.

Digitization has enhanced the utility of cytology in private practice by allowing for rapid sample receipt and analysis, leading to better informed real-time patient care. Despite many advantages of digital cytology, understanding its limitations is required to avoid common pitfalls. A strong foundation in sample preparation and imaging techniques is also required to obtain high-quality diagnostic samples. By optimizing these factors, the benefits of digital cytology are maximized, allowing for the practice of high-quality point-of-care medicine that best addresses the needs of the patient and pet owner in a rapid time frame.

Select Avian Diagnostic Analytes

Inflammation represents a fundamental response to diverse diseases ranging from trauma and infection to immune-mediated disease and neoplasia. As such, inflammation can be a nonspecific finding but is valuable as an indicator of pathology that can itself lead to disease if left unchecked. This article focuses on inflammatory biomarkers that are available and clinically useful in avian species. Inflammatory biomarkers are identified via evaluation of whole blood and plasma and can be divided into acute and chronic, with varying degrees of specificity and sensitivity.

Evaluation of multiple biomarkers may be necessary to identify subclinical disease.

Hugues Beaufrère

Lipids are the main biomolecular constituents of plasma and occupy a central place in the pathophysiology of several common diseases of parrots. Dyslipidemias frequently occur in psittacine birds in relation to a variety of lipid accumulation disorders and female reproductive disorders. The five main lipid classes in the plasma are sterols, fatty acyls, glycerolipids, glycerophospholipids, and sphingolipids. Most lipids are transported in the blood within lipoproteins. Lipidologic diagnostic tests to characterize dyslipidemias and risk factors of lipid disorders include routine biochemical tests such as cholesterol and triglycerides, lipoprotein testing, and newer comprehensive techniques to assess whole lipid pathways using lipidomics.

Clinical Pathology Diagnostic Overviews for Select Reptile Species

Clark Broughton and Kyle Lauren Webb

The bearded dragon (Pogona vitticeps), an omnivorous Agamid lizard native to inland Australia, is one of the most popular reptile pets due to their sociable behavior, tame demeanor, low-maintenance care, and relative ease of breeding. Because they are generally stoic animals, thorough physical examination in conjunction with routine clinicopathologic data can prove invaluable in identifying disease and implementing appropriate therapy in a timely manner. The goal of this article is to assist the practicing clinician, based on literature review, on how to approach the diagnostic challenge encountered in everyday practice when working up various conditions in bearded dragons.

Laura Adamovicz and Matthew C. Allender

Box turtles are commonly presented for veterinary care and clinicopathologic testing is a vital component of case management. This article summarizes recent literature about box turtle clinical pathology and identifies directions for future research.

Cheryl Moller and J. Jill Heatley

Clinicopathologic evaluation of terrestrial tortoises is useful for health assessment and monitoring. There are specific considerations when evaluating data from these species, including sex, age, time of year/season, reproductive status, diet, captive versus wild, geographic location, methodology, and anticoagulant. The authors describe sample collection, hematology, biochemistry, and urinalysis features of terrestrial tortoises and discuss clinical relevance.

Michael F. Rosser

Freshwater turtles are physiologically unique in their adaptations to life on both land and freshwater habitats. Appropriate interpretation of laboratory values specific to these species is important for both conservation efforts in free-ranging populations and in captive populations, especially because these animals become increasingly popular as pets. Although normal physiology has been well characterized, understanding of clinicopathologic changes in response to disease processes in freshwater chelonian species is relatively limited. This article reviews the current knowledge of hematology, plasma biochemistry, and urinalysis specific to freshwater turtles, with correlates to other chelonian species when specific data are unavailable.

Amy N. Schnelle

Hematology and biochemistry testing of boas and pythons is a valuable topic for practicing clinicians and researchers alike. This article reviews blood cell morphology (with accompanying images) and reviews the literature for hematologic and biochemical material clinically relevant to the families Boidae and Pythonidae.

VETERINARY CLINICS OF NORTH AMERICA: EXOTIC ANIMAL PRACTICE

SERIES OF RELATED INTEREST

Veterinary Clinics of North America: Small Animal Practice
Available at: https://www.vetsmall.theclinics.com/

THE CLINICS ARE NOW AVAILABLE ONLINE!
Access your subscription at:
www.theclinics.com

Preface

Somethings Old with Somethings New

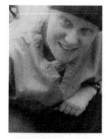 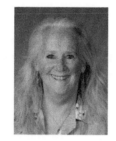

J. Jill Heatley, DVM, MS   Karen E. Russell, DVM, PhD
Editors

We are excited to present another fine issue of the *Veterinary Clinics of North America: Exotic Animal Practice* series. This issue focuses on clinical pathology: diagnostic testing and test interpretation. As you will see, the topics cover a wide range of subject matter and a variety of different species that include, but are not limited to, small mammals; psittacines and other avian species; tortoises, box turtles, and aquatic turtles; bearded lizards and snakes; and other exotic animal species. Some of the articles, such as bile acids, inflammatory markers, lactate, endocrine testing, and hemostatic testing, present information about diagnostic testing and test interpretation that have been available and in use for quite some time. These articles offer a comprehensive review and present current and new information about each respective topic. Other articles discuss newer diagnostic modalities that are becoming more available; these include viscoelastic coagulation testing, blood lipid diagnostics, and digital cytology. Finally, this issue includes several articles that discuss general clinical pathology of species that are becoming more and more popular as pets, such as bearded dragons, box turtles, and tortoises.

In this issue, we have enlisted experts from around the world to share their knowledge in clinical pathologic diagnostic testing and test interpretation in a variety of exotic species. The authors of these articles represent veterinarians and researchers with expertise in internal medicine, zoo medicine, and clinical pathology. In many of the articles, clinicians are partnered with clinical pathologists to bring to you practical and up-to-date information about the use and interpretation of laboratory testing. We sincerely thank all of the authors for their time and willingness to contribute to this issue. They have made this issue what it is.

Although each article contains a wealth of information, you will see an overlying and recurrent theme. There remains a substantial lack of peer-reviewed information for diagnostic testing and interpretation in many of these species; hence more studies

Vet Clin Exot Anim 25 (2022) xiii–xiv
https://doi.org/10.1016/j.cvex.2022.07.001
1094-9194/22/© 2022 Published by Elsevier Inc.

vetexotic.theclinics.com

are desperately needed. Nevertheless, the authors are all to be commended for not only the useful but also the most up-to-date information provided. We hope that you will not only enjoy but also learn from their expertise. We also hope that this may entice some of our readers to consider advancing the knowledge in the subject matter through future studies and research.

In conclusion, we would also like to thank the folks at Elsevier for their support and guidance throughout this process. It has been a great pleasure to have this opportunity.

J. Jill Heatley, DVM, MS
Department of Small Animal Clinical Sciences
College of Veterinary Medicine and
Biomedical Sciences
Texas A&M University
College Station, TX 77843, USA

Karen E. Russell, DVM, PhD
Department of Veterinary Pathobiology
College of Veterinary Medicine &
Biomedical Sciences
Texas A&M University
TAMU-CVM Clinical Pathology
Building 1085, Room 2020
College Station, TX 77843-4457, USA

E-mail addresses:
jheatley@cvm.tamu.edu (J.J. Heatley)
krussell@cvm.tamu.edu (K.E. Russell)

I. Comparative Utility of Select Diagnostics for Exotic Animals

The Utility of Bile Acids for the Diagnosis of Liver Disease in Exotic Animals

Linn Clarizio, DVM[a],*, Nora L. Springer, DVM, PhD, DACVP[b],
Trevor T. Zachariah, DVM, MS, DACZM[c]

KEYWORDS

- Bile acids • Liver • Biochemistry • Avian • Reptile • Amphibian • Small mammals

KEY POINTS

- Measurement of bile acids might aid in the diagnosis of the identification of hepatocellular dysfunction or alterations in portal circulation.
- Enzymatic methods for bile acid quantification are preferred to immunologic methods in veterinary species.
- Bile acids measurement is recommended in birds and ferrets as a standard assessment of liver health, whereas bile acids utility is equivocal in many small mammals and reptiles.

INTRODUCTION

Bile is an excretory and secretory fluid composed of mostly water with numerous dissolved solutes including bile salts, bilirubin and/or biliverdin, phospholipids, and inorganic ions among others. As an excretory fluid, bile is important for the elimination of waste products such as cholesterol, bilirubin, and metabolized xenobiotics. As a secretory fluid, bile is essential for the emulsification and absorption of lipids. Bile is also involved in the secretion of buffers to neutralize the acidic pH from gastric contents entering the duodenum and secretion of IgA for protection against gastrointestinal infections.

Bile acids and/or bile alcohols are derived from cholesterol and make up approximately 85% of the solids found in biliary secretions.[1] These organic molecules are found in all vertebrates and have been used in understanding evolutionary relationships between various taxa.[2] Bile acids carry a carboxyl group in the side chain, as opposed to bile alcohols that carry a hydroxyl group in the side chain. Both bile acids and bile alcohols are classified by the total number of carbon atoms and the number

[a] Kansas State University, College of Veterinary Medicine, 1800 Denison Avenue, Manhattan, KS 66506, USA; [b] University of Tennessee College of Veterinary Medicine, 2407 River Drive, Knoxville, TN 37996, USA; [c] Brevard Zoo, 8225 North Wickham Road, Melbourne, FL 32940, USA
* Corresponding author.
E-mail address: linn.clarizio@gmail.com

Vet Clin Exot Anim 25 (2022) 563–584
https://doi.org/10.1016/j.cvex.2022.05.001
1094-9194/22/© 2022 Elsevier Inc. All rights reserved.

and position of hydroxyl groups added to the "parent cholesterol" steroid nucleus and side chain (**Fig. 1**).[2,3]

Bile acids consisting of 24 carbons (C24 bile acids) are the predominant class of bile acids in people and many mammals, thus, the current understanding of bile acid synthesis and enterohepatic circulation is based on research from C24 bile acids in mammals.[4] In some reptiles, birds, and amphibians, bile acids consist of 27 carbons (C27 bile acids), whereas C27 bile alcohols predominate in few evolutionarily ancient mammals (elephant, manatee, hyrax, rhinoceros).[4] Although C24 bile acids occur in varying proportions in reptiles, birds, and boney fish, relatively little is known about the enterohepatic circulation of bile acids in nonmammalian species.[4,5] While the overall structural composition between species is known for its great diversity, methodology used by most current clinical laboratory diagnostics relies on the enzymatic identification of a well-conserved 3α-hydroxyl group present in many vertebrates.[2]

Biologic Function of Bile Acids

Bile acids are a key source of cholesterol elimination. Biosynthesis of bile acids is an important contributor to stimulating bile flow through the biliary system. Additionally, bile acids have several signaling properties, including providing negative feedback for their biosynthesis and activation of binding proteins needed for enterohepatic transport.[6,7] Bile acids are amphipathic molecules (ie, there is a polar and nonpolar surface) that are essential for the digestion and absorption of dietary fats and oils. The same physical properties that facilitate the breakdown of dietary lipids also negatively impact the ability of bile acids to solubilize normal cell membranes when they accumulate in the liver and other organs.[8]

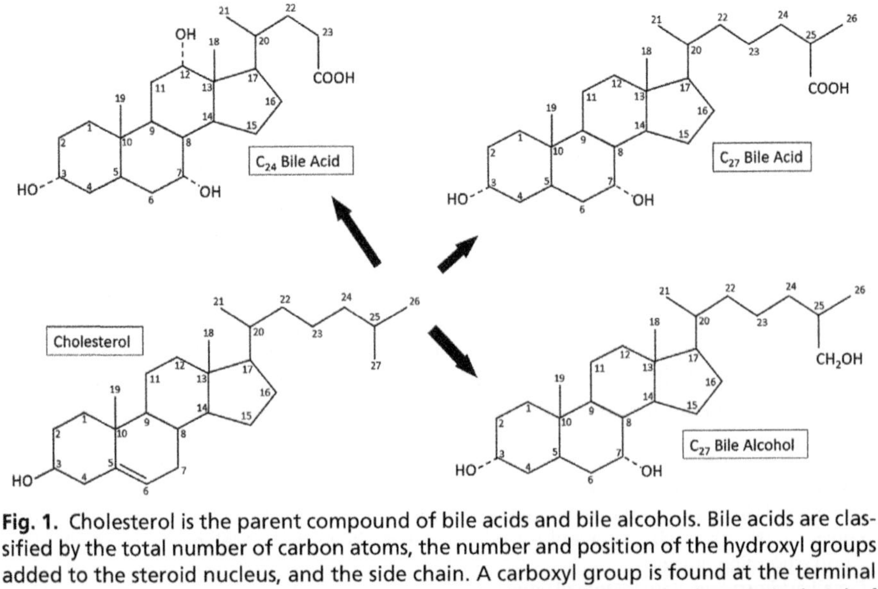

Fig. 1. Cholesterol is the parent compound of bile acids and bile alcohols. Bile acids are classified by the total number of carbon atoms, the number and position of the hydroxyl groups added to the steroid nucleus, and the side chain. A carboxyl group is found at the terminal end of the side chain in bile acids in contrast to the hydroxyl group at the terminal end of the side chain in bile alcohols. Enzymatic assays used for bile acid quantification in current clinical laboratory diagnostics detect the α-hydroxyl moiety on the third carbon of the steroid nucleus.

Bile Acid Synthesis and Elimination

The synthesis of primary bile acids is the primary metabolic pathway for the break-down of insoluble cholesterol into a water-soluble waste product (**Fig. 2**).[7] Primary bile acids are synthesized by hepatocytes via multiple complex enzymatic steps and conjugated to glycine and/or taurine. Conjugation is an important step that converts a newly formed weak acid into a strong acid, enabling bile acids to exist as ionized anions (termed "bile salts") that cannot be passively absorbed into biliary and intestinal epithelial cells.[9,10] In mammals, conjugation of bile acids with glycine is more frequent with a smaller proportion conjugated to taurine, whereas conjugation to taurine is more common in nonmammals.[2]

Most bile salts are absorbed in the ileum by active transport systems. Transformation of the primary bile acid structure occurs in the distal intestine from bacterial enzymes. Deconjugated bile acids in the distal ileum and colon are also absorbed by the portal venous system.[7] Additional bacterial modifications, specifically alterations

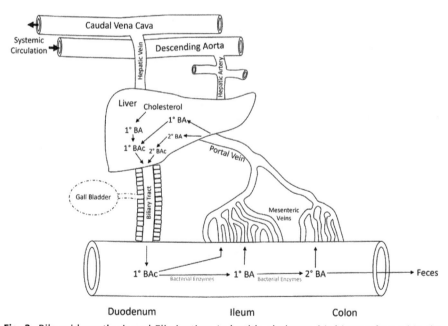

Fig. 2. Bile acids synthesis and Elimination. In health, cholesterol is biotransformed in the liver into primary bile acids (1° BA) and conjugated to an amino acid (commonly glycine or taurine). Conjugated primary bile acids (1° Bac) enter the biliary tract and ultimately secreted into the duodenum. Conjugated primary bile acids have fates in the intestine. The majority of conjugated primary bile acids are efficiently resorbed in the ileum and enter portal circulation whereby they are taken up by the liver and reenter the biliary tract for recycling. Alternatively, conjugated primary bile acids may be deconjugated by bacterial enzymes resulting in unconjugated primary bile acids, which may also be resorbed via portal circulation. Upon uptake by hepatocytes, these unconjugated primary bile acids are then re-conjugated and enter the biliary tract for recycling. Unconjugated primary bile acids may also undergo further transformation via bacterial enzymes into secondary bile acids (2° BA) in the colon. Secondary bile acids may be resorbed by portal circulation for recycling by the liver or small amounts may be passed in feces.

to various hydroxyl groups, resulting in the formation of secondary bile acids (see **Fig. 2**). Small portions of secondary bile acids are resorbed by portal venous circulation and returned to hepatocytes or eliminated in urine. Secondary bile acids that are not resorbed in the colon are excreted by defecation.[7]

Enterohepatic Circulation

Under normal conditions, conjugated bile salts produced by hepatocytes are actively pumped into the biliary canaliculus. Bile salt concentrations in hepatic bile are approximately 1000-fold higher than in portal blood resulting in osmotic forces that draw additional water into the canaliculus.[9] These osmotic forces, in addition to an actin spiral surrounding the canaliculus, result in bile flowing down the biliary tract from canaliculi into biliary ductules and ducts.[4]

In vertebrates that have a gall bladder, entry of bile into the gall bladder is pressure dependent. The function of the gall bladder is similar in most species, in that it serves as an accessory organ for storing and concentrating bile.[11] If the pressure in the common bile duct is greater than the pressure in the cystic duct, bile will enter the gall bladder for storage and later secretion.[6] Ingestion of a meal eventually results in the release of cholecystokinin from endocrine cells of the intestinal mucosa and results in gall bladder contracture and the delivery of bile to the duodenum.[6]

Why only some animals have a gall bladder remains unclear. Some suggest the constant flow of bile from the liver into the intestine is adequate for animals that eat continuously, such as horses, rats, pigeons, and deer.[11] Gall bladder presence is considered a primitive trait found in most fish, adult amphibians, some reptiles and birds, and numerous mammals, although the anatomic position, size, and route in which bile is secreted into the duodenum varies.[11] Vertebrates lacking a gall bladder may compensate for its storage and concentrating functions by modifications to other parts of the biliary tree.[11]

Within the small intestine, bile acids function to solubilize dietary lipids promoting fat absorption by enterocytes. Primary bile acids are transported aborally by the propulsive activity of peristalsis. Conjugated primary bile acids are efficiently ($\sim$95%) resorbed by the ileum into portal circulation and returned to the liver.[12] Hepatocytes are effective at first-pass uptake of conjugated bile acids ($\sim$50–90% depending on bile acid structure) from portal circulation; these conjugated bile acids are then reexcreted into the biliary system.[8,12] Conjugated bile acids not reabsorbed from the ileum then enter the colon and may be deconjugated and dehydroxylated by bacteria to form secondary bile acids that are either recycled or eliminated.[7]

Measurement of Bile Acids

By understanding bile acid synthesis and enterohepatic circulation, clinicians can use the measurement of serum or plasma bile acids to aid in the identification of hepatocellular dysfunction or alterations in portal circulation. Increases in serum or plasma bile acids may be caused by nonspecific hepatocyte dysfunction leading to a reduced capacity to remove bile acids from the portal venous system. Portosystemic shunting results in the delivery of venous portal blood directly into systemic circulation, eliminating the opportunity for the extraction of bile acids by hepatocytes and ultimately, an increase in serum or plasma bile acids. Finally, serum or plasma bile acids will be increased as a consequence of cholestasis. Therefore, the measurement of bile acids may be used as a sensitive test for bile acid clearance and should be interpreted in conjunction with standard indicators of liver function. Additionally, serial bile acid testing may be used to monitor progression or response to therapy in patients with proven hepatic disease.

Analytical Methodology

Bile acids can be measured in biological fluids via several analytical methodologies, including gas–liquid chromatography (GLC), immunoassays (radioimmunoassay [RIA], enzyme-linked immunosorbent assay [ELISA]), and enzymatic assay.

Gas–liquid chromatography

Early studies on the measurement of bile acids in veterinary or laboratory species were performed under research conditions with GLC.[13–15] GLC identifies the composition of individual bile acids by alkaline or enzymatic deconjugation of the glycine or taurine moiety.[16] This methodology requires specialized equipment and is, therefore, impractical for routine diagnostic applications.

Immunoassays

Immunoassays depend on antibodies that have high specificity for the steroid or conjugated moiety of bile acids. Radioimmunoassay and ELISA kits for bile acids developed for humans and have variable results in veterinary species,[17–20] likely based on differences in the specificity, avidity, and affinity of antibodies and linearity of the kit across species.[21] Therefore, only species-specific RIA or ELISA test kits are recommended for use.

Enzymatic tests

Enzymatic assays for bile acid measurement rely on the oxidation of the conserved 3α-hydroxyl group to 3-oxo-bile acids by 3α-hydroxysteroid dehydrogenase. During the oxidative reaction, nicotinamide adenine dinucleotide (NAD) is converted to its reduced form, NADH. Subsequently, NADH is oxidized back to NAD with concurrent reduction of nitro blue tetrazolium salt to formazan resulting in a measurable color change an absorbance of 530 nm (**Fig. 3**). Color intensity is proportional to the concentration of bile acids in the sample. As this assay is directed against a highly conserved residue of bile acids, it is not species-specific and is widely used in diagnostic laboratories.

Preanalytical Considerations

According to a method comparison study in chickens and psittacine birds, bile acids concentration decreases by greater than 50% after 4 days when stored at 4°C.[18] This same study reported that bile acids concentrations in these species are stable when stored at −20°C or −70°C, but the length of time the samples were stable at these temperatures was not provided.[18] The presence of hemolysis, lipemia, or high concentrations of lactate dehydrogenase falsely decreases bile acids concentrations when measured via spectrophotometric enzymatic assays.[18] Sample volume can be limiting depending on methodology and instrumentation.

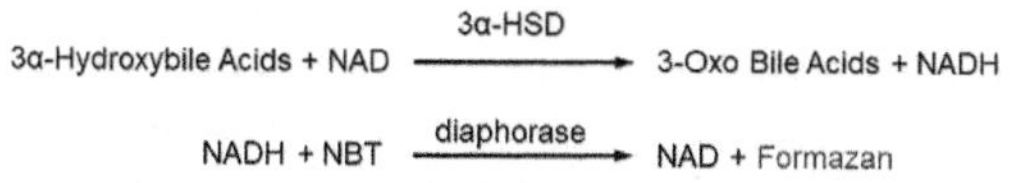

$$3\alpha\text{-Hydroxybile Acids} + \text{NAD} \xrightarrow{\text{3}\alpha\text{-HSD}} \text{3-Oxo Bile Acids} + \text{NADH}$$

$$\text{NADH} + \text{NBT} \xrightarrow{\text{diaphorase}} \text{NAD} + \text{Formazan}$$

Fig. 3. Enzymatic methodology for the measurement of bile acid concentration. Oxidation of bile acids to 3-oxo bile acids is catalyzed by 3α-hydroxysteroid dehydrogenase (3α-HSD). During this reaction, an equimolar quantity of nicotinamide adenine dinucleotide (NAD) is reduced to NADH. Subsequently, NADH is oxidized to NAD with concurrent reduction of nitro blue tetrazolium salt (NBT) to formazan by the catalytic action of diaphorase. Formazan color intensity is measured at 530 nm and is directly proportional to bile acid concentration in the sample.

Reference Versus Point-of-Care Assays

Handheld or small benchtop point-of-care biochemical analyzers have advantages including smaller sample volume and ease of use in the field or general practice. The performance of these analyzers should be compared with standard reference methods found in commercial or academic veterinary diagnostic laboratories. Bile acids measurement for exotic species has been assessed on the VetScan VS2 (Abaxis North America, Union City, CA) in Hispaniolan amazon parrots (*Amazonia ventralis*), [22] Strigiformes, [23] American flamingos (*Phoenicopterus ruber*) [24] loggerhead sea turtles (*Caretta caretta*), [25] and various reptiles, [25–30] likely because it has been marketed with tho Avian/Reptilian Profile Plus (ARP) rotor that requires 100 uL of whole blood, serum, or plasma to measure 11 analytes. Bile acids concentrations using the ARP rotor are linear within 35 to 200 umol/L.[31] Many healthy birds and reptiles have plasma bile acid concentrations that are below this concentration, resulting in several studies reporting plasma bile acids as less than 35 umol/L.[22–25,28–30,32,33] Interestingly, the VetScan Mammalian Liver Profile (MLP) rotor is linear over ranges between 1 and 140 umol/L and may be better suited for the measurement of lower concentrations of plasma bile acids as seen in many birds and reptiles.[34] Lower plasma bile acid concentrations in common chameleons, *Chameleo chameleon,* and green iguanas, *Iguana iguana,* were quantifiable using the MLP rotor, whereas the ARP rotor was unable to provide a quantitative value below the detection limit or was not reported.[28,35] When clinical suspicion of liver disease is high in nonmammalian species, clinicians are encouraged to use enzymatic assay methods with physiologically relevant lower limits of detection. Similarly, the creation of reference intervals for bile acids of many of these species may be better served via the use of the VetScan MLP rotor.

Bile Acids in Small Mammalian Species

Published reference values of circulating bile acids concentrations for ferrets *Mustela putorius furo,* rabbits, *Oryctolagus cuniculus,* and a variety of rodent species are available.[36–39] In general, the diagnostic use of bile acids is not common in rabbits[40] and may not be as sensitive as hepatocellular (ie, ALT, AST, SDH) and biliary (ie, ALP, GGT, total bilirubin) analytes to evaluate for hepatic pathology in rodents.[41] However, bile acids concentration has been reported to be a sensitive and specific indicator of liver disease in hystricomorph rodents (eg, guinea pigs, *Cavia porcellus,* chinchillas, *Chinchilla lanigera,* degus, *Octodon degus*).[39]

One study has evaluated differences in pre and postprandial bile acid concentrations in a rodent species, the Syrian hamster, *Mesocricetus auratus.*[20] In both healthy animals and those affected by chronic hepatitis, there was no difference in bile acids in relation to fasting status. Fasting of small mammals for diagnostic sample collection is problematic, and generally not recommended in rodents. Catabolism may be induced in small patients with high metabolic rates.[42] The feeding strategy of some species (eg, cecotrophy) can prevent a true fasting state.[43,44] Likewise, rabbit and rodent gastrointestinal physiology can prevent complete emptying of the stomach.[20,44] Ferrets may be fasted, but a period of greater than 4 hours is not recommended.[42,45]

Increases in circulating bile acids concentrations in small mammals are reported to occur with many hepatic diseases, including cholestasis, decreased functional liver mass, and vascular shunts.[38,46,47] Decreases in the enterohepatic circulation of bile acids (eg, ileal malabsorption) may result in concomitant serum decreases.[47] However, studies evaluating the association of bile acids with hepatic or other diseases are limited. Rabbits with chronic cholestatic disease induced by the administration of sex steroids (methyltestosterone or ethinyl estradiol) had increased bile acids starting at 8

- 14 weeks (ethinyl estradiol administered rabbits, 8 weeks = 117 ± 26 uM/L and methyltestosterone administered rabbits, 14 weeks = 75 ± 12 uM/L) and persisting through the end of the experiment (ethinyl estradiol administered rabbits, 20 weeks = 159 ± 40 uM/L; methyltestosterone administered rabbits, 20 weeks = 152 ± 58 uM/L).[48] In rats and mice, increases in bile acids were found with liver necrosis secondary to the administration of various hepatotoxic chemicals.[49] When toxic compounds were used to induce bile duct hyperplasia, total bile acids did not increase. However, specific bile acid concentrations did change, suggesting that individual bile acids may be more sensitive indicators of biliary hyperplasia and able to differentiate between types of hepatic pathology. Guinea pigs with induced ketotic states had a moderate and positive correlation between bile acids concentrations and histologic evidence of liver damage from hepatic lipidosis, although descriptive statistics regarding bile acids concentrations were not provided for this dissertation.[50] Finally, guinea pigs with ascorbic acid (vitamin C) deficiency were found to have minor decreases (2.63 ± 0.87 mg/dL) in circulating bile acids.[51]

The recommendation to use serum or plasma bile acids concentrations to investigate hepatic function and disease in small mammal species is equivocal. When the collected sample volume is sufficient, the addition of bile acids to a biochemical panel is suggested. In most species, fasting is not necessary or possible. However, comparing fasted and postprandial samples in ferrets is recommended, and interpretation of bile acid values can be conducted in a manner similar to that used for domestic dogs and cats.

Bile Acids in Avian Species

The clinical use of circulating bile acids concentrations for disease diagnosis in birds was not present in the scientific literature before the late 1980s.[52] Since that time, reference values for a limited number of species have been determined, including parrots,[19,53–57] pigeons (*Columba livia*),[55,58] Galliformes,[18,59,60] mallard ducks (*Anas platyrhynchos*),[61] and falcons (*Falco peregrinus, F. rusticollis, F. cherrug*).[62]

Similar to mammals, postprandial changes in bile acids occur in birds and are not dependent on the presence of a gall bladder.[55,61,63,64] Most studies have found that these changes are increases, though one study reported that postprandial changes were decreased in 5 psittacine species.[55] Due to these findings, fasting before blood sample collection is generally suggested, with a period of 12 hours for many species and 24 hours for raptors.[17,21] However, fasting may not be possible in all circumstances. Smaller or debilitated birds may not be able to tolerate it, sick birds commonly have crop stasis, and crop emptying times are variable by taxa.[21] Additionally, fasting may not always be necessary. Differentiation between postprandial increases in bile acid concentrations and those induced by hepatobiliary disease may be possible. Increases related to hepatobiliary disease are commonly 5- to 10-fold greater than the upper limit of reference values, while postprandial bile acids increases are not as great.[65] One study of psittacine species found that bile acids concentrations during random food consumption were intermediate to those during fasting and postprandial periods.[55]

Bile acid concentration is a useful measure of liver function and a specific clinical analyte for hepatic disease in avian species.[17] Its sensitivity, however, varies greatly with the type and chronicity of hepatic disease present.[66,67] Peracute to acute liver pathology may not induce detectable changes in plasma bile acids concentrations,[57,66] while chronic liver disease associated with cirrhosis or scarring may result in decreased bile acids concentrations due to decreased production.[68] Physical injury to the liver via endoscopy (biopsy or crushing) and surgery (6% or 18% hepatectomy) does not alter bile acids concentrations[69,70] Severe increases are commonly associated with biliary hyperplasia and hepatic fibrosis.[66] Published cases demonstrating these findings in *Amazona* spp. suggest that aflatoxin could play a role.[71,72] Aflatoxin is a known hepatotoxin, particularly in domestic fowl.[71,73] Experimental studies in pigeons and cockatiels (*Nymphicus hollandicus*) have found bile acids increases after aflatoxin toxicosis, though the increases were sometimes only mild to moderate.[64,74] Hepatotoxicity experimentally induced by other chemicals, such as α-naphthyl isothiocyanate, ethylene glycol, and D-galactosamine, has been associated with increased plasma bile acids concentrations.[58,59] Other liver diseases reported to cause moderate to severe increases in bile acids are lipidosis, amyloidosis, and congestion secondary to heart failure.[00,07,75,76]

Several retrospective studies have attempted to determine the utility of plasma bile acid concentrations for antemortem diagnosis of hepatic disease in psittacine birds with histologically confirmed liver pathology. Increased bile acids were a highly significant indicator of hepatic disease in psittacines.[19] Abnormal bile acid concentrations occurred in 80% (74% increased, 6% decreased) of the cases with hepatic disease. Association of bile acid concentrations with histologic lesions is variable. One study reported that increased bile acids were present in 47% of cases with hepatic lesions, while any abnormal bile acids values (increases and decreases) were present in 61% of cases.[67] However, another study found that only 12.5% of cases with liver pathology had associated increased bile acids concentrations and concluded that changes in bile acids are not a significant indicator of hepatic disease.[77] The contradictory findings among these studies are likely explained by the amount of information available for cases (eg, timeline of the disease process), differing methodologies, and the relatively small numbers of cases included (ie, 25–38 individual birds).

Bile acids should be included as part of a standard plasma biochemical panel for clinical diagnostic investigations in birds, especially when liver pathology is suspected. Fasted samples are beneficial to avoid the influence of recent diet consumption. Bile acid reference values for a small number of avian species are available (**Table 1**). However, the best practice is to compare previous bile acid measurements from the same individual taken during a normal state of health.

Bile Acids in Reptilian and Amphibian Species

Bile acid concentrations have been reported in several species of chelonians,[25,30,32,33,78–86] few lizards,[27–29,35,87–92] and even fewer snakes[93,94] (**Tables 2 and 3**).

The utility of fasting vs postprandial measurement of bile acids in reptiles is mixed and may be affected by variable gastrointestinal transit times seen in reptiles. One study investigated fasting (48 hours) and postprandial (at 3 and 7.5 hours) plasma bile acids in 11 healthy male green iguanas.[89] Preprandial, fasted bile acids ranged from 2.6 to 30.3 umol/L with a mean of 7.5 umol/L. At 3 hours, values significantly increased in all but one animal. The plasma bile acid concentration of this outlier had decreased and delayed gastric emptying was suspected. At 7 and a half hours, bile acid concentrations were significantly increased in all animals relative to the preprandial concentration. Another study assessed fasting (10 days) and postprandial (at 8, 2, and 48 hours) serum bile acids in red-eared terrapins (*Trachemys scripta elegans*) and found no significant difference between fasting and postprandial samples.[86] Although gastrointestinal transit times likely affect the optimal time for postprandial collection for bile acids testing in reptiles, studies assessing gastrointestinal transit times for reptilian taxa are sparsely reported and are affected by ambient temperature and feeding strategy (eg, herbivory, omnivory, carnivory).[95,96]

Table 1
Select published plasma bile acid values for various pet bird species

Species	N	Sexes	Fasting Status	Method	Mean	SD	Median	Interval	Range	Reference
Cockatiel (Nymphicus hollandicus)	70 samples from 32 birds	Not given	Not fasted	Enzymatic	—	—	<15	—	<15–139	Battison et al,[54] 1996
	Minimum 100 birds	Not given	Not given	Radioimmunoassay	—	—	—	20–85[b]	—	Cray et al,[19] 2008
	50 birds	Not given	Not given	Enzymatic	43.5	14.3	—	—	—	Cray et al,[18] 2003
	50 birds	Not given	Not given	Radioimmunoassay	38.3	10.4	—	—	—	Cray et al,[18] 2003
African gray (Psittacus erithacus)	103 birds	Not given	Not given	Enzymatic	39	17.8	35	18–71[c]	16–120	Lumeij and Overduin[53] 1990
	15 birds[a]	Not given	Not fasted	Enzymatic	—	—	—	19–68[c]	—	Flammer[55] 1994
	Minimum 100 birds	Not given	Not given	Radioimmunoassay	—	—	—	13–90[b]	—	Cray et al,[19] 2008
	50 birds	Not given	Not given	Enzymatic	35.7	19.8	—	—	—	Cray et al,[18] 2003
	50 birds	Not given	Not given	Radioimmunoassay	33.1	17.1	—	—	—	Cray et al,[18] 2003
Amazona spp.	99 birds	Not given	Not given	Enzymatic	63	48	52	19–144[c]	11–186	Lumeij and Overduin[53] 1990
	Minimum 100 birds	Not given	Not given	Radioimmunoassay	—	—	—	18–60[b]	—	Cray et al,[18] 2003
	50 birds	Not given	Not given	Enzymatic	33.5	23.4	—	—	—	Cray et al,[18] 2003
	50 birds	Not given	Not given	Radioimmunoassay	27.8	19.8	—	—	—	Cray et al,[18] 2003
Orange-winged Amazon (Amazona amazonica)	15 birds[a]	Not given	Not fasted	Enzymatic	—	—	—	34–131[c]	—	Flammer[55] 1994
Blue-fronted Amazon (Amazona aestiva)	15 birds[a]	Not given	Not fasted	Enzymatic	—	—	—	19–87[c]	—	Flammer[55] 1994
Ara spp.	16 birds	Not given	Not given	enzymatic	47	11.8	50	—	25–71	Lumeij and Overduin[53] 1990
	Minimum 100 birds	Not given	Not given	Radioimmunoassay	—	—	—	6–35[b]	—	Cray et al,[19] 2008
	50 birds	Not given	Not given	Enzymatic	21.4	13.9	—	—	—	Cray et al,[18] 2003
	50 birds	Not given	Not given	Radioimmunoassay	21.2	13.6	—	—	—	Cray et al,[18] 2003

(continued on next page)

Table 1
(continued)

Species	N	Sexes	Fasting Status	Method	Mean	SD	Median	Interval	Range	Reference
Cacatua spp.	27 birds	Not given	Not given	Enzymatic	41	17.8	37	23-70[c]	16-84	Lumeij and Overduin[53] 1990
	Minimum 100 birds	Not given	Not given	Radioimmunoassay	-	-	-	25-87[b]	-	Cray et al,[19] 2008
	50 birds	Not given	Not given	Enzymatic	31.8	17.5	-	-	-	Cray et al,[18] 2003
	50 birds	Not given	Not given	Radioimmunoassay	28.3	17.3	-	-	-	Cray et al,[18] 2003
Goffin's cockatoo (*Cacatua goffiniana*)	15 birds[a]	Not given	Not fasted	Enzymatic	-	-	-	21-144[c]	-	Flammer[55] 1994
Conures (*Aratinga* spp. and *Nandayus nenday*)	Minimum 100 birds	Not given	Not given	Radioimmunoassay	-	-	-	15-55[b]	-	Cray et al,[19] 2008
Eclectus parrot (*Eclectus roratus*)	Minimum 100 birds	Not given	Not given	Radioimmunoassay	-	-	-	10-61[b]	-	Cray et al,[19] 2008
Quaker parrot (*Myiopsitta monachus*)	Minimum 100 birds	Not given	Not given	Radioimmunoassay	-	-	-	25-65[b]	-	Cray et al,[19] 2008
Pigeon (*Columba livia*)	15 birds[a]	Not given	Not fasted	Enzymatic	-	-	-	29-56[c]	-	Flammer[55] 1994
	Not given	Approximately half male, half female	Not given	Enzymatic	-	-	-	22-60[c]	-	Lumeij and Wolfswinkel[58] 1988
	9 birds	Not given	Fasted	Enzymatic	35.4	18.1	31	-	17-71	Lumeij[61] 1991
Mallard (*Anas platyrhynchos*)	8 birds	Not given	Fasted	Enzymatic	27.8	7.6	27.5	-	17-40	Lumeij[61] 1991
Domestic chicken (*Gallus domesticus*)	27 birds	Not given	Not given	Enzymatic	6.7	5.8	-	-	-	Cray et al,[18] 2003
	27 birds	Not given	Not given	Radioimmunoassay	7.5	7.8	-	-	-	Cray et al,[18] 2003

All values are presented with the units of umol/L.

Abbreviation: SD, standard deviation.

[a] Bile acid concentration measured in serum.

[b] Mean ± 2 SD.

[c] Inner limits of the percentiles P2.5 - P97.5 with a 90% probability.

Table 2
Published bile acids values for various chelonians

Species	n	Sexes	Fasting Status	Method	Mean	SD	Median	Interval	Range	Reference
New Guinea Snapping Turtle (*Elseya novaeguineae*)	29	Not given	Fasted[b] 48 h	Enzymatic	–	–	5	0–41[c]	0–44	Anderson et al,[81] 1997
				Enzymatic	–	–	8[a]	0–44[c,a]	0–50[a]	
Loggerhead Sea Turtle (*Caretta caretta*)	100	Not given	Not given	Enzymatic	<35 (LOD)	–	–	–	–	Atkins et al,[25] 2010
				Enzymatic	0.85	–	–	0–1.7[c]	0–6	
Desert Tortoise (*Gopherus agassizii*)	98 - winter	47 male; 51 female	Not given	Enzymatic	–	–	1.5	0–44.0[c]	–	Christopher et al,[82] 1999
	98 - spring	47 male; 51 female	Not given	Enzymatic	–	–	0.7	0–18.0[c]	–	
	[b]8 - summer	47 male; 51 female	Not given	Enzymatic	–	–	0	0–55.0[c]	–	
	98 - fall	47 male; 51 female	Not given	Enzymatic	–	–	1.5	0–37.0[c]	–	
	25	Male	Not given	Enzymatic	2.2	–	–	0–5.1[c]	–	Dickinson et al,[83] 2002
	36	Female	Not given	Enzymatic	2.1	–	–	0–5.4[c]	–	
Sulcata (African Spurred) Tortoise (*Centrochelys sulcata*)	60	Not given	Not given	Enzymatic	<35 (LOD)	–	–	–	–	Eshar et al,[32] 2016
Chinese Three-Striped Box Turtle (*Cuora trifasciata*)	38	Males	Not fasted	Enzymatic	<35 (LOD)	–	–	–	<35 (LOD) - 61	Grioni et al,[33] 2014
	48	Females	Not fasted	Enzymatic						
Red-Eared Terrapin (*Trachemys scripta elegans*)	10	Female	Fasted[b]10 d	Enzymatic	8.69	5.11	7.87	–	1.27–43.7	Knotkova et al,[86] 2008
Hermann's Tortoises (*Testudo hermanni*)	30	50% female; 50% male	Not given	Enzymatic	–	–	4.0	1.0–12.0[c]	–	Scope et al,[78] 2013
	148 - spring	Male	Not given	Enzymatic	4.3	2.7	4	–	0.8–11.9	Leineweber et al,[84] 2019
	148 - summer		Not given	Enzymatic	3.8	2.1	3.7	1.1–6.9[d]	0.8–9.6	
	148 - fall		Not given	Enzymatic	3.0	2	2.9	0.6–5.4[d]	0-9.8	
	108 - spring	Female	Not given	Enzymatic	2.6	1.9	2.3	0.5–4.7[d]	0.2–8.7	
	108 - summer		Not given	Enzymatic	2.0	1.4	1.7	0.5–4.1[d]	0.05–6.7	
	108 - fall		Not given	Enzymatic	2.0	1.8	1.8	0.3–5.1[d]	0.02–7.9	
	32	Not given	Not given	Enzymatic	17.6	–	–	0–44.9[b]	–	Montesinos et al,[79] 2002

(continued on next page)

Table 2
(continued)

Species	n	Sexes	Fasting Status	Method	Mean	SD	Median	Interval	Fange	Reference
Greek Tortoise (*Testudo graeca*)	30	Not given	Not given	Enzymatic	17.86	–	–	0–33.2[b]	–	Montesinos et al,[79] 2002
Hinged Back Tortoise (*Kinixiz belliana*)	8	Not given	Not given	Enzymatic	6.0	–	–	5.9–6.1[b]	–	Montesinos et al,[79] 2002
Russian Tortoise (*Agronnemmys horsfieldii*)	8	Not given	Not given	Enzymatic	20.0	–	–	0–44.7[b]	–	Montesinos et al,[79] 2002
Radiated Tortoise (*Geochelone radiata*)	6 - winter	Male	Not given	Enzymatic	12.7	14.0	–	–	8.3–31.3	Zaias et al,[85] 2006
	4 - summer				10.4	8.0	–	–	3.3–18.0	
	7 - winter	Female	Not given	Enzymatic	4.5	4.0	–	–	.1–11.6	
	7 - summer				7.3	4.0	–	–	3.1–12.5	
Santa Cruz Galapagos Tortoise (*Chelonoidis porteri*)	210	Not given	Not given	Enzymatic	<35 (LOD)	–	–	–	–	Nieto-Claudin et al,[30] 2021
Blanding's turtle (*Emydoidea blandingii*)	349	254.103.36	Not given	Enzymatic	3.6	3.1	3	1.0–10.6[c]	0.6–39.9	Mumm et al,[80] 2019

All values are presented with the units of umol/L.
Abbreviation: SD, standard deviation.
[a] Bile acid concentration measured in serum.
[b] Mean ± 2 SD.
[c] Inner limits of the percentiles P2.5 - P97.5 with a 90% probability.
[d] Nonparametric method (10th–90th percentiles).

Table 3
Published bile acids values for various squamates

Species	N	Sexes	Fasting Status	Method	Mean	SD	Median	Interval	Range	Reference
Leopard Gecko (*Eublepharis macularius*)	22	Not given	Fasted -24 h	Enzymatic	–	–	2	0.6–37.5[b]	0.8–21	Cojean et al,[27] 2020
Crested Gecko (*Rhacodactylus ciliatus*)	30	21 male 19 female	Not given	Enzymatic	–	–	43	<35 (LOD) –44.0[b]	<35 (LOD) –89.0	Mayer et al,[29] 2011
Gila monster (*Heloderma suspectum*)	16	Not given	Not given	Enzymatic	16.2	13.3	12.4	–	2.6–55.1	Cooper-Bailey et al,[87] 2011
Common chameleon (*Chameleo chamaeleon*)	41	Not given	Not given	Enzymatic	<35	–	–	–	–	Eshar et al,[28] 2018
	26	Not given	Not given	Enzymatic	3	2	3	0–7[a]	0–6	
Green Iguana (*Iguana iguana*)	25	Male	Fasted - 12 h	Enzymatic	4.55	–	–	–	1.15–15.97	Grant et al. 2009
	21	Female	fasted - 12 h	Enzymatic	3.83	–	–	–	0.47–18.16	
	11	Male	Fasted - 28 h	Enzymatic	7.5	7.8	5.5	–	2.6–30.3	McBride et al,[89] 2006
			3 h postprandial	Enzymatic	33.3	22	–	–	5.2–71.5	
			7.5 h post prandial	Enzymatic	32.5	8.4	–	–	15.2–44.1	
Panther Chameleon (*Furcifer pardalis*)	27 - January	Male	Not given	Enzymatic	6.7	0.4	–	2.4–15.5[a]	1.7–23.2	Laube et al. 2018
	32 - August	Male	Not given	Enzymatic	4.6	1.7	–	1.0–10.6[a]	0.9–14.9	
	40 - January	Female	Not given	Enzymatic	6.7	1.7	–	1.6–16.2[a]	1.3–21.9	
	36 - August	Female	Not given	Enzymatic	4.9	1.4	–	0.4–14.0[a]	0.2–20.6	

(continued on next page)

Table 3
(continued)

Species	N	Sexes	Fasting Status	Method	Mean	SD	Median	Interval	Range	Reference
Allen Cays rock iguana (*Cyclura cychlura inornata*)	37	20 male 17 female	Not given	Enzymatic	10.6	20.2	–	–	0.9–38.3	James et al,[90] 2006
Ricord's iguana (*Cyclura ricordii*)	23	10 adult male 5 adult female 5 juvenile male 2 juvenile female 1 male hatchling	Not given	Enzymatic	7	7	4.6	–	0–27	Maria et al,[91] 2007
El Hierro giant lizard (*Gallotia sp*)	23	Males and females	Not given	Enzymatic	32	25.4	–	–	–	Martinez-Silvestre et al. 2004
Louisiana Pine snake (*Pituphis ruthveni*)	11	6 - adults 5 - juveniles	Not given Not given	Enzymatic Enzymatic	9.7 3	4.4 2.1	10 2	– –	3–15 1–7	Giori et al. 2019
Viperid Snakes	31	Not given	Not given	Enzymatic	–	–	–	–	12–128.1	Dutton & Taylor[93] 2003

All values are presented with the units of umol/L.

Abbreviation: SD, standard deviation.

[a] Inner limits of the percentiles P2.5 - P97.5 with a 90% probability.

[b] Nonparametric method (10th–90th percentiles).

Increased bile acid concentrations in reptiles are reported with nonspecific hepato-biliary disease. A case report following a Pacific gopher snake (*Pituophis catenifer*) with recurrent cholecystitis documented a fasted (13 days) plasma bile acids of 11.8 umol/L and a marked increase 24-h after the consumption of a meal (postprandial = 94.8 umol/L).[97] A markedly increased plasma bile acid concentration was demonstrated in a green iguana with hepatocellular carcinoma.[98] In a case of imidazole-induced hepatotoxicity secondary to treatment for pulmonary candidiasis in a Greek tortoise (*Testudo graeca*), bile acid concentrations were increased (95 umol/L) after 9 days of ketoconazole treatment (15 mg/kg p.o. SID) and resolved with the withdrawal of the medication.[99] Hepatotoxicity associated with significant cannabis consumption with increased AST and bile acids is also reported in three green iguanas.[100]

Circulating bile acid concentrations may be difficult to interpret in reptiles given the paucity of species-specific reference values and incomplete understanding of bile acid metabolism in reptiles. In some cases, bile acids concentrations did not correlate with liver disease documented at postmortem or surgical biopsy.[101–105] Discordantly low bile acids concentrations have been attributed to lowered production secondary to extensive hepatocellular loss, delayed gastric emptying, and poor analytical sensitivity.[102–104] Additionally, gall bladder contracture secondary to pressure associated with manual restraint may cause increased values in animals with no other evidence of liver disease.[89]

Few reference interval studies have been performed on amphibians. At least 2 studies have used the VetScan ARP rotor; however, bile acids were not included in the published reports.[106,107] Published reports involving increased bile acids in amphibians were not identified at the time of writing this article.

The utility of measuring serum or plasma bile acids concentrations to assess for hepatobiliary disease in reptiles is unclear. The low bile acid concentrations in some reptiles confound interpretation, particularly if concentrations are below the detection limit of the analyzer. Comparing fasted and postprandial bile acids concentrations in green iguanas may be helpful while in other species there does not seem to be a significant difference.[81,99]

SUMMARY

Based on knowledge derived from humans, dogs, and cats, measurement of bile acid concentrations is expected to aid in the diagnosis of liver disease as it is a sensitive indicator of hepatocellular dysfunction or altered portal circulation. Although reference values have been reported in numerous exotic animal species, summarized in **Tables 1, 2, and 3**, based on available evidence, bile acid diagnostic utility is somewhat equivocal. In many exotic animal species, sensitivity of bile acid concentrations to rule out liver disease seems to be poor, and bile acid concentrations do not correlate well to histologic evidence of liver disease. However, current evidence is based on studies that are retrospective in nature, have small sample sizes, or use immunologic versus the preferred enzymatic assay methodology. Current challenges also include sample volume constraints, lack of species- and analyzer-specific reference intervals, and incomplete knowledge of bile acids metabolism in many nonmammalian species. Standardization of methodology for future studies, as well as prospective and multi-institutional data collection to improve sample numbers, will be necessary to further evaluate bile acid utility in exotic animal species. Until then, bile acid concentrations should be interpreted in context with other liver function parameters and assessed serially or against intraindividual baseline values, when possible.

CLINICS CARE POINTS

- The evidence for the clinical utility of bile acids for the diagnosis of liver disease is strongest in birds and ferrets with equivocal evidence in rodents, rabbits, and reptiles.
- In many exotic animal species, sensitivity of bile acid concentrations to rule out liver disease seems to be poor, and bile acids concentrations do not correlate well to histologic evidence of liver disease.
- The utility of fasting and measurement of postprandial bile acid concentrations is variable among species. Fasting before sample collection may not be necessary or possible depending on the species.
- Enzymatic assays detect a highly conserved residue of bile acids that is not species specific.
- Hemolysis, lipemia, or high concentrations of lactate dehydrogenase can interfere with the enzymatic measurement of bile acid concentrations.
- Using assays with a lower limit of detection may be helpful for species with low physiologic concentrations of bile acids.

DISCLOSURE

The authors have nothing to disclose.

REFERENCES

1. Center SA. Serum bile acids in companion animal medicine. Vet Clin North Am 1993;23(3):625–57.
2. Hofmann AF, Hagey LR, Krasowski MD. Bile salts of vertebrates: structural variation and possible evolutionary signifi cance. J Lipid Res 2010;51(2):226–46.
3. Anwer MS, Meyer DJ. Bile acids in the diagnosis, pathology, and therapy of hepatobiliary diseases. Vet Clin North Am 1995;25(2):503–17.
4. Hofmann AF. The enterohepatic circulation of bile acids in mammals: form and functions. Front Biosci 2009;14:2584–9.
5. Thakare R, Alamoudi JA, Gautam N, et al. Species differences in bile acids II. bile acid metabolism. J Appl Toxicol 2018;38(10):1336–52.
6. Hofmann AF. Bile acids: the good, the bad, and the ugly. News Physiol Sci 1999; 14:24–9.
7. Hofmann AF, Hagey LR. Key discoveries in bile acid chemistry and biology and their clinical applications: history of the last eight decades. J Lipid Res 2014; 55(8):1553–95.
8. Monte MJ, Marin JJG, Antelo A, et al. Bile acids: chemistry, physiology, and pathophysiology. World J Gastroenterol 2009;15(7):804–16.
9. Kullak-Ublick GA, Stieger B, Meier PJ. Enterohepatic bile salt transporters in normal physiology and liver disease. Gastroenterology 2004;126(1 SUPPL. 1): 322–42.
10. Washabau RJ. Integration of gastrointestinal function. biology of the gastrointestinal tract, pancreas, and liver. In: Washabau RJ, Day MJ, editors. Canine and feline gastroenterology. St. Louis (MO): Elsevier, Inc.; 2013. p. 15–6.
11. Oldham-Ott CK, Gilloteaux J. Comparative Morphology of the gallbladder and biliary tract in vertebrates: variation in structure, homology in function and gallstones. Microsc Res Tech 1997;38(6):571–97.

12. Meyer DJ. Laboratory approach - liver. diagnostic approach to gastrointestinal, pancreatic, and hepatobiliary problems. In: Washabau RJ, Day MJ, editors. Canine and feline gastroenterology. St. Louis (MO): Elsevier, Inc.; 2013. p. 195–9.

13. Kothari R, Godbole N, Vaidya V. Separation and identificatoin of bile acids in some reptiles using thing layer chromatography. Biochem Biophys Res Commun 1972;49(3):736–9.

14. Davis AE, Imary CHE, Minoura T, et al. Gas liquid chromotography (GLC) analysis of hamster conjugated biliary bile acids. Biochem Soc Trans 1991;19:171S.

15. Sheriha GM, Waller GR, Chan T. Composition of bile acids in ruminants. Lipids 1967;3(1):72–8.

16. Tolman K, Reg R. Liver function. In: Burtis CA, Ashwood E, editors. Tietz textbook of clinical chemistry. Philadelphia (PA): W.B. Saunders Company; 1999. p. 1125–77.

17. Hoefer HL. Bile acid testing in psittacine birds. Semin Avian Exot Pet Med 1994; 3(1):33–7.

18. Cray C, Andreopoulos A. Comparison of two methods to determine plasma bile acid concentrations in healthy birds. J Avian Med Surg 2003;17(1):11–5.

19. Cray C, Gautier D, Harris DJ, et al. Changes in clinical enzyme activity and bile acid levels in psittacine birds with altered liver function and disease. J Avian Med Surg 2008;22(1):17–24.

20. Brunnert S, Altman NH. Laboratory assessment of chronic hepatitis in Syrian hamsters. Lab Anim Sci 1991;41:559–62.

21. Harr KE. Clinical chemistry of companion avian species: A review. Vet Clin Pathol 2002;31(3):140–51.

22. Greenacre CB, Flatland B, Souza MJ, et al. Comparison of avian biochemical test results with abaxis VetScan and Hitachi 911 analyzers. J Avian Med Surg 2008;22(4):291–9.

23. Ammersbach M, Beaufrère H, Gionet Rollick A, et al. Laboratory blood analysis in Strigiformes-Part II: Plasma biochemistry reference intervals and agreement between the Abaxis Vetscan V2 and the Roche Cobas c501. Vet Clin Pathol 2015;44(1):128–40.

24. Gancz AY, Eshar D, Beaufrère H. Paired biochemical analysis of pigmented plasma samples from zoo-kept American flamingos (*Phoenicopterus ruber*) using a point-of-care and a standard wet chemistry analyzer. J Zoo Wildl Med 2019;50(3):619–26.

25. Atkins A, Jacobson E, Hernandez J, et al. Use of a portable point-of-care (Vetscan Vs2) biochemical analyzer for measuring plasma biochemical levels in free-living loggerhead sea turtles (*Caretta caretta*). J Zoo Wildl Med 2010;41(4): 585–93.

26. McCain SL, Flatland B, Schumacher JP, et al. Comparison of chemistry analytes between 2 portable, commercially available analyzers and a conventional laboratory analyzer in reptiles. Vet Clin Pathol 2010;39(4):474–9.

27. Cojean O, Alberton S, Froment R, et al. Determination of leopard gecko (*Eublepharis macularius*) packed cell volume and plasma biochemistry reference intervals and reference values. J Herpetol Med Surg 2020;30(3).

28. Eshar D, Ammersbach M, Shacham B, et al. Venous blood gases, plasma biochemistry, and hematology of wild-caught common chameleons (*Chamaeleo chamaeleon*). Can J Vet Res 2018;82(2):106–14.

29. Mayer J, Knoll J, Wrubel KM, et al. Characterizing the hematologic and plasma chemistry profiles of captive crested geckos (*Rhacodactylus ciliatus*). J Herpetol Med Surg 2012;21(2):68.

30. Nieto-Claudín A, Palmer JL, Esperón F, et al. Haematology and plasma biochemistry reference intervals for the critically endangered western Santa Cruz Galapagos tortoise (*Chelonoidis porteri*). Conserv Physiol 2021;9(1).

31. *VetScan ® avian reptilian profile Plus* technical data sheet. Abaxis North America; 2007.

32. Eshar D, Gancz AY, Avni-Magen N, et al. Selected plasma biochemistry analytes of healthy captive sulcata (African spurred) tortoises (*Centrochelys sulcata*). J Zoo Wildl Med 2016;47(4):993–9. https://doi.org/10.1638/2016-0051.1.

33. Grioni A, Ho KKY, Karraker NE, et al. Blood clinicla biochemistry and packed cell volume of th echines three-striped box turtle, *Cuora trifasciata* (Reptilia: Geoemydidae). J Zoo Wildl Med 2014;45(2):228–38.

34. *VetScan ® mammalian liver profile* technical data sheet. Abaxis North America; 2006.

35. Grant KR, Thode HP III, Connor S, et al. Establishment of plasma biochemical reference values for captive green iguanas, *Iguana Iguana*, using a point-of-care biochemistry analyzer. J Herpetol Med Surg 2009;19(1):23–8.

36. Wyre NR, Eshar D. Serum bile acids concentration in captive black-tailed prairie dogs (*Cynomys ludovicianus*). Comp Clin Path 2016;25(1):47–51. https://doi.org/10.1007/s00580-015-2137-5.

37. Fudge AM. Laboratory reference ranges for selected avian, mammalian, and reptilian species. In: Fudge A, editor. Laboratory medicine: avian and exotic pets. Philadelphia (PA): W.B. Saunders Company; 2000. p. 375–400.

38. Kusmeirczyk J, Kling M, Kier A. Rats and mice. In: Heatley J, Russell K, editors. Exotic animal laboratory diagnosis. 1st edition. Hoboken (NJ): John Wiley and Sons, Inc.; 2020. p. 81–112.

39. Rettenmund C, Heatley J. Hystricomorph rodents. In: Heatley J, Russell K, editors. Exotic animal laboratory diagnosis. 1st edition. Hoboken (NJ): John Wiley and Sons, Inc.; 2020. p. 129–44.

40. Oglesbee B. Rabbits. In: Heatley J, Russell K, editors. Exotic animal laboratory diagnosis. 1st edition. Hoboken (NJ): John Wiley and Sons, Inc.; 2020. p. 63–79.

41. Siegel A, Walton R. Hematology and biochemistry of small mammals. In: Ferrets, rabbits, and rodents: clinical medicine and surgery. 4th edition. St. Louis (MO): Elsevier, Inc.; 2021. p. 569–82.

42. Hawkins M, Pascoe P. Anesthesia, analgesia, and sedation of small mammals. In: Quesenberry K, Orcutt C, Mans C, et al, editors. Ferrets, rabbits, and rodents: clinical medicine and surgery. 4th edition. St. Louis (MO): Elsevier, Inc.; 2021. p. 536–58.

43. Washington IM, Van Hoosier G. Clinical Biochemistry and Hematology. In: The laboratory rabbit, Guinea pig, hamster, and other rodents. Elsevier Inc.; 2012. p. 57–116. https://doi.org/10.1016/B978-0-12-380920-9.00003-1.

44. Jenkins J. Rabbit and ferret liver and gastrointestinal testing. In: Fudge A, editor. Laboratory medicine: avian and exotic pets. Philadelphia (PA): W.B. Saunders Company; 2000. p. 291–304.

45. Greenacre C. Ferrets. In: Heatley J, Russell K, editors. Exotic animal laboratory diagnosis. 1st edition. Hoboken (NJ): John Wiley and Sons; 2020. p. 17–44.

46. Huynh M, Laloi F. Diagnosis of liver disease in domestic ferrets (*Mustela putorius*). Vet Clin North Am Exot Anim Pract 2013;16(1):121–44.

47. Weidmeyer C. Evaluation of hepatic function and injury. In: Kurtz D, Travlos G, editors. The clinical chemistry of laboratory animals. 3rd edition. Boca Raton (FL): CRC Press; 2018. p. 367–406.

48. Tennant BC, Balazs T, Baldwin BH, et al. Assessment of hepatic function in rabbits with steroid-induced cholestatic liver injury. Fundam Appl Toxicol 1981;1: 329–33.

49. Luo L, Schomaker S, Houle C, et al. Evaluation of serum bile acid profiles as biomarkers of liver injury in rodents. Toxicol Sci 2014;137(1):12–25.

50. Schmid N. Investigation on the development, diagnosis and therapy of ketosis in non-gravid and non-lactating guinea pigs. Switzerland: Doctoral dissertation, University of Zurich; 2019.

51. Holloway DE, Rivers JM. Influence of chronic ascorbic acid deficiency and excessive ascorbic acid intake on bile acid metabolism and composition in the guinea pig. J Nutr 1981;111:412–24.

52. Lumeij JT, Westerhof I. Blood chemistry for the diagnosis of hepatobiliary disease in birds. A review. Vet Q 1987;9(3):255–61.

53. Lumeij JT, Overduin LM. Plasma chemistry references values in psittaciformes. Avian Pathol 1990;19(2):235–44.

54. Battison AL, Buckzowski S, Archer FJ. Plasma bile acid concentration in the cockatiel. Can Vet J 1996;37:233–4.

55. Flammer K. Serum bile acids in psittacine birds. In: Proc Annu Conf Assoc avian Vet. Reno: NV); 1994. p. 9–12.

56. Altman R, Clubb S, Dorrestein G. Hematology/biochemical reference ranges. In: Altman R, Clubb S, Dorrestein G, editors. Avian medicine and surgery. Philadelphia (PA): W.B. Saunders Company; 1997. p. 1004–23.

57. Tully T. Psittaciformes. In: Heatley J, Russell K, editors. Exotic animal laboratory diagnosis. 1st edition. Hoboken (NJ): John Wiley and Sons, Inc.; 2020. p. 483–502.

58. Lumeij JT, Meidam M, Wolfswinkel J, et al. Changes in plasma chemistry after drug-induced liver disease or muscle necrosis in racing pigeons (*Columba livia domestica*). Avian Pathol 1988;17(4):865–74.

59. Bromidge ES, Wells JW, Wight PAL. Elevated bile acids in the plasma of laying hens fed rapeseed meal. Res Vet Sci 1985;39:378–82.

60. Cook J, Heatley J, Galliformes. In: Heatley J, Russell K, editors. Exotic animal laboratory diagnosis. 1st edition. Hoboken (NJ): John Wiley and Sons, Inc.; 2020. p. 503–41.

61. Lumeij JT. Fasting and postprandial plasma bile acid concentrations in racing pigeons (*Columba Livia Domestica*) and mallards (*Anas Platyrhynchos*). J Assoc Avian Veterinarians 1991;5:197–200.

62. Jones M, Chitty J. Raptors. In: Heatley J, Russell K, editors. Exotic animal laboratory diagnosis. 1st edition. Hoboken (NJ): John Wiley and Sons, Inc.; 2020. p. 437–82.

63. Lumeij JT, Remple JD. Plasma bile acid concentrations in response to feeding in peregrine falcons (*Falco peregrinus*). Avian Dis 1992;36:1060–2.

64. Carpenter J, Bossart G, Bachues K. Use of serum bile acids to evaluate hepatobiliary function in the cockatiel (Nymphicus hollandicus). In: Proc Annu Conf Assoc avian Vet. Tampa (FL), August 24-27, 1996:73-75.

65. Lumeij JT. Hepatology. In: Ritchie B, Harrison G, Harrison L, editors. *Avian medicine: principles and application*. Delray Beach (FL). HBD International, Inc.; 1994. p. 522–37.

66. Fudge A. Avian liver and gastrointestinal testing. In: Fudge A, editor. Laboratory medicine: avian and exotic pets. Philadelphia (PA): W.B. Saunders Company; 2000. p. 47–55.

67. Vergneau-Grosset C, Beaufrere H, Ammerbach M. Clinical biochemistry. In: Speer B, editor. Current therapy in avian medicine and surgery. 1st edition. St. Louis (MO): Elsevier, Inc.; 2016. p. 486–501.

68. Hochleithner M. Biochemistries. In: Ritchie B, Harrison G, Harrison L, editors. *Avian medicine: Principles and application.* Delray Beach (FL). HBD International, Inc.; 1994. p. 223–45.

69. Jaensch SM, Raidal SR. Assessment of liver function in galahs (*Eolophus roseicapillus*) after partial hepatectomy: a comparison of plasma enzyme concentrations, serum bile acid levels, and galactose clearance tests. J Avian Med Surg 2000;14(3):164–71.

70. Williams SM, Holthaus L, Barron HW, et al. Improved clinicopathologic assessments of acute liver damage due to trauma in Indian ring-necked parakeets (*Psittacula krameri manillensis*). J Avian Med Surg 2012;26(2):67–75.

71. Clyde VL, Orosz SE, Munson L. Severe hepatic fibrosis and bile duct hyperplasia in four amazon parrots. J Avian Med Surg 1996;10:252–7.

72. Lee S-Y, Kim Y, Park H-M. Hepatic fibrosis and bile duct hyperplasia in a young orange winged Amazon parrot (*Amazona amazonica*). J Vet Clin 2011;28: 617–20.

73. Dumonceaux G, Harrison G. Toxins. In: Ritchie B, Harrison G, Harrision L, editors. Avian medicine: Principles and application. Delray Beach (FL): HBD International, Inc.; 1994. p. 1030–52.

74. Hadley TL, Grizzle J, Rotstein DS, et al. Determination of an oral aflatoxin dose that acutely impairs hepatic function in domestic pigeons (*Columba livia*). J Avian Med Surg 2010;24(3):210–21.

75. James Stephanie B, Raphael, Bonnie L, et al. Diagnosis and treatment of hepatic lipidosis in a barred owl (*Strix varia*). J Avian Med Surg 2000;14(4):268–72.

76. Samour J, Naldo J. The use of serum bile acids in the assessment of hepatobiliary function in saker falcons (*Falco cherrug*) in Saudi Arabia. In: Proc Eur Assoc avian Vet. Spain: Tenerife; 2003. p. 292–5.

77. Hung C, Sladakovic I, Divers SJ. Diagnostic value of plasma biochemistry, haematology, radiography and endoscopic visualisation for hepatic disease in psittacine birds. Vet Rec 2019. https://doi.org/10.1136/vetrec-2018-105214.

78. Scope A, Schwendenwein I, Schauberger G. Characterization and quantification of the influence of season and gender on plasma chemistries of Hermann's tortoises (*Testudo hermanni*). Res Vet Sci 2013;95(1):59–68.

79. Montesinos A, Martínez R, Jiménez A. Plasma bile acids concentration in tortoises: reference valaues and histopathologic findings of importance for interpretation. Proc WSAVA Congress 2002. Granada; Spain, October 3-5.

80. Mumm LE, Winter JM, Andersson KE, et al. Hematology and plasma biochemistries in the Blanding's turtle (*Emydoidea blandingii*) in Lake County, Illinois. PLoS One 2019;14(11):1–15.

81. Anderson NL, Wack RF, Hatcher R. Hematology and clinical chemistry reference ranges for clinically normal, captive new guinea snapping turtle (*Elseya novaeguineae*) and the effects of temperature, sex, and sample type. J Zoo Wildl Med 1997;28:394–403.

82. Christopher MM, Berry KH, Wallis IR, et al. Reference intervals and physiologic alterations in hematologic and biochemical values of free-ranging desert tortoises in the mojave desert. J Wildl Dis 1999;35(2):212–38.

83. Dickinson VM, Jarchow JL, Trueblood MH. Hematology and plasma biochemistry reference range values for free-ranging desert tortoises in Arizona. J Wildl Dis 2002;38(1):143–53.

84. Leineweber C, Stöhr AC, Öfner S, et al. Changes in plasma chemistry parameters in Hermann's tortoises (*Testudo hermanni*) influenced by season and sex. J Herpetol Med Surg 2019;29(3–4):113.

85. Zaias J, Norton T, Fickel A, et al. Biochemical and hematologic values for 18 clinically healthy radiated tortoises (*Geochelone radiata*) on St Catherines Island, Georgia. Vet Clin Pathol 2006;35(3):321–5.

86. Knotkova Z, Dorrestein GM, Jekl V, et al. Fasting and postprandial serum bile acid concentrations in 10 healthy female red-eared terrapins (*Trachemys scripta elegans*). Vet Rec 2008;163(17):510–4.

87. Cooper-Bailey K, Smith SA, Zimmerman K, et al. Hematology, leukocyte cytochemical analysis, plasma biochemistry, and plasma electrophoresis of wild-caught and captive-bred Gila monsters (*Heloderma suspectum*). Vet Clin Pathol 2011;40(3):316–23.

88. Laube A, Altherr B, Clauss M, et al. Reference intervals for bile acids and protein electrophoresis in plasma of captive panther chameleons (*Furcifer pardalis*): a first approach. J Herpetol Med Surg 2019;28(3–4):99–101.

89. Mcbride M. Preliminary evaluation of pre-and post-prandial 3α-hydroxy-bile-acids in the green iguana (*Iguana iguana*). J Herpetol Med Surg 2006;4:129–34.

90. James SB, Iverson J, Greco V, et al. Health assessment of Allen Cays rock iguana, *Cyclura cychlura inornata*. J Herpetol Med Surg 2006;16:93–8.

91. Maria R, Ramer J, Reichard T, et al. Biochemical reference intervals and intestinal microflora of free-ranging Ricord's iguanas (*Cyclura ricordii*). J Zoo Wildl Med 2007;38(3):414–9.

92. Martínez AS. Hepatic lipidosis in reptiles. Proceedings, southern European veterinary conference, Barcelona, Spain, October 17-19, 2013.

93. Dutton CJ, Taylor P. A comparison between pre-and posthibernation morphometry, hematology, and blood chemistry in viperid snakes. J Zoo Wildl Med 2003; 34:53–8.

94. Giori L, Stacy NI, Ogle M, et al. Hematology, plasma biochemistry, and hormonal analysis of captive Louisiana pine snakes (*Pituophis ruthveni*): effects of intrinsic factors and analytical methodology. Comp Clin Path 2020;29(1):145–54.

95. Smith D, Dobson H, Spence E. Gastrointestinal studies in the green iguana; technique and reference values. Vet Radiol Ultrasound 2001;42:515–20.

96. González-Paredes D, Ariel E, David MF, et al. Gastrointestinal transit times in juvenile green turtles: An approach for assessing digestive motility disorders. J Exp Mar Bio Ecol 2021;544:151616.

97. Kinney ME, Chinnadurai SK, Wack RF. Cholecystectomy for the treatment of mycobacterial cholecystitis in a Pacific gopher snake (*Pituophis cate nifer*). J Herpetol Med Surg 2013;23:10–4.

98. Knotek Z, Dorrestein GM, Hrdá A, et al. Hepatocellular carcinoma in a green iguana - a case study. Acta Vet Brno 2011;80(3):243–7.

99. Hernandez-Divers SJ. Pulmonary candidiasis caused by *Candida albicans* in a Greek tortoise (*Testudo graeca*) and treatment with intrapulmonary amphotericin B. J Zoo Wildl Med 2001;32:352–9.

100. Girling SJ, Fraser MA. Cannabis intoxication in three Green iguanas (*Iguana iguana*). J Small Anim Pract 2011;52(2):113–6.

101. Naples LM, Langan JN, Mylniczenko ND, et al. Islet Cell Tumor in a Savannah Monitor (*Varanus exanthematicus*). J Herpetol Med Surg 2011;19(4):97.

102. Perpiñán D, Addante K, Driskell E. Gastrointestinal Disturbances in a Bearded Dragon (*Pogona vitticeps*). J Herpetol Med Surg 2010;20:54–7.
103. Wilson GH, Fontenot DK, Brown CA, et al. Pseudocarcinomatous biliary hyperplasia in two green iguanas, *Iguana iguana*. J Herpetol Med Surg 2004;14:12–8.
104. Parkinson LA, Kierski K, Mans C. Coagulopathy secondary to chronic hepatopathy in three lizards. J Herpetol Med Surg 2021;31(4):296–301.
105. Giuseppe M Di, Oliveri M, Morici M, et al. Hepatic encephalopathy in a redtailed boa (*Boa constrictor imperator*). J Exot Pet Med 2017;26(2):96–100.
106. Brady S, Burgdorf-Moisuk A, Kass PH, et al. Hematology and plasma biochemistry intervals for captive-born california tiger salamanders (*Ambystoma californiense*). J Zoo Wildl Med 2016;47(3):731–5.
107. Takami Y, Une Y. Blood Clinical Biochemistries and Packed Cell Volumes for the Mexican Axolotl *(Ambystoma mexicanum)*. J Herpetol Med Surg 2017;27: 104–10.

Diagnostic Use of Lactate in Exotic Animals

Jane Merkel, RVT, MS, VTS (Zoo)[a],
Sathya K. Chinnadurai, DVM, MS, DACZM, DACVAA, DACAW[b,c],*

KEYWORDS

- Lactate • Avian • Reptile • Exotic • Hypoperfusion

KEY POINTS

- Point-of-care (POC) lactate meters are inexpensive, rapid, and easy to use.
- An increased concentration of blood lactate allows the recognition of hypoperfusion.
- Prolonged or extremely increased blood lactate concentrations can be predictive of mortality.
- Serial lactates are much more helpful than a single lactate reading.
- Reference ranges for lactate have yet to be established for most exotic species.

INTRODUCTION

Lactate is produced during anaerobic metabolism, and lactate concentrations often increase in cases of hypoperfusion. Other causes of increased lactate concentrations include mitochondrial dysfunction, drug reactions, and decreased clearance due to liver or kidney disease. Human critical care settings use lactate concentrations to assess the severity of shock and provide prognostic guidelines; higher concentrations of lactate and prolonged elevation lead to a poorer prognosis.[1] Point-of-care (POC) lactate meters are easy to use, quick, and require a small patient sample, allowing serial use even with small patients. Many tools are available for monitoring ill or anesthetized exotic patients: blood pressure, capillary refill time, mucous membrane color, oxygen saturation, and expired carbon dioxide. Determination of patient-side blood lactate concentrations provides an excellent addition to this arsenal, allowing quick assessment of perfusion status. Blood lactate concentrations often reflect a change in patient status before changes in vital signs. Lactate has been studied in domestic animals, particularly in horses, dogs, and in certain disease processes as a standard for the assessment of prognosis, notably gastric dilatation in dogs.[2] In exotic animals,

[a] Department of Animal Health, Saint Louis Zoo, One Government Drive, St Louis, MO 63110, USA; [b] Department of Animal Health, Saint Louis Zoo, St Louis, MO 63110, USA; [c] Chicago Zoological Society, Brookfield, IL 60513, USA
* Corresponding author. Chicago Zoological Society, Brookfield, IL 60513.
E-mail address: schinnadurai@yahoo.com

Vet Clin Exot Anim 25 (2022) 585–596
https://doi.org/10.1016/j.cvex.2022.05.006
1094-9194/22/© 2022 Published by Elsevier Inc.

many studies have focused on animals in a field study setting; however, due to the stress of handling and capture these animals may demonstrate higher lactate values than companion mammals. Lactate studies of exotic animals and animals in a zoologic setting are becoming more common, allowing for some generalities regarding lactate to be deduced, although much research remains to be conducted. Exotic animals present their own set of anesthetic challenges and monitoring of lactate values can help increase the standard care provided.

Lactate

Lactate occurs in 2 isomers l-lactate, the form measured by POC devices, and created when the body undergoes anaerobic metabolism and d-lactate which is generated by bacteria in the gut. Increased d-Lactate concentrations occur in ruminal acidosis and in humans with short gut syndrome.[3] L-Lactate is produced at low concentrations by the red blood cells, brain, and skeletal muscles. Lactate concentrations can increase due to overproduction or failure of clearance and are primarily metabolized by the liver, and secondarily by the kidneys.

Lactate concentrations can increase due to intense exercise, stress, sepsis, drug reactions, and mitochondrial dysfunction. Importantly, during critical emergencies or during anesthetic events, lactate can indicate hypoperfusion. Increased lactate concentration origins can be categorized as hypoxic (Type A) or nonhypoxic (Type B) (**Box 1**). A patient with high or increasing lactate concentrations should be evaluated holistically, as a critically ill patient may have mixed origins of an elevated blood lactate concentration (Type A and Type B). An example of mixed causes of increased lactate is a trauma patient with concurrent hepatic disease.

Methods of Measuring Lactate

Point-of-care lactate meters are inexpensive, easy to use, provide rapid results and require only miniscule blood sample volumes. Similar to blood glucose handheld monitors, POC lactometers require minimal training to use. The use of a POC meter allows for patient-side results and the small amount of blood needed for testing allows for repeated sampling with minimal harm to the patient. In comparison, benchtop analyzers are large, expensive, and impractical in many veterinary settings. Comparisons of benchtop analyzers and multiple brands of handheld lactate meters demonstrate good agreement.[4] However, the Accutrend Plus model of lactate meter (Roche Diagnostics, Indianapolis IN 46256) lacks acceptable agreement with other handheld units and benchtop analyzers.[5]

Box 1
Classification of Type A and B causations of increased blood lactate concentrations

Type a Hypoxic Lactate Elevation – All Caused by Shock	Type B Non-hypoxic Lactate Elevation – Reasons Other than Shock
• Obstructive shock (eg, thrombus)	• Disease (liver disease, sepsis, neoplasia)
• Cardiogenic shock (heart cannot pump enough blood)	• Medications or toxins (acetaminophen, cyanide, propofol)
• Distributive shock (anaphylactic or septic)	• Inborn errors of metabolism (disorder of pyruvate metabolism, mitochondrial errors)
• Hypovolemic (hemorrhagic and nonhemorrhagic)	

Normal Lactate Concentrations

In mammals, with a few exceptions, less than 2.0 mmol/L is within the normal range of lactate, 2.0 to 4.0 mmol/L is considered hyperlactatemia, and greater than 4.0 mmol/L with a pH of less than 7.35 is considered lactic acidosis.

Importance of Monitoring Lactate

Lactate concentrations are valuable in critical cases, in long-term hospitalized patients, in patients undergoing anesthesia, or to measure probable outcomes. Serial lactates are more valuable than a single data point as trends give actionable information. Some species may initially demonstrate a high lactate concentration (>4.0 mmol/L) due to the stress of handling or capture; this value should decrease over time, if not, compensatory stages of hypoperfusion may be assumed if other causes of elevated lactate have been ruled out. Many species of birds and mammals are susceptible to exertional myopathy and may initially have an elevated lactate concentration based on the exertion and stress of a capture. These patients should be diligently monitored for a falling lactate concentration.[6] High lactate concentrations (>4.0 mmol/L) which remain high over an extended period of time can be a grave prognosticator when coupled with a pH of less than 7.35, as this indicates lactic acidosis. Lactate measurement is important as it is an early indicator of compensatory shock and this value will often change before changes in indirect blood pressure, mucous membrane color, capillary refill time, heart rate, and pulse intensity. Early detection of increasing lactate concentrations is important to establish resuscitative measures before the patient sliding into noncompensatory shock and lactic acidosis which is much more challenging to reverse.

Sample Collection

Arterial blood is the gold standard for measuring lactate concentrations; however, in view of the different anatomies of exotic patients this is not always practical. Differences in lactate concentrations between an arterial blood draw and venous blood draw commonly have an acceptable agreement, and trends can be followed in the individual patient.[7] After an initial lactate value is established, continued use of the same vessel for the determination of subsequent lactate concentrations is recommended. Minor differences occur in lactate concentrations obtained from cephalic, saphenous, and jugular veins.[8] If another vessel must be used, monitor trends within the patient rather than absolute values, as differences between the 2 vessels may be clinically irrelevant. Lactate concentrations of the basilic vein and jugular vein in boat-tailed grackles (*Quiscalus major*) were comparable; however, these comparisons were based on samples obtained from different birds rather than from within one bird.[9] In the early stages of shock, collection of a blood sample for lactate concentration from both a central and peripheral vein is recommended to determine if blood is being shunted to internal organs. Large discrepancies between lactate concentrations from a central and peripheral site indicate that peripheral tissue may be affected by compartment syndrome or regional hypoperfusion. Prolonged region ischemia could lead to irreversible tissue damage and necrosis.

Bodily fluids, other than blood, can be used for lactate measurements. In horses with colic, peritoneal fluid lactate concentrations changed more quickly than blood samples.[10] Saliva has been used to measure lactate concentrations, with inconsistent results.[11,12] Saliva lactate validation is promising for small exotic animals as blood samples are often needed for other tests.

Issues that May Alter Lactate Results

Lactate concentrations can be artificially increased for a number of reasons, including with the use of certain drugs.[13] Neonates often have higher lactate concentrations than their adult counterparts; puppies have elevated lactate for up to 70 days[14] and baboons less than 6 week old have lactate concentrations higher than adults.[15] Lactated ringers solution (LRS) can elevate lactate concentrations, blood collected from an intravenous catheter delivering LRS necessitates discarding the first portion of the blood before sample collection for the determination of lactate. Tourniquets, while once thought to create lactate elevation were found to be of little consequence unless left in place for an extended period of time.[16] Red blood cells continue to produce lactate postcollection in tubes containing Ethylenediaminetetraacetic acid (EDTA) or heparin. Immediate application of blood to the testing strip, postblood draw, will avoid this effect. Whole blood transfusions of stored red blood cells can increase blood lactate concentrations; however, this generally requires a large volume transfusion.[17] Time is of the essence when processing samples for lactate concentrations, 15 minutes at room temperature or an hour in the refrigerator will cause an increase in lactate concentrations.[18]

Gloves are recommended to prevent the contamination of lactate test strips by sweat from handling. Lactate is concentrated in human sweat to up 40 times that that found in the body.[19]

Lactate in Domestic Versus Exotic Animals

Many studies have been performed on dogs, horses and to a lesser extent, cats.[2,20] In dogs with gastric dilatation-volvulus lactate concentrations can be used as a predictor of mortality.[2] Lactate is well studied in horses both in relation to disease and performance.[21,22]

Although animals as diverse as white rhino, flamingos, and grasshoppers have been the subject of lactate evaluation studies, few reference ranges have been validated.[23–25] Given the number of species and the diverse physiologies and life histories represented, further research is warranted. At the moment normal lactate values must be extrapolated from what is known in domestic animals. Almost all research to date has been performed in field settings, under varying conditions. Studies have included anesthetized, stressed, sick or hibernating animals and this will all add a layer of complexity to the extrapolation of a normal lactate range from a wild animal to exotic taxa in human care.

As with many things in exotic medicine, trends within a patient and within species matter more than a single datum point. Serial lactate concentrations are, therefore, much more important for monitoring a patient than a single lactate concentration.

Mammals

Lactate is well described in the human literature and to a lesser extent in companion and laboratory animals; therefore, extrapolation of lactate concentrations to other mammals is easier than in the case of reptiles and birds. Again, due to the wide variety of gas analyzers and treatments of animals in these studies, lactate values should be used as a rough guideline rather than an absolute range. Animals frequently used in laboratories have been more extensively studied than companion mammals via large benchtop analyzer. Guinea pigs of the Short hair English (SHE) and Duncan-Hartley (DH) variety, had lactate values of 0.11 to .56 mmol/L (SHE) and 0.003 to 0.73 mmol/L (DH).[26] Female mice had normal lactate concentrations of 0.04 mmol/L–0.08 mmol/L, while normal in males were 0.04 to 1.09 mmol/L.[26] Rats had higher concentrations of lactate with males 1.9 to 5.61 mmol/L and females 1.15 to 5.42 mmol/L.[26] Sedated, healthy ferrets had lactate concentrations of 0.3 to 1.5 mmol/L when performed on portable analyzers.[27]

White rhino (Ceratotherium simum) lactate concentrations decreased during prolonged anesthesia from t = 0 at 2.5 mmol/L to t = 20 at 0.89 mmol/L. This finding supports that stressed animals often have higher lactate early in an anesthetic event, which should continue to drop. A failure to observe a downward trend in lactate concentration is caused to reevaluate the anesthetized patient. In this study, rhinos were contained in a boma (enclosure) which may have lessened capture stress. Thus, initial lactate concentrations may have been lower than wild counterparts who may experience more exertion during capture.[23]

Neonatal giraffe with hyperlactatemia greater than 5.0 mmol/L that resolves with fluid therapy was attributable to illness and neonatal status.[28] Antelope are often volatile and prone to capture myopathy and should have lactate concentrations determined at time zero postcapture and at least one additional time during a capture/ anesthesia procedure to ensure a progressive decrease of blood lactate concentrations. Although lactate concentrations in this taxon may initially be relatively high they should trend downward during the course of anesthesia.

Rabbits, are unusual, in that ill rabbits with higher lactate concentrations have a higher probability of surviving than their low lactate counterparts. This deviation of lactate concentrations from what occurs in other mammals may be linked to cecatrophy.[29,30] Lactic acid metabolism within rabbits seems to differ and much higher blood lactate concentrations occur in rabbits compared with other species.

Birds

Birds, in contrast to reptiles, seem to have lactate values that are more similar to mammals, this may at least in part be due to the endothermic nature of both birds and mammals. True reference values for avian patients have yet to be established and most studies have been performed under field circumstances (**Box 2**). In the absence of reference values, perform serial lactate concentrations both within individuals and across species. Research conducted on lactate concentrations in birds has measured lactate concentrations post–mist-netting, under physical restraint, with and without sedation, birds held in pillowcases, and unconditioned versus conditioned flight; all of these parameters can induce stress in birds and have an impact on lactate concentrations.

A large study of passerine birds, more than 100 individuals from 11 families, under field conditions, measured lactate with both sedated and unsedated protocols. In general, the sedated birds had decreased lactate mean concentrations [2.79 mmol/L] compared with unsedated birds [4.39 mmol/L].[31] In an additional study on another large group of passerines, adult birds had a mean lactate of 4.4 mmol/L as opposed to juveniles whereby the mean was 5.048 mmol/L.[32] Higher lactate concentrations in young passerine birds mirrors previous findings in mammals, as mammalian neonates have relatively increased concentrations of lactate.

Studies on the effect of mist netting on 3 species of birds found that all 3 species had a reduction in the concentration of lactate if birds were allowed to calm after release from a mist net before blood was collected. Mourning doves (Zenaida macroura) immediately postmist net release (7.72 mmol/L), to delayed of 4.83 mmol/L, House sparrows (Passer domesticus) immediately postmist net release (4.77 mmol/ L), to a delayed value of 3.14 mmol/L.[9] Boat-tailed grackles (Q. major) immediately postmist net release (5.61 mmol/L) to a delayed value of 2.62 mmol/L.[9] Although this was true in these 3 species, bird taxa will likely react differently to being placed

Box 2		
Avian lactate concentrations under various conditions		
Species	Lactate Level Mean mmol/L	Conditions
Flamingo (Phoenicopterus ruber)	8.61 mmol/L	Hand capture, restraint Delay in testing[24]
Boat-tailed grackle (Quiscalus major)	5.61 mmol/L	Immediately after release from mist net[9]
Boat-tailed grackle (Quiscalus major)	2.62 mmol/L	Allowed to calm after release from mist net[9]
House sparrow	4.77 mmol/L	Immediate postrelease from mist net[9]
House sparrow	3.14 mmol/L	Allowed to calm after release from mist net[9]
Mourning dove	7.72 mmol/L	Immediate postrelease from mist net[9]
Mourning dove	4.83 mmol/L	Allowed to calm after release from mist net[9]
Raptor	22.2 mmol/L	Unconditioned postflight lactate level[33]
Raptor	5.5–8.8 mmol/L	Conditioned postflight lactate level[33]
Penguin (Aptenodytes forsteri)	1.2 mmol/L– 2.7 mmol/L	Lactate was measured predive[34]
Passerines (11 families)	2.79 mmol/L	With Midazolam sedation[31]
Passerines (11 families)	4.39 mmol/L	Without midazolam sedation[31]
Passerine chicks	5.04 mmol/L	No sedation[32]

in a pillowcase as some species may experience higher stress levels that parallel the amount of time in restraint.

A study of flamingos found that an increased lactate concentration correlated to the amount of time the bird was held postcapture, but not to the capture difficulty.[24] This study found a higher mean lactate concentration, 8.61 mmol/L than has been found in other taxa of birds. The birds were confined to a boma before testing with some animals not processed for over an hour. The unit designated as the gold standard for this study was the ABL-750 gas analyzer. Three types of lactate units were used with 3 different processing methodologies; the iStat produced the highest lactate values and the ABL-750 intermediate and VetTest the lowest values. Although all three units returned different lactate concentration values were strongly correlated.[24] This study clarifies the need for the lack of interchangeability of lactate values provided from different analyzers and the need to standardize the analyzer used.

Lactate concentrations have been used to assess the ability of raptors to be returned to the wild after rehabilitation, after flying unconditioned raptors could reach lactate concentrations of 22.2 mmol/L, while conditioned birds had lactate concentrations of 5.55 to 8.88 mmol/L.[33]

Emperor penguins (Aptenodytes forsteri) and penguins in general, differ greatly from other taxa of birds and have the ability to stay submerged when feeding for up to 8 minutes.[34] In a study of the aerobic dive limit in Emperor penguins, submersion beyond 5 minutes was needed to begin to increase lactate concentrations with lactate concentrations increasing substantially after 7 to 8 minutes. Predive lactate concentrations in Emperor penguins (A forsteri) were 1.2 mmol/L–2.7 mmol/L.[34]

Reptiles

Reptiles constitute a large group of animals with vastly different physiologies. As ectotherms, reptiles rely more on anaerobic metabolism than endotherms, even during relatively short bursts of activity. Reptiles have evolutionary adaptations to survive in anoxic conditions including slow metabolic rates and ability to sequester and buffer lactate. Reptiles may have a much higher lactate tolerance and the associated acidosis, than other taxa. Unfortunately, the few studies available of reference ranges in reptiles and studies assessing lactate concentrations used vastly differing study methodologies (**Box 3**).

Early laboratory studies on lizards demonstrated that Iguana (*Iguana iguana*) had a resting lactate of 2.1 mmol/L, while after an intense treadmill run had a lactate of 16.5 mmol/L and *Varanus exanthematicus*, a larger bodied lizard had a resting lactate of 1.6 mmol/L and after the same run had a blood lactate concentration of 20.5 mmol/L.[35]

Lava lizards (*Microlophus bivittatus*), an endemic species of the Galapagos islands, had lactate concentrations of 17.08 mmol/L for men and 17.04 mmol/L in women, with animals handled for 5 to 10 minutes before sampling, which may account for the higher concentrations than seen in some other reptile species.[36]

Painted turtles (*Chrysemys picta*) who spend long periods of time submerged in anoxic conditions and demonstrate remarkable adaptations.[37] A lowered metabolic rate contributes to slowing the rate of lactate production, and this species has very high concentrations of bicarbonate (HCO 3-) in extracellular fluid, to include the pericardial space.[37] This species can also buffer and sequester lactic acid in the shell and bones.[38] Painted turtles can tolerate concentrations of lactic acid as high as 150 to 200 mmol/L. Tolerance to high concentrations of lactate also occurs in other species of freshwater turtle; species with harder shells seem able to tolerate lactate buildup more than soft-shelled turtles (*Apalone spinifera*).[39]

As in many vertebrates, disease and capture time correlated to a rise in lactate concentrations in a study on box turtles (*Terrapene carolina carolina*).[40]

Free-ranging Eastern copperheads (*Agkistrodon contortrix*) and Eastern rat snakes (*Pantherophis alleghaniensis*) were captured, bled immediately, then processed for morphometric measurements and resampled, between immediate and postprocessing lactate concentrations both species had a rise in lactate. Although both species

---

Box 3
Reptile lactate concentrations under various conditions

Species	Lactate Level Mean mmol/L	Conditions
Eastern Copperhead (*Agkistrodon contortrix*)	10.9 mmol/L	Field, shortly after capture[41]
Eastern Copperhead (*A. contortrix*)	12.7 mmol/L	Field, resampled after morphometric measurement[41]
Eastern rat snake (*Pantherophis alleghaniensis*)	10.3 mmol/L	Field, shortly after capture[41]
Eastern rat snake (*P. alleghaniensis*)	17.4 mmol/L	Field, resampled after morphometric measurement[41]
Lava Lizard (*Microlophus bivattatus*)	17.08 (m) 17.04 (f)	Field, handled for ~10 min before sample[36]
Nile crocodile (*Crocodylus niloticus*)	4.0 mmol/L	Electrostunned[42]
Nile Crocodile (*C niloticus*)	10.2 mmol/L	Noosed[42]
Galapagos marine iguanas (*Amblyrhynchus cristatus*)	6.63 mmol/L	Field, captured and quickly sampled[43]
Galapagos green turtles (*Chelonia mydas*)	3.73 mmol/L	Field, captured and quickly sampled[45]

had relatively increased lactate concentrations in the second sample, rat snakes had significantly higher concentrations of lactate at the second reading than the copperheads. Immediate sampling for the copperheads provided a mean lactate concentration of 10.9 mmol/L with the second sample of 12.7 mmol/L. For rat snakes, immediate mean lactate concentrations were 10.3 mmol/L and 17.4 mmol/L for the second sample.[41]

When farmed Nile crocodiles were subjected to electro-stunning and noosing, electro-stunned animals had a mean lactate of 4.0 mmol/L and the noosed animals had a mean lactate of 10.2 mmol/L. These findings are expected as noosed crocodiles often struggle violently, thereby increasing blood lactate concentrations.[42]

Wild Galapagos marine iguanas (*Amblyrhynchus cristatus*) were captured and processed for blood samples within a few minutes, the mean lactate of this species was 6.63 mmol/L.[43] As the only lizard which forages in the ocean, marine iguanas differ greatly from land lizards, but do not use the anaerobic capacity to forage underwater.[44]

Galapagos green turtles (*Chelonia mydas*) sampled within 5 minutes of capture had lactate concentrations of 3.73 mmol/L.[45] Lactate concentrations, determined 2 to 3 days post event, increased significantly in cold-stunned Kemp's Ridley sea turtles (*Lepidochelys kempii*), and were presumed linked to perfusion status.[46]

Amphibians

The ability to use both pulmonary and cutaneous respiration, allows amphibians to use both aerobic and anaerobic metabolism to meet energy needs. During times of high energy demand or low oxygen availably the reliance on the anerobic metabolism does result in elevated lactate concentrations, similar to other taxa.[47] In bullfrogs (*Bufo americanus*), approximately 20% of the energy expended during activity is derived from anaerobic metabolism and 80% from aerobic metabolism. After periods of intense exertion, lactate concentrations quickly exceed 5 to 20 times resting concentrations, but may take an hour or more to return to resting concentrations postactivity.[48] Studies on the clinical utility of lactate measurement during anesthesia or disease in amphibian patients are lacking.

Treatment

Increased blood lactic acid concentrations have an underlying cause which has resulted in hypoperfusion. While the resolution of the inciting cause must be managed, some supportive care is appropriate. Symptomatic treatments include increasing oxygenation, inotropes, vasopressors, and resuscitative fluid therapy. In reptiles, the use of lactate-free fluids is recommended to alleviate a presumed high burden of lactate; the use of lactated ringers is not recommended. Treatment of lactic acidosis with sodium bicarbonate alone will not alleviate the primary problem, only the symptom, and may be injurious. Bicarbonate can cause intracellular acidosis and potentially exacerbate the acidosis.[49,50]

SUMMARY

Reference values have yet to be established for many species but generalizations can be made particularly with mammals and birds. Reptiles and amphibians may demonstrate highly variable lactate concentrations compared with mammals or birds but trends within a patient make lactate a valuable analyte to assess.

Increased lactate concentrations may indicate early, compensatory stages of shock (hypoperfusion). Vital signs and clinical appearance of the patient may not change in silent or occult hypoperfusion (early compensatory shock). Thus, monitoring lactate concentrations provides an early indication that the patient requires additional support. Rapid response to a patient in compensatory shock prevents the patient from moving toward noncompensatory shock and lactic acidosis, a course much harder to reverse. Early recognition and correction of hypoperfusion increases the likelihood of a favorable positive patient outcome and improves the level of care administered. Although a patient may recover and seem clinically normal after an event or procedure that may have included some level of ischemia; each subsequent event increases patient vulnerability to ischemia. Thus, the use of patient-side lactate meters allows for simple, rapid, and cost-conscious improvement of patient care.

CLINICS CARE POINTS

- Rabbits have higher lactate values than other mammalian species.
- Lactate should be incorporated into a robust anesthetic monitoring protocol.
- Lactate values can vary in different parts of the body, indicating poor regional perfusion.
- Mixed reasons for lactate elevations can occur in complex cases.
- Lactate values can change quickly, patient-side processing of samples is essential.
- Collecting samples from venous catheters while administering lactated ringer's solution can cause artificially elevated lactate measurement

DISCLOSURE

The authors have nothing to disclose.

REFERENCES

1. Stevenson CK, Kidney B, Duke T, et al. Serial blood lactate concentrations in systemically ill dogs. Vet Clin Pathol 2007;36(3):234–9.
2. De Papp E, Drobatz KJ, et al. Plasma lactate concentration as a predictor of gastric necrosis and survival among dogs with gastric dilatation-volvulus: 102 cases (1995-1998). J Am Vet Med Assoc 1999;215(1):49–52.
3. Ewaschuk JB, Naylor JM, Zello GA. D-lactate in human and ruminant metabolism. J Nut 2005;135(7):1619–25.
4. Acierno MJ, Mitchell MA. Evaluation of four point-of-care meters for rapid determination of blood lactate concentrations in dogs. J Am Vet Med Assoc 2007; 230(9):1315–8.
5. Acierno MJ, Johnson ME, Eddelman LA, et al. Measuring statistical agreement between four point of care (POC) lactate meters and a laboratory blood analyzer in cats. J Feline Med Surg 2008;10(2):110–4.
6. Breed D, Meyer LC, Steyl JC, et al. Conserving wildlife in a changing world: Understanding capture myopathy—A malignant outcome of stress during capture and translocation. Conservation Physiol 2019;7(1):coz027.
7. Pang DS, Boysen S. Lactate in veterinary critical care: pathophysiology and management. J Am Anim Hosp Assoc 2007;43(5):270–9.
8. Hughes D, Rozanski E, Shofer F, et al. Effect of sampling site, repeated sampling, pH, and PCO2 on plasma lactate concentration in healthy dogs. Am J Vet Res 1999;60(4):521–4.
9. Harms CA, Jinks MR, Harms RV. Blood gas, lactate, and hematology effects of venipuncture timing and location after mist-net capture of mourning doves

(*Zenaida macroura*), boat-tailed grackles (*Quiscalus major*), and house sparrows (*Passer domesticus*). J Wildl Dis 2016;52(2s):S54–64.

10. Hashimoto-Hill S, Magdesian KG, Kass PH. Serial measurement of lactate concentration in horses with acute colitis. J Vet Intern Med 2001;25(6):1414–9.

11. Lindner A, Marx S, Kissenbeck S, et al. Saliva collection and relationship between lactate concentration in blood and saliva of exercising horses. J Equine Vet Sci 2000;20(1):52–4.

12. Contreras-Aguilar MD, Cerón JJ, Muñoz A, et al. Changes in saliva biomarkers during a standardized increasing intensity field exercise test in endurance horses. Animal 2021;15(6):100236.

13. Andersen LW, Mackenhauer J, Roberts JC, et al. Etiology and therapeutic approach to elevated lactate levels. Mayo Clin Proc 2013;88(10):1127–40.

14. McMichael MA, Lees GE, Hennessey J, et al. Serial plasma lactate concentrations in 68 puppies aged 4 to 80 days. J Vet Emerg Crit Care 2005;15(1):17–21.

15. Levitsky LL, Fisher DE, Paton JB, et al. Fasting plasma levels of glucose, acetoacetate, d-β-hydroxybutyrate, glycerol, and lactate in the baboon infant: correlation with cerebral uptake of substrates and oxygen. Pediatr Res 1977;11(4): 298–302.

16. Balakrishnan V, Wilson J, Taggart B, et al. Impact of phlebotomy tourniquet use on blood lactate levels in acutely ill patients. Can J Emerg Med 2016;18(5): 358–62.

17. Woehlck HJ, Boettcher BT, Dorantes RP. Clinical use of lactate measurements: Comment. Anesthesiology 2021;35(4):765–6.

18. Calatayud O, Tenias JM. Effects of time, temperature and blood cell counts on levels of lactate in heparinized whole blood gas samples. Scand J Clin Lab Invest 2003;63(4):311–4.

19. Onor M, Gufoni S, Lomonaco T, et al. Potentiometric sensor for noninvasive lactate determination in human sweat. Anal Chim Acta 2017;989:80–7.

20. Tynan B, Kerl ME, Jackson ML, et al. Plasma lactate concentrations and comparison of two point-of-care lactate analyzers to a laboratory analyzer in a population of healthy cats. J Vet Emerg Crit Care 2015;25(4):521–7.

21. Kubo K, Takagi S, Murakami M, et al. Heart rate and blood lactate concentration of horses during maximal work. Bull Equine Res Inst 1984;21:39–45.

22. Muñoz A, Castejón-Riber C, Riber C, et al. Current knowledge of pathologic mechanisms and derived practical applications to prevent metabolic disturbances and exhaustion in the endurance horse. J Equine Vet Sci 2017;51:24–33.

23. Buss P, Olea-Popelka F, Meyer L, et al. Evaluation of cardiorespiratory, blood gas, and lactate values during extended immobilization of white rhinoceros (*Ceratotherium simum*). J Zoo Wildl 2015;46(2):224–33.

24. Burgdorf-Moisuk A, Wack R, Ziccardi M, et al. Validation of lactate measurement in American flamingo (*Phoenicopterus ruber*) plasma and correlation with duration and difficulty of capture. J Zoo Wildl 2012;43(3):450–8.

25. Harrison JF, Phillips JE, Gleeson TT. Activity physiology of the two-striped grasshopper, Melanoplus bivittatus: gas exchange, hemolymph acid-base status, lactate production, and the effect of temperature. Physiol Zool 1991;64(2): 451–72.

26. Boehm O, Zur B, Koch A. et al. Clinical chemistry reference database for Wistar rats and C57/BL6 mice. 2007;547-554.

27. Yuschenkoff D, Graham J, Sharkey L, et al. Reference interval determination of venous blood gas, hematologic, and biochemical parameters in healthy sedated, neutered ferrets (*Mustela putorius furo*). J Exot Pet Med 2021;36:25–7.

28. Dixon CE, Bedenice D, Restifo M, et al. Neonatal intensive care of 10 hospitalized giraffe calves (*Giraffa camelopardalis*) requiring hand-rearing. J Zoo Wildl Med 2021;52(1):57–66.

29. Ardiaca M, Dias S, Montesinos A, et al. Plasmatic l-lactate in pet rabbits: association with morbidity and mortality at 14 days. Vet Clin Pathol 2016;45(1):116–23.

30. Langlois I, Planché A, Boysen SR, et al. Blood concentrations of d-and l-lactate in healthy rabbits. J Small Anim Pract 2014;55(9):451–6.

31. Heatley JJ, Cary J, Kingsley L, et al. Midazolam sedates Passeriformes for field sampling but affects multiple venous blood analytes. Vet Med Res Rep 2015; 6:61.

32. Heatley JJ, Cary J, Russell KE, et al. Clinicopathologic analysis of Passeriform venous blood reflects transitions in elevation and habitat. Vet Med Res Rep 2013;4:21.

33. Chaplin SB, Mueller LR, Degernes LA. Physiological assessment of rehabilitated raptors prior to release. In: Redig PT, Cooper JE, Remple JD, et al, editors. Raptor Biomedicine. Minneapolis (MN): University of Minnesota Press; 1993. p. 167–73.

34. Ponganis PJ, Kooyman GL, Starke LN, et al. Post-dive blood lactate concentrations in emperor penguins, Aptenodytes forsteri. J Exp Biol 1997;200(11):1623–6.

35. Gleeson TT, Bennett AF. Acid-base imbalance in lizards during activity and recovery. J Exp Biol 1982;98(1):439–53.

36. Arguedas R, Steinberg D, Lewbart GA, et al. Haematology and biochemistry of the San Cristóbal Lava Lizard (*Microlophus bivittatus*). Conserv Physiol 2018; 6(1):coy046.

37. Jackson DC. Hibernating without oxygen: physiological adaptations of the painted turtle. J Physiol 2002;543(3):731–7.

38. Jackson DC, Taylor SE, Asare VS, et al. Comparative shell buffering properties correlate with anoxia tolerance in freshwater turtles. Am J Physiol Regul Integr Comp Physiol 2007;292(2):R1008–15.

39. Reese SA, Jackson DC, Ultsch GR. Hibernation in freshwater turtles: softshell turtles (*Apalone spinifera*) are the most intolerant of anoxia among North American species. J Comp Physiol B 2003;173(3):263–8.

40. Klein K, Adamovicz L, Phillips CA, et al. Blood lactate concentrations in eastern box turtles (*Terrapene carolina carolina*) following capture by a canine search team. J Zoo Wildl 2021;52(1):259–67.

41. Cerreta AJ, Cannizzo SA, Smith DC, et al. Venous hematology, biochemistry, and blood gas analysis of free-ranging Eastern Copperheads (*Agkistrodon contortrix*) and Eastern Ratsnakes (*Pantherophis alleghaniensis*). PLoS One 2020;15(2): e0229102.

42. Pfitzer S, Ganswindt A, Fosgate GT, et al. Capture of farmed Nile crocodiles (*Crocodylus niloticus*): comparison of physiological parameters after manual capture and after capture with electrical stunning. Vet Rec 2014;175(12):304.

43. Lewbart GA, Hirschfeld M, Brothers JR, et al. Blood gases, biochemistry and haematology of Galápagos marine iguanas (*Amblyrhynchus cristatus*). Conserv Physiol 2015;3(1):cov034.

44. Gleeson TT. Lactic acid production during field activity in the Galapagos marine iguana, *Amblyrhynchus cristatus*. Physiol Zool 1980;53(2):157–62.

45. Lewbart GA, Hirschfeld M, Denkinger J, et al. Blood gases, biochemistry, and hematology of Galapagos green turtles (*Chelonia mydas*). PLoS One 2014;9(5): e96487.

46. Innis CJ, Tlusty M, Merigo C, et al. Metabolic and respiratory status of cold-stunned Kemp's ridley sea turtles (*Lepidochelys kempii*). J Comp Physiol B 2007;177(6):623–30.
47. Bennett AF, Licht P. Anaerobic metabolism during activity in amphibians. Comp Biochem Physiol A Physiol 1974;48(2):319–27.
48. Withers PC, Lea M, Solberg TC, et al. Metabolic fates of lactate during recovery from activity in an anuran amphibian, Bufo americanus. J Exp Zool 1988;246(3): 236–43.
49. Rudnick MR, Blair GJ, Kuschner WG, et al. Lactic acidosis and the role of sodium bicarbonate: a narrative opinion. Shock 2020;53(5):528–36.
50. Mathieu D, Neviere R, Billard V, et al. Effects of bicarbonate therapy on hemody-namics and tissue oxygenation in patients with lactic acidosis: a prospective, controlled clinical Care. Med 1991;19(11):1352–6.

Viscoelastic Coagulation Testing in Exotic Animals

Charles O. Cummings, DVM[a],*, Jessica Eisenbarth, DVM[b],
Armelle deLaforcade, DVM, DACVECC[b]

KEYWORDS

- Thromboelastography • Thromboelastometry • Sonoclot • Zoological medicine
- Hemostasis • Clotting • Coagulopathy

KEY POINTS

- Whole-blood viscoelastic coagulation testing (VCT) evaluates global hemostatic pathways, considering clotting factors, cellular contributions, and fibrinolysis.
- VCT assays can be interpreted both quantitively and qualitatively to identify thrombotic or bleeding tendencies.
- Most VCT research in exotic animals has centered on a few model organisms: rats, rabbits, and chickens.
- Lack of standardized protocols limits interpretability of VCT in exotic animals.
- As point-of-care viscoelastic coagulation monitors become increasingly available, their potential for use in exotic animal medicine grows.

INTRODUCTION

Although uncommon in zoological medicine due to a lack of reference intervals,[1] coagulation testing is widely used in human and domestic animal medicine for the detection of bleeding and/or thrombotic tendencies Supplementary Data. The most common of these diagnostics in veterinary medicine are platelet/thrombocyte counts, prothrombin time (PT), activated partial thromboplastin time (aPTT), and fibrinogen concentration, used especially in large animal medicine. In critical care settings, other assays, such as D-dimers and fibrin degradation products (FDPs), are also used. Although useful, each of these assays only evaluate a single component of hemostasis. Platelet/thrombocyte count and buccal mucosal bleeding time evaluate platelet/thrombocyte number, form, and function, whereas PT and aPTT evaluate the function of the extrinsic and intrinsic clotting factor cascades. D-dimers and FDPs are used in the assessment of fibrinolysis and can be used, in combination with other tests, to diagnose thrombotic diseases such as disseminated intravascular coagulation (DIC).

---

[a] Tufts Clinical and Translational Science Institute, Tufts Medical Center, 35 Kneeland Street Suite 8, Boston, MA 0211, USA; [b] Department of Clinical Sciences, Cummings School of Veterinary Medicine at Tufts University, 200 Westboro Road, North Grafton, MA 01536, USA
* Corresponding author.
E-mail address: cummings3793@gmail.com

Vet Clin Exot Anim 25 (2022) 597–612
https://doi.org/10.1016/j.cvex.2022.06.001
1094-9194/22/© 2022 Elsevier Inc. All rights reserved.
vetexotic.theclinics.com

Abbreviations	
TEG	Thromboelastography
TEM	Thromboelastometry

In the last 2 decades, viscoelastic coagulation assays including thromboelastography (TEG), thromboelastometry (TEM), and Sonoclot have gained traction in human and veterinary medicine. Viscoelastic coagulation testing (VCT) allows the assessment of cellular (platelet/thrombocyte, erythrocyte, leukocyte) and plasma contributions (fibrinogen and other clotting factors) to clot formation and fibrinolysis, providing the greatest global assessment of coagulation currently available. Viscoelastic assays are able to visually display clot kinetics in the form of a clot curve. The shapes of different clot curves often reveal the underlying clotting problem and suggests an appropriate therapy (fibrinogen, plasma, fresh whole blood). These assays have been used in domestic animals to diagnose DIC and to make decisions on anticoagulant and antiplatelet therapy in a wide array of systemic conditions. In zoological medicine, these assays have been used for evaluation of elephant endotheliotropic herpesviruses in elephants,[2–4] cold stress/stunning in manatees[5,6] and sea turtles,[7–9] and verminous pneumonia in red pandas[10] and seals.[11] This article focuses on the use of VCT in exotic companion animals.

THROMBOELASTOGRAPHY AND THROMBOELASTOMETRY

In thromboelastography and thromboelastometry analyzers, a pin is suspended in a sample cup of recalcified whole blood. Then, either the pin (TEM) or the cup (TEG) starts to rotate or oscillate (**Fig. 1A, B**). As a clot begins to form, fibrin strands between the pin and the sample cup cause the pin to be deflected from its expected position. This is detected with an electromechanical transducer (TEG) or optical detector (TEM). The amplitude of this deflection continues to increase as the clot becomes larger and stronger. Eventually, as fibrinolysis occurs, this amplitude decreases.

From this curve, there are 5 main parameters that are reported (**Fig. 2A**). The first is a measure of initial fibrin formation, defined as a 2-mm amplitude deflection. This value is called R, or reaction time, in TEG and clotting time (CT) in TEM. Prolonged R or CT values can indicate factor deficiencies, whereas rapid R/CT values indicate hypercoagulability. The next parameter is called K in TEG and clot formation time (CFT) in TEM. Both are measurements of the time it takes for a clot to attain a fixed degree of viscoelasticity; K/CFT are defined as the time from a 2-mm deflection (R/CT) to a 20-mm deflection. A related measure in TEG and TEM is the alpha angle (α°), which measures the rate of clot formation. Alpha angle and K/CFT measurements are heavily affected by the concentration of fibrinogen. Insufficient fibrinogen results in prolonged K/CFTs and smaller clotting angles. Conversely, if fibrinogen is markedly elevated, K/CFTs can be decreased and α° increased, indicating hypercoagulability. Maximum amplitude (MA) in TEG or maximum clot firmness (MCF) in TEM refer to the largest amplitude of pin deflection that is achieved. MA and MCF are thought to reflect mostly platelet number and function, so, in some human medical algorithms, MAs less than a certain threshold may trigger a platelet transfusion. Lysis at 30 minutes (LY30 for TEG and LI30 for TEM) is expressed as a percentage reduction in MA/MCF. These parameters can allow the detection of hyperfibrinolysis. Importantly, although all of these parameters are similarly defined, they are not directly comparable between TEG and TEM due to differences in pin/cup materials and activators.[12]

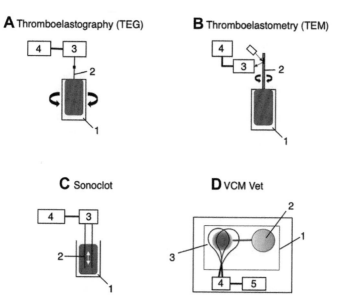

Fig. 1. Viscoelastic coagulation monitors. (*A*) Thromboelastography (TEG): rotating sample cup (1), pin and torsion wire (2), electromechanical transducer (3), data processor (4). (*B*) Thromboelastometry (TEM): stationary sample cuvette (1), rotating pin and rotating axis (2), electromechanical signal detector using light source and mirror mounted on rotating axis (3), data processor (4). (*C*) Sonoclot: stationary sample cuvette (1), oscillating probe (2), electromechanical transducer (3), data processor (4). (*D*) VCM Vet: cartridge (1), sample well (2), oscillating glass plates (3), oscillating plate-arm driver and electromechanical transducer (4), data processor (5).

These assays are customizable to answer different clinical questions. They can be run using different activators to trigger extrinsic or intrinsic clotting cascades. They can also be run using platelet inhibitors or fresh frozen plasma, which measures functional fibrinogen. Fresh frozen plasma TEG/TEM is more common in zoological medicine, as these analyzers are not commonly found outside of universities and referral hospitals.

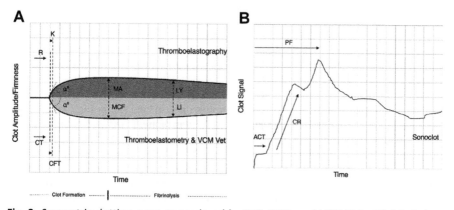

Fig. 2. Symmetric clotting curve as produced by TEG, TEM, and VCM Vet with labeled parameters (*A*). Sonoclot Signature with labeled parameters (*B*).

SONOCLOT

Sonoclot differs from TEG and TEM in that it neither uses the same "pin in cup" technology nor provides the same kind of clot curve. Instead, a hollow, open-ended probe, connected to a transducer, is suspended in the sample (**Fig. 1**C) and oscillates up and down. As a clot begins to form, the impedance of the probe's motion is detected by the transducer, and a Sonoclot Signature (clot curve) is generated (**Fig. 2**B).

The parameters generated by Sonoclot are activated clotting time (ACT), clot rate (CR), and platelet function (PF). Activated clotting time is defined as the time point that the clot curve viscosity measurement increases by one Clot Signal unit. Clot rate is defined as the maximum slope of the Sonoclot Signature during initial fibrin gel formation and is conceptually similar to alpha angles. Platelet function is given as an automated result that quantifies the quality of clot retraction. A PF of 0 represents no platelet function, whereas a value of 5 represents high platelet function. Sonoclot assays are similarly customizable as TEG/TEM.

VCM VET AND OTHER NEXT-GENERATION VISCOELASTIC COAGULATION MONITORS

The VCM Vet is a novel, cartridge-based, viscoelastic coagulation monitor that is gaining use in small animal emergency and critical care settings.[13–16] Although it provides a similar clot curve to TEG/TEM, VCM Vet does not use the same "pin in cup" technology. Instead, the whole blood sample is suspended between 2 glass plates that oscillate across one another (**Fig. 1**D). As the clot begins to form between the 2 plates, an optical sensor detects the mechanical displacement of the plates, resulting in a clot tracing. Although it uses similar conventions of TEM for naming its parameters, VCM Vet is not directly comparable to TEM or TEG.[16]

Several other technologies are being used to improve ease of use and portability of viscoelastic coagulation monitoring.[17] These systems are also cartridge based and designed with austere settings in mind, such as helicopters.[17] Cartridge-based systems are likely to improve ease of use and interoperator error relative to open systems but that may come at the expense of customizability.

VISCOELASTIC COAGULATION TESTING IN SMALL MAMMALS

Few studies have evaluated the use of VCT in small exotic companion mammals for veterinary medicine, but these animals can serve as models for human disease. Blood volume limitations in the smallest species have led to the use of other larger models, such as pigs and sheep, being preferred. Nonetheless, normal TEG values have been published for rats,[18–21] mice,[19] guinea pigs,[22] and rabbits,[19,23] normal TEM values for rabbits[24,25] and rats,[25,26] normal Sonoclot values for rabbits,[27] and normal VCM Vet values for mice[28] (**Table 1**).

There remains much to learn regarding optimal sample handling and how different variables may affect VCT results in exotic mammals. In one study that established reference intervals for the VCM Vet in mice, MCF was higher in females with no differences found in the other main parameters.[28] In one mouse study, venipuncture site (facial vein vs cardiac puncture) did not affect TEG results,[29] whereas in another rat study, different venipuncture sites (femoral artery vs cardiac puncture) resulted in different TEG parameters.[21] It should be noted, however, that, in any difficult venipuncture requiring multiple attempts, VCT results could be altered through premature tissue factor activation. In rabbits, there was no difference in TEM results between samples that were allowed to rest at room temperature for 30 minutes when compared

Table 1
Viscoelastic coagulation assay values for clinically healthy, exotic companion mammals

Species	N	Method	Activator	Sample	Temperature (C°)	R/CT (s)	K/CFT (s)	α°/CR (°)	MA/MCF (mm/VCM units)	LY30/LI30 (%)	Notes
Norway Rat[20] (*Rattus norvegicus*)	35	TEG	None	Citrated blood	37	198–438	66–210	48–72	54–71	0	—
Norway Rat[26] (*R. norvegicus*)	43	TEM (mini-cup)	TF	Citrated blood	37	18–77	20–80	73–86	53–70	0–2	Reference Interval
House Mouse[28] (*Mus musculus*)	63	VCM Vet™	None	Fresh blood	37	43–353	49–138	54–62	38–63	0	Reference Interval
Guinea Pig[22] (*Cavia porcellus*)	30	TEG	NR	Citrated blood	37	142–374	54–161	NR	56–79	NR	—
European Rabbit[31] (*Oryctolagus cuniculus*)	15	TEG	None	Fresh blood	37	88–449	31–114	63–82	55–76	NR	—
Species	**N**	**Method**	**Activator**	**Sample**	**Temperature (C°)**	**ACT (s)**		**CR (Units/min)**	**PF (PF units)**		**Notes**
European Rabbit[27] (*O. cuniculus*)	18	Sonoclot	None	Citrated blood	37	160–296	—	8–24	2–5	—	Allowed to rest at room temperature

Data are reported as a range of mean ± 1.96*standard deviation. R/CT and K/CFT had a minimum limit of 0 s, whereas α° had a maximum limit of 90°. Refer to the bottom row for Sonoclot parameter names. PF had a minimum limit of 0 and maximum limit of 5. For normal values using alternative VCT modalities and protocols, see S1.

with warmed samples, suggesting that resting samples at room temperature is acceptable.[30] Conversely, another study of rabbits using Sonoclot found that resting temperature and citration had a dramatic impact on the results.[27] Analysis temperature is also an important consideration, as blood from hypothermic rabbits may exhibit a normal VCT (TEG and Sonoclot) tracing when analyzed at 37°C but is markedly hypocoagulable when measured at the hypothermic patient's body temperature.[31] Failure to consider this can lead to the false impression of normal coagulation ability. Unfortunately, even with established optimal protocols, animals can sometimes show systematically different VCT parameters for seemingly nonclinical reasons, such as stress from exposure to construction noise.[32]

Although considerably more research is needed, VCT has the potential to be an excellent ancillary diagnostic modality in exotic companion mammals. In rats and rabbits with carcinomas (squamous cell carcinoma in rats), TEG parameters indicated the presence of a paraneoplastic hypercoagulable state.[33,34] In rats, this hypercoagulability was even shown to resolve following complete, but not partial, tumor excision.[34] Rats chronically exposed to known hepatotoxins were hypocoagulable on TEG compared with controls.[35] Thus, VCT could potentially be used, along with measurement of glucose/albumin/bile acids, to monitor liver function in rats with hepatopathies. Rats injected with scorpion venom (tityustoxin) were hypercoagulable relative to controls, although different toxins may result in hypocoagulability.[36] Red pandas infected with novel metastrongyloid nematode similar to *Angiostrongylus vasorum* (known to cause bleeding tendencies) had mildly prolonged R and K, but similar alpha angles and MAs, compared with healthy controls.[10] Lastly, VCT is frequently used in the monitoring of snakebite envenomation in humans and domestic animals and may have similar utility in exotic companion mammals.

Viscoelastic coagulation testing has recently been gaining traction in human medicine for use in trauma patients, and data exist regarding exotic mammals and coagulopathy associated with trauma.[37–39] In a rabbit model of hypothermia and hemodilution, TEG was shown to be a more sensitive indicator of coagulopathy than the conventional PT assay.[37] In multiple studies using a rat model of uncontrolled hemorrhagic shock, aggressive fluid therapy was found to result in coagulopathy, whereas hypothermia alone had minimal impact on coagulation.[38,39] In rats with an induced triad of death—acidosis, hypothermia, and coagulopathy—rewarming resulted in improved Sonoclot parameters but not necessarily improved survival.[40]

VISCOELASTIC COAGULATION TESTING IN BACKYARD POULTRY AND COMPANION BIRDS

Backyard poultry and companion birds are susceptible to an array of bleeding conditions: hepatic lipidosis/hemorrhagic liver syndrome in poultry,[41,42] polytetrafluoroethylene toxicosis in all birds,[43,44] and aflatoxicosis in poultry.[45,46] In addition, wild birds of prey are affected by anticoagulant rodenticide toxicoses around the world.[47–52] Aberrant thrombosis, although not as prevalent as in mammals due to differences in platelet versus thrombocyte aggregation,[53] may also occur in some disease processes such as pit viper envenomation.[54]

Some conventional coagulation assays, such as PT, can work well in avian species, but they require avian-specific reagents (eg, tissue thromboplastin prepared from chick brains) in order to produce similar times and precision to mammalian assays.[55] Another conventional assay, aPTT, can be unreliable depending on the activator used and generally results in greatly prolonged times compared with mammals (>200s), likely due to a diminished or absent contact/intrinsic clotting cascade in avian species.[46,56]

In avian VCT, a similar trend is found in which unactivated or intrinsically activated samples have prolonged R/CT, K/CFT, and ACT relative to mammals.[46,57–59] When using mammalian tissue factor (TF) as an extrinsic activator at standard dilutions for mammals, TEG reaction times were markedly delayed relative to undiluted TF.[59]; this may be the result of either a greatly reduced affinity for mammalian TF compared with mammals, or running viscoelastic assays at a temperature (37°) less than body temperature, or a combination of both factors.[59]

Most of the VCT in birds has been performed using chickens (*Gallus gallus*) as a model organism; this is the only species for which normal values are available for TEG, TEM, VCM Vet, and Sonoclot (**Table 2**, S2).[46,58–60] Hispaniolan Amazon parrots have been evaluated with TEG and VCM Vet (Tully 2021, personal communication).[57] Other species, including Amazon parrots (*Amazonas spp*), American flamingos (*Phoenicopterus ruber*), scarlet ibises (*Eudocimus ruber*), Humboldt penguins (*Spheniscus humboldti*), and helmeted guineafowl (*Numida meleagris*) have been evaluated with TEG alone (see **Table 2**).[59]

In healthy chickens, several different VCT protocols have been used, comparing analyzers, activators, different additives, assay temperatures, and fresh versus citrated blood. In one study, fresh blood, unactivated VCM Vet parameters were imprecise and similar to unactivated and kaolin-activated TEG parameters (unpublished data, Eisenbarth et al. 2021). Inconsistencies with VCM Vet clot curve generation were noted in Hispaniolan Amazon parrots (Tully 2021, personal communication). When using undiluted mammalian TF as an activator, however, VCM Vet resulted in similar values to TF-activated TEG (unpublished data, Eisenbarth et al. 2021). One study, using TEM, found that a homologous extrinsic activator (tissue thromboplastin prepared from chick brains) resulted in more rapid CT and greater MCF than using TEM's standard extrinsic activator (EXTEM/mammalian TF).[60] In one TEG study, undiluted mammalian TF-activated TEG resulted in much greater qualitative consistency in generating clot curves, reduced R and K, and greater alpha angles compared with kaolin-activated and native blood TEG (unpublished data, Eisenbarth et al. 2021). Using Sonoclot, one study found differences in ACT, CR, and PF between fresh blood and citrated blood samples using different acitvators.[58] In addition to differences between assay protocols, there can be differences between chicken subgroups.[46] One study, using TEG, found that R and K were prolonged and alpha angles decreased in mature laying hens compared with 2-, 4-, and 6-week-old broiler chickens (S2).[46]

Thromboelastography and thromboelastometry have also been used to experimentally evaluate the effects of different toxins, drugs, and diseases on chicken coagulation.[46,60] Dicoumarol, a naturally occurring warfarin-like anticoagulant, was administered to growing broiler chickens in feed. Those fed the highest concentrations were hypocoagulable relative to controls.[46] With much more potent anticoagulants responsible for rodenticide toxicoses in birds of prey, these data speak to the potential utility of VCT in identifying rodenticide toxicoses in raptors. Mature layer hens fed aflatoxins, a common feed contaminant,[45] had prolonged K and decreased alpha angle and MA relative to controls.[46] Broiler chickens that were administered sulfaquinoxaline, a coccidiostat associated with hemorrhagic disease in chickens and domestic mammals,[61–63] in water or feed were found to be markedly hypocoagulable compared with controls in one study, but no difference was found in another.[60,64] These conflicting results may be attributable to different dosing regimens and use of different TEG protocols. Other sulfa drugs, sulfamethazine and sulfadimethoxine, were not found to affect TEG profiles.[64] Chickens experimentally infected with *Streptococcus equi zooepidemicus* displayed increased alpha angles and MA at 3 and 6 days postinfection relative to baseline values and sham-infected controls.[65] Fibrinogen

Table 2
Values for mammalian tissue factor–activated thromboelastography in clinically healthy birds

Species	N	Method	Activator	Sample	Temperature (C°)	R/CT (s)	K/CFT (s)	α° (°)	MA/MCF (mm)	LY30 (%)
Amazon parrot spp. (Amazona spp.)[59]	9	TEG	20 µL Undiluted Mammalian TF	Citrated blood	37	0–517	0–552	26–85	31–57	0–5
American Flamingo (Phoenicopterus ruber)[59]	13	TEG	20 µL Undiluted Mammalian TF	Citrated blood	37	0–736	0–445	28–88	43–60	0
Humboldt penguins (Spheniscus humboldti)[59]	6	TEG	20 µL Undiluted Mammalian TF	Citrated blood	37	0–1216	0–516	13–90	49–66	0
Scarlet Ibis (Eudocimus ruber)[59]	13	TEG	20 µL Undiluted Mammalian TF	Citrated blood	37	51–309	25–119	64–81	49–73	0
Helmeted Guineafowl (Numida meleagris)[59]	16	TEG	20 µL Undiluted Mammalian TF	Citrated blood	37	0–1067	0–32	37–90	53–80	0
Domestic Chicken (Gallus gallus)[59]	16	TEG	20 µL Undiluted Mammalian TF	Citrated blood	37	12–624	13–107	66–88	57–74	0

Data are reported as a range of mean ± 1.96*standard deviations; R and K had a minimum limit of 0 s, whereas α° had a maximum limit of 90°. For normal values using alternative VCT modalities and protocols, see S2.

concentrations were also elevated in experimentally infected birds and likely accounts for the relative hypercoagulability seen.

Viscoelastic assays, especially TEG, have demonstrated utility in identifying hypocoagulable and hypercoagulable states in birds; however, many questions remain to be answered about their use in everyday practice.[46,61,66–69] Currently, the most widely used and recommended VCT protocol in birds is citrated whole blood analyzed with TEG at 37°C with undiluted mammalian TF as an activator at 0.5 to 2 hours after blood collection.[59]

VISCOELASTIC COAGULATION TESTING IN POIKILOTHERMS

Comparatively little work has been done to investigate VCT in poikilotherms (S3). Much of the recent work that has been done has focused on developing a TEG protocol for use in sea turtles.[7,8] Other work has examined the effects of different activators on VCT in rattlesnakes,[70] the comparative coagulotoxicity of snake venoms to different prey classes (mammalian vs avian vs amphibian),[69,71–73] and the effect of stress and traumatic venipuncture on VCT in fish.[74,75] Unfortunately, there has been no published research into VCT in common exotic companion poikilotherms.

SOURCES OF VARIABILITY

As noted earlier, different VCT sampling protocols can result in markedly different results. Most of these differences are due to variation in activator type and amount and analysis temperature. More troubling, however, is that anemia causes TEGs to seem artifactually hypercoagulable; this is problematic because coagulopathic patients are often anemic, and it means that finding an appropriate comparator may be difficult or impossible in some clinical scenarios.

CLINICAL UTILITY OF VISCOELASTIC COAGULATION TESTING IN EXOTIC ANIMAL PRACTICE

Although suboptimal, a lack of reference intervals for healthy individuals of a given species does not necessarily preclude the use of VCT in that species; this is the daily reality for exotic animal veterinarians for most diagnostics. Instead, viscoelastic coagulation testing can be used to qualitatively evaluate differences in the shape of clot curves from a sick individual and a single healthy (or small number of) conspecific. The sensitivity and specificity for such a test is unclear and would depend on the patient's illness severity and a lack of subclinical disease in the comparison animal.

Nonetheless, VCT has proved useful in the authors' and others' experience. In one case at an investigator's institution, a ferret was transfused during an open liver biopsy and common bile duct stenting. The following morning, however, it was found to have a hemoabdomen with a markedly decreased PCV. When PT and aPTT were determined to be normal, however, a TEG was performed. Although no healthy ferret TEGs were available to review, a healthy ferret TEM curve was available in the literature.[76] For a qualitative rather than quantitative comparison, this TEM curve was considered an acceptable comparator. Based on this comparison, the ferret was diagnosed as hyperfibrinolytic. This real-time ability to assess fibrinolysis was extremely beneficial, as it enabled the medical management of hyperfibrinolysis with aminocaproic acid, preventing unnecessary exploratory surgery to address continued bleeding.

This is just one example of how VCT can be a useful aid in clinical decision-making. Nonetheless, there will remain a high degree of uncertainty in understanding how to interpret these assays in nondomestic species. Most importantly, aside from limitations to interpretability, the benefits of VCT need to be weighed against the costs to the patient and the owner. Clinicians should consider *a priori* how different degrees of hyper- or hypocoagulability would affect their treatment or diagnostic plan. If VCT results would not change the plan, the test should not be performed. Even when clinicians would benefit from VCT results, the blood volume needed or risk of hemorrhage may preclude sampling, especially in small exotics.

In addition to diagnostic use, VCT has potential for use in therapeutic monitoring. As with reference ranges, the ideal dosages for anticoagulant and antiplatelet drugs are unknown for most species, and VCT offers a way to therapeutically monitor coagulation-related drugs in an individual patient. Because these treatments can have narrow therapeutic indices, dosages can be titrated over the course of days/weeks to attain optimal control. In thrombocytopenic rabbits, TEG has been used to evaluate recombinant activated human coagulation factor VII with recipients showing improvements in clotting parameters.[77] Another study in rabbits found that TEG was more sensitive compared with aPTT and activated clotting time for monitoring changes in circulating heparin activity.[23]

FUTURE DIRECTIONS

Viscoelastic coagulation testing has great potential in exotic animal medicine as a diagnostic tool and as a means to monitor coagulation-related treatments. The most pressing current research needs are the establishment of standardized VCT protocols (fresh or citrated blood, type and amount of activator, time between sample collection and analysis, analysis temperature) in different higher order taxa for each VCT device. Ideally, these protocols would use citrated blood to permit transportation of the sample to the laboratory, commercially available reagents, and an analysis temperature consistent with a species' normal temperature or within that species' preferred optimum temperature zone in the case of poikilotherms. With established protocols, the generation of new reference intervals is made easier. Lastly, the diagnostic utility of VCT should be evaluated in specific disease conditions that could plausibly lead to hemostatic derangements, for example, hepatic torsion in rabbits.

SUMMARY

Coagulation abnormalities are almost certainly underdiagnosed in exotic companion animals; this is due to a lack of appropriate reference ranges and a lack of widespread availability of ideal reagents and analyzers for both conventional and viscoelastic coagulation analyzers. Crucially, viscoelastic assays have major advantages over conventional coagulation tests because they assess both factor and cellular contributions to clotting and fibrinolysis. Although subject to substantial variation when different protocols are used, VCT assays have been shown to be useful tools to diagnose bleeding or thrombotic tendencies, both quantitatively and qualitatively, in humans, domestic, and zoo animals when appropriate comparators are available. Exotic companion animals should be no different.

Clinics Care Points

Viscoelatic coagulation testing (VCT) can be useful in identifying functional deficits of both platelets and clotting factors.

There are very few reference intervals for viscoelastic coagulation assays in exotic species. These reference intervals can also vary widely when generated using different VCT protocols (analyzer, activator, temperature, etc).

VCT clot curves can be used qualitatively to diagnose clotting and fibrinolytic abnormalities in sick patients compared to healthy, control animals.

VCT may be useful in titrating antiplatelet and anticoagulant drug doses in exotic species that lack sufficient pharmokinetic and pharmacodynamic data.

CLINICS CARE POINTS

- Viscoelatic coagulation testing (VCT) can be useful in identifying functional deficits of both platelets and clotting factors.
- There are very few reference intervals for viscoelastic coagulation assays in exotic species. These reference intervals can also vary widely when generated using different VCT protocols (analyzer, activator, temperature, etc).
- VCT clot curves can be used qualitatively to diagnose clotting and fibrinolytic abnormalities in sick patients compared to healthy, control animals.
- VCT may be useful in titrating antiplatelet and anticoagulant drug doses in exotic species that lack sufficient pharmokinetic and pharmacodynamic data.

ACKNOWLEDGMENTS

This work was supported by the National Center for Advancing Translational Sciences, National Institutes of Health Award Number TL1TR002546. The content is solely the responsibility of the authors and does not necessarily represent the official views of the NIH nor any listed employer.

DISCLOSURE

All authors have previously received support from Entegrion, the manufacturer of VCM Vet, in the form of consumable cartridges for use in research projects. No financial support was provided by Entegrion. The authors have no other disclosures.

SUPPLEMENTARY DATA

Supplementary data related to this article can be found online at https://doi.org/10.1016/j.cvex.2022.06.001.[78-80]

REFERENCES

1. Gerlach TJ, Barratclough A, Conner B. Coagulation assessment: underutilized diagnostic tools in zoo and aquatic animal medicine. J Zoo Wildl Med 2017; 48(4):947–53.
2. Kaye S, Abou-Madi N, Fletcher DJ. Effect of e-aminocaproic acid on fibrinolysis in plasma of Asian elephants (Elephas maximus). J Zoo Wildl Med 2016;47(2): 397–404.
3. Perrin K.L., Kristensen A.T., Krogh A.K.H., et al. Thromboelastography-guided diagnosis and therapy in a case of elephant endotheliotropic herpesvirus hemorrhagic disease. In: Proceedings of the American Association Of Zoo Veterinarians. Portland (OR): Sept 26 - Oct 02, 2015. p. 84–85.
4. Perrin KL, Krogh AK, Kjelgaard-Hansen M, et al. Thromboelastography in the healthy Asian elephant (Elephas maximus): reference intervals and effects of storage. J Zoo Wildl Med 2018;49(1):54–63.
5. Barratclough A, Conner BJ, Brooks MB, et al. Identifying coagulopathies in the pathophysiology of cold stress syndrome in the Florida manatee Trichechus manatus latirostris. Dis Aquat Organ 2017;125(3):179–88.

6. Barratclough A, Floyd RF, Reep RL, et al. Thromboelastography in wild Florida manatees (Trichechus manatus latirostris). Vet Clin Pathol 2018;47(2):227–32.

7. Barratclough A, Hanel R, Stacy NI, et al. Establishing a protocol for thromboelastography in sea turtles. Vet Rec Open 2018;5(1):e000240.

8. Barratclough A, Tuxbury K, Hanel R, et al. Baseline plasma thromboelastography in Kemp's ridley (Lepidochelys kempii), green (Chelonia mydas) and loggerhead (Caretta caretta) sea turtles and its use to diagnose coagulopathies in cold-stunned Kemp's ridley and green sea turtles. J Zoo Wildl Med 2019;50(1):62–8.

9. Harms CA, Ruterbories LK, Stacy NI, et al. Safety of multiple-dose intramuscular ketoprofen treatment in loggerhead turtles (Caretta caretta). J Zoo Wildl Med 2021;52(1):126–32.

10. Willesen JL, Meyland-Smith F, Wiinberg B, et al. Clinical implications of infection with a novel metastrongyloid species in the red panda (Ailurus fulgens). J Zoo Wildl Med 2012;43(2):283–8.

11. Kaye S, Johnson S, Arnold RD, et al. Pharmacokinetic study of oral e-aminocaproic acid in the northern elephant seal (Mirounga angustirostris). J Zoo Wildl Med 2016;47(2):438–46.

12. Ganter MT, Hofer CK. Coagulation monitoring: current techniques and clinical use of viscoelastic point-of-care coagulation devices. Anesth Analg 2008;106(5):1366–75.

13. Buriko Y, Drobatz K, Silverstein DC. Establishment of normal reference intervals in dogs using a viscoelastic point-of-care coagulation monitor and its comparison with thromboelastography. Vet Clin Pathol 2020;49(4):567–73.

14. Fudge JM, Cano KS, Page B, et al. Comparison of viscoelastic test results from blood collected near simultaneously from the jugular and saphenous veins in cats. J Feline Med Surg 2021;23(6):598–603.

15. Fudge JM, Page B, Mackrell A, et al. Blood loss and coagulation profile in pregnant and non-pregnant queens undergoing elective ovariohysterectomy. J Feline Med Surg 2021;23(6):487–97.

16. Rosati T, Jandrey KE, Burges JW, et al. Establishment of a reference interval for a novel viscoelastic coagulometer and comparison with thromboelastography in healthy cats. Vet Clin Pathol 2020;49(4):660–4.

17. Hartmann J, Murphy M, Dias JD. Viscoelastic hemostatic assays: moving from the laboratory to the site of care—a review of established and emerging technologies. Diagnostics 2020;10(2):118.

18. Kaspereit F, Doerr B, Dickneite G. The effect of fibrinogen concentrate administration on coagulation abnormalities in a rat sepsis model. Blood Coagul Fibrinolysis 2004;15(1):39–43.

19. Jankun J, Selman SH, Keck RW, et al. Very long half-life plasminogen activator inhibitor type 1 reduces bleeding in a mouse model. BJU Int 2010;105(10):1469–76.

20. Wohlauer MV, Moore EE, Harr J, et al. A standardized technique for performing thromboelastography in rodents. Shock 2011;36(5):524–6.

21. Huby M del P, Cardenas JC, Baer LA, et al. Establishment of methods for performing thrombelastography and calibrated automated thrombography in rats. Shock 2014;42(1):27–30.

22. Kaspareit J, Messow C, Edel J. Blood coagulation studies in guineapigs (Cavia porcellus). Lab Anim 1988;22(3):206–11.

23. Nielsen VG. The detection of changes in heparin activity in the rabbit: a comparison of anti-xa activity, thrombelastography, activated partial thromboplastin time, and activated coagulation time. Anesth Analg 2002;95(6):1503–6.

24. Lechner R, Helm M, Müller M, et al. In-vitro study of species-specific coagulation differences in animals and humans using rotational thromboelastometry (RO-TEM). J R Army Med Corps 2019;165(5):356–9.

25. Siller-Matula JM, Plasenzotti R, Spiel A, et al. Interspecies differences in coagulation profile. Thromb Haemost 2008;100(3):397–404.

26. Cruz MV, Luker JN, Carney BC, et al. Reference ranges for rotational thromboelastometry in male Sprague Dawley rats. Thromb J 2017;15(1):31.

27. Brandão J., Sypniewski L., Kanda I., et al. The effects of citrate and rest time temperature on dynamic viscoelastic coagulometry (Sonoclot®) in New Zealand White rabbits (Oryctolagus cuniculus). In: AEMV and ARAV Proceedings. Dallas (TX): Sept 23 - Sept 27, 2017. p. 56.

28. Rigor RR, Schutzman LM, Galante JM, et al. Viscoelastic coagulation monitor (VCM Vet) reference intervals and sex differences in mature adult mice. Acta Haematol 2021;144(6):633–40.

29. Kaur H, Fisher K, Othman M. Thromboelastography testing in mice following blood collection from facial vein and cardiac puncture. Blood Coagul Fibrinolysis 2019;30(7):366–9.

30. Studer KA, Hanzlicek A, Di Girolamo N, et al. Effect of rest temperature on rotational thromboelastometry in New Zealand White rabbits. J Vet Diagn Invest 2021; 33(1):47–51.

31. Shimokawa M, Kitaguchi K, Kawaguchi M, et al. The influence of induced hypothermia for hemostatic function on temperature-adjusted measurements in rabbits. Anesth Analg 2003;96(4):1209–13.

32. Toukh M, Gordon SP, Othman M. Construction noise induces hypercoagulability and elevated plasma corticosteroids in rats. Clin Appl Thromb Hemost 2014; 20(7):710–5.

33. Raina S, Spillert CR, Greenstein SM, et al. Effect of surgery on tumor-induced accelerated coagulation in a rat carcinoma. J Surg Res 1985;38(2):138–42.

34. Haid M, Zuckerman L, Caprini JA, et al. Thromboelastographic changes in carcinoma: an animal model. J Med 1976;7(3–4):189–216.

35. Cerrati A, Fenda E, Italiano D, et al. Thromboelastographic behaviour in rats submitted to experimental liver intoxication. Riv Med Aeronaut Spaz 1977;40(3–4): 296–300.

36. Lisboa TA, Andrade MVM, Rezende-Neto JB, et al. Effects of Tityus serrulatus scorpion venom on thromboelastogram in rats. Toxicon 2015;94:45–9.

37. Kheirabadi BS, Crissey JM, Deguzman R, et al. In vivo bleeding time and in vitro thrombelastography measurements are better indicators of dilutional hypothermic coagulopathy than prothrombin time. J Trauma Acute Care Surg 2007; 62(6):1352–61.

38. Iwamoto S, Takasu A, Sakamoto T. Therapeutic mild hypothermia: effects on coagulopathy and survival in a rat hemorrhagic shock model. J Trauma 2010;68(3): 669–75.

39. Nishi K, Takasu A, Shinozaki H, et al. Hemodilution as a result of aggressive fluid resuscitation aggravates coagulopathy in a rat model of uncontrolled hemorrhagic shock. J Trauma Acute Care Surg 2013;74(3):808–12.

40. Nishi K, Takasu A, Shinozaki H, et al. Hypothermia does not hasten death during uncontrolled hemorrhagic shock presenting as the "triad of death" in rats. Acute Med Surg 2015;2(1):29–34.

41. Gazdzinski P, Squires EJ, Julian RJ. Hepatic lipidosis in turkeys. Avian Dis 1994; 38(2):379–84.

42. Trott KA, Giannitti F, Rimoldi G, et al. Fatty liver hemorrhagic syndrome in the backyard chicken: a retrospective histopathologic case series. Vet Pathol 2014; 51(4):787–95.

43. Shuster KA, Brock KL, Dysko RC, et al. Polytetrafluoroethylene toxicosis in recently hatched chickens (Gallus domesticus). Comp Med 2012;62(1):49–52.

44. Wells RE, Slocombe RF, Trapp AL. Acute toxicosis of budgerigars (Melopsittacus undulatus) caused by pyrolysis products from heated polytetrafluoroethylene: clinical study. Am J Vet Res 1982;43(7):1238–42.

45. Fernandez A, Verde MT, Gomez J, et al. Changes in the prothrombin time, haematology and serum proteins during experimental aflatoxicosis in hens and broiler chickens. Res Vet Sci 1995;58(2):119–22.

46. Miller BL. Characterization of blood coagulation in chickens by thromboelastography. Athens (GA): Ph.D., University of Georgia; 1999.

47. Mendenhall VM, Pank LF. Secondary poisoning of owls by anticoagulant rodenticides. Wildl Soc Bull 1980;8(4):311–5.

48. Murray M. Anticoagulant rodenticide exposure and toxicosis in four species of birds of prey presented to a wildlife clinic in Massachusetts, 2006–2010. J Zoo Wildl Med 2011;42(1):88–97.

49. Murray M. Anticoagulant rodenticide exposure and toxicosis in four species of birds of prey in Massachusetts, USA, 2012–2016, in relation to use of rodenticides by pest management professionals. Ecotoxicology 2017;26(8):1041–50.

50. Pay JM, Katzner TE, Hawkins CE, et al. Endangered Australian top predator is frequently exposed to anticoagulant rodenticides. Sci Total Environ 2021;788: 147673.

51. Roos S, Campbell ST, Hartley G, et al. Annual abundance of common Kestrels (Falco tinnunculus) is negatively associated with second generation anticoagulant rodenticides. Ecotoxicology 2021;30(4):560–74.

52. Thomas PJ, Mineau P, Shore RF, et al. Second generation anticoagulant rodenticides in predatory birds: probabilistic characterisation of toxic liver concentrations and implications for predatory bird populations in Canada. Environ Int 2011;37(5):914–20.

53. Schmaier AA, Stalker TJ, Runge JJ, et al. Occlusive thrombi arise in mammals but not birds in response to arterial injury: evolutionary insight into human cardiovascular disease. Blood 2011;118(13):3661–9.

54. Tian H, Liu M, Li J, et al. Snake c-type lectins potentially contribute to the prey immobilization in Protobothrops mucrosquamatus and Trimeresurus stejnegeri venoms. Toxins 2020;12(2). https://doi.org/10.3390/toxins12020105.

55. Dickson AJ, Belthoff JR, Mitchell KA, et al. Evaluating a rapid field assessment system for anticoagulant rodenticide exposure of raptors. Arch Environ Contam Toxicol 2020;79(4):454–60.

56. Guddorf V, Kummerfeld N, Mischke R. Methodical aspects of blood coagulation measurements in birds applying commercial reagents–a pilot study. Berl Munch Tierarztl Wochenschr 2014;127(7–8):322–7.

57. Keller KA, Guzman DS-M, Acierno MJ, et al. Thromboelastography values in Hispaniolan amazon parrots (Amazona ventralis): a pilot study. J Avian Med Surg 2015;29(3):174–80.

58. Rodenbaugh CI, Lyon SD, Hanzlicek AS, et al. Dynamic viscoelastic coagulometry of blood obtained from healthy chickens. Am J Vet Res 2019;80(5):441–8.

59. Strindberg S, Nielsen TW, Ribeiro ÂM, et al. Thromboelastography in selected avian pecies. J Avian Med Surg 2015;29(4):282–9.

60. Thomazini CM. Aplicação da tromboelastometria na avaliação hemostática em frangos de dorte. São Paulo, Brazil: Master's, Universidade Estadual Paulista; 2012.
61. Bietner JK. Factors affecting Hematology and Growth of the chick and their relation to the hemorrhagic syndrome. Columbus, OH: Ph.D., The Ohio State University; 1958.
62. Neer TM, Savant RL. Hypoprothrombinemia secondary to administration of sulfaquinoxaline to dogs in a kennel setting. J Am Vet Med Assoc 1992;200(9):1344–5.
63. Patterson JM, Grenn HH. Hemorrhage and death in dogs following the administration of sulfaquinoxaline. Can Vet J 1975;16(9):265–8.
64. Folden K. Investigations on four antibiotics for possible use against E. coli in broiler chickens. Athens, GA: Master's, University of Georgia; 2003.
65. Roy K, Bertelsen MF, Pors SE, et al. Inflammation-induced haemostatic response in layer chickens infected with Streptococcus equi subsp. zooepidemicus as evaluated by fibrinogen, prothrombin time and thromboelastography. Avian Pathol 2014;43(4):364–70.
66. Bernardoni JL, Sousa LF, Wermelinger LS, et al. Functional variability of snake venom metalloproteinases: adaptive advantages in targeting different prey and implications for human envenomation. PLOS One 2014;9(10):e109651.
67. Oguiura N, Kapronezai J, Ribeiro T, et al. An alternative micromethod to access the procoagulant activity of Bothrops jararaca venom and the efficacy of antivenom. Toxicon 2014;90:148–54.
68. Prezoto BC, Tanaka-Azevedo AM, Marcelino JR, et al. A functional and thromboelastometric-based micromethod for assessing crotoxin anticoagulant activity and antiserum relative potency against Crotalus durissus terrificus venom. Toxicon 2018;148:26–32.
69. Sousa LF, Zdenek CN, Dobson JS, et al. Coagulotoxicity of Bothrops (lancehead pit-vipers) venoms from Brazil: differential biochemistry and antivenom efficacy resulting from prey-driven venom variation. Toxins 2018;10(10):411.
70. Vieira CO. Mecanismo hemostático da serpente Crotalus durissus terrificus (Ophidia: Viperidae, Crotalinae). São Paulo: Doutorado em Fisiologia Geral, Universidade de São Paulo; 2014.
71. Rodrigues CFB, Zdenek CN, Bourke LA, et al. Clinical implications of ontogenetic differences in the coagulotoxic activity of Bothrops jararacussu venoms. Toxicol Lett 2021;348:59–72.
72. Sousa LF, Bernardoni JL, Zdenek CN, et al. Differential coagulotoxicity of metalloprotease isoforms from Bothrops neuwiedi snake venom and consequent variations in antivenom efficacy. Toxicol Lett 2020;333:211–21.
73. Youngman NJ, Chowdhury A, Zdenek CN, et al. Utilising venom activity to infer dietary composition of the Kenyan horned viper (Bitis worthingtoni). Comp Biochem Physiol C Toxicol Pharmacol 2021;240:108921.
74. van Vliet KJ, Smit GL, Pieterse JJ, et al. A thrombelastographic study of the effect of stress on the blood coagulation in Cyprinus carpio (Cyprinidae) and Oreochromis mossambicus (Cichlidae). Comp Biochem Physiol A Comp Physiol 1985; 82(1):23–7.
75. van Vliet KJ, Smit GL, Pleterse JJ, et al. Thrombelastographic diagnosis of blood coagulation in two freshwater fish species. Comp Biochem Physiol A Comp Physiol 1985;82(1):19–21.
76. Krigsfeld GS, Savage AR, Billings PC, et al. Evidence for radiation-induced disseminated intravascular coagulation as a major cause of radiation-induced death in ferrets. Int J Radiat Oncol Biol Phys 2014;88(4):940–6.

77. Tranholm M, Rojkjaer R, Pyke C, et al. Recombinant factor VIIa reduces bleeding in severely thrombocytopenic rabbits. Thromb Res 2003;109(4):217–23.
78. Kuznik BI, Tsybikov NN. The state of blood clotting in bursectomized cocks: effect of blood loss. Bull Exp Biol Med 1981;92(6):1700–2.
79. op den Brouw B, Coimbra FCP, Bourke LA, et al. Extensive variation in the activities of Pseudocerastes and Eristicophis viper venoms suggests divergent envenoming strategies are used for prey capture. Toxins 2021;13(2):112.
80. Ghidalia W, Vendrely R, Montmory C, et al. Overall study of the in vitro plasma clotting system in an invertebrate, Liocarcinus puber (crustacea decapoda): Considerations on the structure of the crustacea plasma fibrinogen in relation to evolution. J Invertebr Path 1989;53(2):197–205.

Hemostatic Testing in Companion Exotic Mammals

Sarrah Kaye, DVM, DiplACZM[a],*, Tracy Stokol, BVSc, PhD, DiplACVP[b]

KEYWORDS

- Coagulation • Diagnostic test • Fibrinolysis • Partial thromboplastin time
- Prothrombin time • Viscoelastic test

KEY POINTS

- Pathways of primary and secondary hemostasis are highly conserved across mammalian species. Diagnostic methods used in human and domestic animal medicine can be applied to exotic mammal species.
- Indications for hemostatic testing include mucosal hemorrhage, frank hemorrhage from an orifice, petechiae or ecchymoses, cavitary hemorrhage, patients presenting with hepatopathy, or history of exposure to certain drugs and toxins.
- Challenges of sample collection from small species and limited test validation and species-specific reference intervals have made hemostatic testing an underutilized tool in exotic animal practice.
- Diagnosis of hemostatic disorders requires interpretation of a panel of diagnostic tests, as no single test provides information about the entire hemostatic system.
- Hemostatic test results are impacted by many preanalytical and analytical variables, complicating interpretation. Standardized sample collection and handling, and establishment of in-house reference intervals or patient baselines for use of reference change values are recommended to improve quality and interpretation of results.

DEFINITIONS

- Hemostasis: Hemostasis is the prevention of hemorrhage following blood vessel injury. Primary hemostasis refers to the function of platelets, which rapidly activate to "plug" small vessel tears. Secondary hemostasis refers to the activation of the coagulation cascade to produce fibrin.
- Coagulation: Coagulation is the formation of the fibrin clot and is used interchangeably with the term secondary hemostasis. Historically it was described as a branched enzymatic cascade, with the intrinsic or contact pathway on one side, and the extrinsic or tissue factor pathway on the other. The two

[a] Staten Island Zoo, 614 Broadway, Staten Island, NY 10310, USA; [b] Cornell University, Upper Tower Road, Ithaca, NY 14853-6401, USA
* Corresponding author.
E-mail address: skaye@statenislandzoo.org

Vet Clin Exot Anim 25 (2022) 613–630
https://doi.org/10.1016/j.cvex.2022.06.005

pathways both produce activated factor X (FXa), which is the initiator of the common pathway that produces thrombin and fibrin. These distinct pathways can be useful in understanding the information provided by different diagnostic tests, and the terms are still frequently used when discussing test interpretation. However, the concept of two distinct pathways running as isolated reaction chains is not representative of in vivo hemostasis. The cell-based model of coagulation incorporates the role of tissue factor-bearing cells as the site of clot initiation reactions and the platelet membrane as the site of clot amplification reactions (**Fig. 1**). These reactions occur simultaneously and concurrently with primary hemostasis, with several positive and negative feedback loops between pathways.

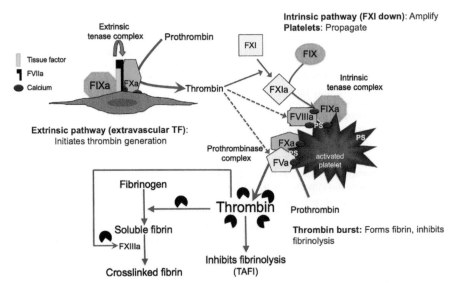

Fig. 1. Formation of crosslinked fibrin in secondary hemostasis. Secondary hemostasis is initiated by activation of factor VII (FVII) by a tissue factor-bearing cell, such as a perivascular fibroblast, which is exposed on vessel injury. Once bound to tissue factor, FVIIa forms an auto-activating complex, also called the extrinsic tenase, because it activates factor X (FX) on the fibroblast surface. The FXa then generates a small amount of thrombin from prothrombin. Thrombin then amplifies its own production by activating factor XI (FXI) of the intrinsic pathway and the cofactors, factors VIII (FVIII) and V (FV) of the intrinsic and common pathways, respectively (*dashed arrows*). The FXIa then activates FIXa on the platelet surface. Generation of FIXa on the activated platelet forms the intrinsic tenase (a complex of FIXa, calcium, FVIIIa and phosphatidylserine or PS) activating FX on the platelet surface. With the aid of its cofactor, FVa, FXa on the platelet surface then generates the thrombin burst. The large amount of thrombin generated on the propagating platelet surface is sufficient to cleave fibrinogen to soluble fibrin, activate FXIII, which then crosslinks soluble fibrin, and inhibits fibrinolysis, by activating thrombin activatable fibrinolysis inhibitor (TAFI). The tissue factor-FVIIa complex can also activate FIX on the fibroblast surface (so-called alternate pathway), which can then move from the fibroblast to the platelet surface to participate in the thrombin burst, but the fibroblast-bound FXa is rapidly inhibited if it dissociates, requiring FXa to be produced on the platelet surface to form the thrombin burst. Note that platelets are activated after adhesion to subendothelial matrix and by thrombin, ensuring there are activated platelets for supporting thrombin generation in the vicinity of the injury. (*From* eClinPath.com, Cornell University, https://eclinpath.com/hemostasis/physiology/secondary-hemostasis/; accessed December 2021.)

- Fibrinolysis is the process of clot dissolution, primarily mediated by plasmin. Elements of secondary hemostasis (contact pathway factors) stimulate release of tissue plasminogen activator (tPA) from the endothelium, which cleaves plasminogen to plasmin. Thus, some degree of fibrinolysis occurs simultaneously with coagulation.
- Disseminated intravascular coagulation (DIC) is a syndrome of widespread, inappropriate coagulation in small blood vessels. Following an initial hypercoagulable and hypofibrinolytic phase (thrombotic phase), the consumption of coagulation factors and endothelial dysfunction leads to a hypocoagulable state and frank hemorrhage. This end stage is often referred to as decompensated or hemorrhagic DIC. Induced by a range of systemic conditions, including sepsis, systemic inflammatory response syndrome (SIRS), trauma, neoplasia, vasculitis, viral infections, drug reactions, and immune-mediated disorders, DIC is never a primary disorder. Therefore, appropriate and life-saving treatment demands not only a diagnosis of DIC but diagnosis and rectification of the underlying causative disorder.

Physiology of Mammalian Hemostasis

Most hemostatic enzymes are highly conserved across vertebrate species, with most factors evolving from components of the innate immune system; some factors, such as factor XII, have evolved from digestive enzymes and thus show greater variability across vertebrate taxa.[1] Models of coagulation developed in the medical field are largely applicable to veterinary medicine. Rabbits and rodents are common biomedical models of hemostasis and DIC, and knock-out and transgenic mice have provided substantial insight into the roles of coagulation factors in hemostasis and innate immunity and tissue-related differences in hemostasis.[2–4]

Mammalian hemostasis is initiated by vessel trauma and exposure of circulating blood components to the subendothelial matrix and extravascular tissue factor (TF). Endothelial matrix constituents, such as collagen and von Willebrand factor, bind to and activate platelets, inducing shape change and altering membrane adhesion properties, resulting in the formation of the platelet plug.[5] Thrombin, arachidonic acid, and adenosine diphosphate serve as additional endogenous platelet activators, with variable platelet sensitivity to these agonists across species in platelet aggregation assays.[6,7]

Simultaneous with platelet plug formation, circulating factor VII binds to exposed TF-bearing cells (perivascular fibroblasts and smooth muscle cells) in a calcium-dependent manner, becoming optimally activated. The factor VIIa–TF complex, called the "extrinsic tenase," then activates factor X to Xa. A positive feedback loop increases activation of factor VII at the site of injury. Factor Xa complexes with factor V, calcium and cell membrane phospholipids to cleave prothrombin to thrombin. This short cascade occurs rapidly at the injury site to initiate the fibrin clot; the small amount of thrombin produced activates platelets and feeds positively into amplification reactions on the platelet membrane, producing the thrombin burst, which is required for formation of crosslinked fibrin from fibrinogen (see **Fig. 1**).[8]

The amplification pathway on the activated platelet surface involves several enzymes of the traditional intrinsic pathway. Extrinsic tenase-generated thrombin activates factor XI to XIa; factor XIa then cleaves factor IX to form IXa. The TF-FVIIa complex can also activate factor IX to factor IXa in the alternate pathway. Factor IXa and its cofactor, factor VIII, complex with platelet membrane phospholipid and calcium to form the "intrinsic tenase" complex, which activates factor X to Xa. This process yields large quantities of thrombin, which is required for producing fibrin and activating factor XIII, which crosslinks fibrin, stabilizing and strengthening the resulting clot. Simultaneously, fibrinolysis is inhibited by thrombin-mediated activation of thrombin activatable fibrinolysis inhibitor (TAFI) (see **Fig. 1**).

Several feedback loops and plasmatic and membrane-bound inhibitors regulate this process and initiate fibrinolysis. Coagulation reactions require binding with specific membrane phospholipids, particularly phosphatidylserine, and are anchored to activated cells at the site of injury.[6] Activated clotting factors that diffuse away from the site of injury are inactivated by plasma proteins, such as antithrombin, to prevent disseminated coagulation.[6] Extrinsic tenase is rapidly inactivated by tissue factor pathway inhibitor and cannot generate the thrombin burst without the intrinsic pathway-platelet positive feedback loop. Thrombin downregulates its own production in a negative feedback loop, by binding to thrombomodulin on endothelial surfaces and activating protein C, which inhibits the activity of activatedfactors VIII and V, co-factors for the thrombin burst. At the site of clot formation, factor XII and kallikrein generate bradykinin, which induces tPA release from the endothelium. Released tPA then cleaves plasminogen to plasmin, initiating fibrinolysis, forming a negative feedback loop to clot formation. Diminishing thrombin concentrations facilitate fibrinolysis via reduced TAFI activation. Plasmin activity is also spatially restricted to the clot by plasminogen, which binds to lysine residues in fibrin; non-fibrin bound plasmin is inactivated by antiplasmin and other protease inhibitors. Fibrinolysis is also inhibited by plasminogen inactivators, such as plasminogen activator inhibitor-1. Thus, numerous checks and balances act to localize clot formation and dissolution to a site of injury and prevent disseminated clotting.

Hemostatic disorders can arise from the failure of any component of this system, including disordered coagulation, pathologies affecting blood flow and endothelial integrity, or the loss or dysfunction of inhibitory and fibrinolytic proteins. Hypercoagulation and hypofibrinolysis can result in infarction, tissue damage, and organ failure. Hypocoagulation and/or hyperfibrinolysis results in uncontrolled hemorrhage. The dynamic and reactive nature of hemostatic pathways may result in multiple conditions occurring in different combinations and at different timepoints in the same disease process.

Diagnosis of Hemostatic Disorders

Common diagnostic tests for the evaluation of hemostatic function include platelet counts,prothrombin time (PT), activated thromboplastin time (APTT), fibrin(ogen) degradation product (FDP), and D-dimer concentrations. There are also the point-of-care tests: activated coagulation time (ACT), bleeding time, and viscoelastic-based global hemostasis testing. These tests evaluate different aspects or arms of the hemostatic process, and are often interpreted together, although viscoelastic-based testing is not widely available. Even in domestic species, test interpretation can be challenging, and this challenge is exacerbated in exotic animals. Published reference intervals are available for ferrets and rabbits,[8,9] but many historical intervals are published without sufficient data on the reference population and may not meet current standards of reference interval development.[10] Additionally, some reference intervals are reported for analyzers without species-specific validation; without a validation process, the performance of the test in a clinical patient is uncertain. In many cases, test accuracy decreases at very low or high ends of the analyte range. Validation procedures evaluate test precision and accuracy across a range of analyte values, and improve interpretation of results that fall below or above published reference limits. Despite these limitations, hemostasis tests can have value to the exotic animal practitioner, especially if evaluated in comparison to an individual's baseline measurement and interpreted in conjunction with anamnestic and clinicopathologic findings.

Anamnesis: Certain aspects of patient history could raise the index of suspicion for coagulopathy. These could include owner-reported bleeding tendencies, such as bleeding from the gums, epistaxis, or prolonged bleeding associated with nail trims or trauma. However, in many cases signs of frank hemorrhage will be absent, and a thorough patient history and establishment of a differential diagnosis list is required to identify the need for hemostatic testing. Certain medications can be associated with altered coagulation or thrombocytopenia, such aspirin, chloramphenicol, or benzimidazoles. Possible exposure to certain toxins, including rodenticides and aflatoxins (ie, from moldy food), should also raise an index of suspicion for coagulopathy. Patients with chronic hepatic, renal, or neoplastic disease presenting with worsening disease may have developed coagulopathic sequelae.

Physical examination: Clinical signs of primary hemostatic disorders include petechiation, ecchymosis, and mucosal hemorrhage, which can include epistaxis, gingival bleeding, gastrointestinal hemorrhage and melena, and hematuria. Prolonged bleeding from surgical incisions or venipuncture sites can be observed. Disorders of secondary hemostasis tend to result in hemorrhage into body cavities or joints, and animals may present with larger bleeds, such as hematomas, and nontraumatic hemoabdomen, hemothorax, hemopericardium, or hemarthrosis. In consumptive coagulopathies, including DIC, both primary and secondary hemostasis are impaired and clinical signs can include a combination of the above. Thrombosis and thrombotic sequelae of DIC are more difficult to recognize clinically.

Importantly, patients may present with only nonspecific signs such as lethargy, weakness, anorexia, abdominal pain, mucosal pallor, tachycardia, tachypnea, or hypotension. Thus, animals presenting in shock, anemia, or with a patient history consistent with that outlined above could benefit from an evaluation of hemostatic function. For these patients, screening tests may identify hemostatic abnormalities and allow for early intervention.

Platelet count: Reference intervals for platelet count are available for several exotic companion mammals although the reference population is not specified in all cases, with information on count methodology, patient sample size, breed, sex and age distribution, and health status not provided (**Table 1**). These counts can be provided by automated hematology analyzers, but immediate evaluation of a blood smear is also recommended. From a small volume of native or EDTA-anticoagulated whole blood, smears can be prepared and reviewed for a manual platelet estimate; one

Table 1
Platelet reference intervals for select exotic companion mammals

Species	Platelet Count, Automated (10^3/mL)	Study Population Size (n)
Ferret, *Mustela furo*[66]	172–1280	106
Rabbit, *Oryctolagus cuniculus*[54]	134–567	54
Rat, *Rattus rattus*[67]	923–1580	140
Mouse, *Mus musculus*[68]	900–1600	Unknown
Gerbil, *Meriones unguiculatus*[69]	432–830	Unknown
Syrian hamster, *Mesocricetus auratus*[70]	200–590	Unknown
Guinea pig, *Cavia porcella*[71]	259–800	143
Chinchilla, *Chinchilla laniger*[72]	300–600	16

recommended method is to count platelets in the monolayer across ten 100× objective oil-immersion fields, calculate the average, and multiply by 15,000 to yield an estimate of platelets in thousands/μL ($\times 10^6$/mL).[11] However, the latter is dependent on the field of view.[12] Platelet clumping will lower platelet counts obtained via smear estimate or automated counts. Thus, regardless of the method of platelet counting, a smear should be evaluated for platelet clumps, which usually occur along the feathered edge but may also appear in the body of the smear. Platelet clumping increases with storage time, particularly at refrigerated temperatures, so perform platelet counts as soon as possible after blood sampling.[13] Sample quality and choice of anticoagulant also affect platelet counts and appearance.[13,14] Humans with platelet counts of less than 10,000/μL are at risk of spontaneous hemorrhage, with certain patient populations at risk of hemorrhage with higher counts of 30,000 to 50,000/ μL.[15] In laboratory mice, prolonged bleeding times occurred when the platelet count was reduced to less than 25,000 platelets per μL, or 2.5% of the normal mouse platelet count.[16] For most exotic species, the relationship between platelet count and risk of hemorrhage has not been explicitly studied. Therefore, monitoring platelet counts sequentially (e.g. every 24-48 hours) for declining counts may be the most beneficial and practical method for detecting clinically relevant thrombocytopenia.

Platelet function: Available platelet function assays include flow cytometry to identify activated platelets, optical- or impedance-based platelet aggregometry, and platelet mapping using thromboelastography (TEG). Descriptions of electrical impedance aggregometry to evaluate platelet function in rats,[17] Rhesus macaques,[18] and pigs[19] are available in biomedical research, but application of these assays to evaluate clinical problems of exotic companion animals have not been published.

The bleeding time is a subjective and nonspecific, but quick and accessible, method to assess platelet function. In small animal medicine, the buccal mucosa is the most common site employed. For the buccal mucosal bleeding time (BMBT), a standard lancet delivers a laceration of specific size and depth, improving consistency of the test. After lancing, the blood is blotted just below the wound with filter paper and the time to cessation of hemorrhage is reported. The presence of thrombocytopenia would negate the need for this test in small animals, and thus it is usually employed to screen for thrombopathia (disorders of platelet function) and von Willebrand disease. Methods and reference data for the BMBT in exotic small mammals have not been reported. In laboratory animals, tail bleed assays are often employed but are not widely standardized;[20] ear incision bleeding times, using standard lancets, have been used in laboratory rabbits,[21] but clinical utility has apparently not been investigated.

Activated clotting time (ACT): This is a test of the common and intrinsic pathways, but is now considered less sensitive and more subjective than other available assays. However, as no analyzer equipment is required, it can be performed patient-side and can be a valuable screening test for general severe coagulopathies, such as anticoagulant rodenticide toxicosis. Fresh whole blood, with no anticoagulant, is added to specialized tubes containing a clot activator; historically this was diatomaceous earth, but currently a contact activator such as kaolin or celine–kaolin–glass combinations are used. This test cannot be run using citrated whole blood as the patient's calcium is required for the reaction. Patient platelets are also required and thrombocytopenia will result in ACT prolongation. Reference intervals are species and tube-specific, due the variation in type and quantity of activator in the tube, and very limited information on this test is available for exotic mammals (**Table 2**).

Prothrombin time (PT): The PT evaluates the extrinsic (factor VII) and common (factors X, V and II or prothrombin) pathways. The test adds rabbit brain thromboplastin (a mixture of calcium, phospholipid, and tissue factor) to platelet-poor plasma from the

Table 2
Published reference data on coagulation screening times for select companion exotic mammals

Species	Assay	N	Sample Type	PT (sec)	APTT (sec)	ACT (sec)
Ferret, *Mustela putorius furo*[8,35]	Antech Diagnostic Laboratories	12	Whole blood	12 ± 1.5	18 ± 2	
	Symbiotics SCA2000	12	Whole blood	20 ± 1	52 ± 19	
	Fibrometer	18	Plasma	12.3 ± 0.3	18.7 ± 0.9	
	ACL3000 (Photooptical)	18	Plasma	10.9 ± 0.3	18.1 ± 1.1	
Sprague-Dawley Rat *Rattus norvegicus*[61,73]	MLA Electra 800	20	Plasma	16.3 ± 0.7	19.2 ± 2.2	
	MedTronic Hemotec	50	Whole blood			48.0 ± 2.2
Syrian golden hamster, *Mesocricetus auratus*[73]	MedTronic Hemotec	48	Whole blood			42.5 ± 2.4
Rabbit *Oryctolagus cuniculus*[9,58]	MS QuickVet Coag Combo	33	Whole blood	17.2–28.5	103.2–159.2	
	Idexx Coag DX	33	Whole blood	10.0–14.8	104.3–159.1	
	Hemochron Response	11	Whole blood			177 ± 17
Guinea pig, *Cavia porcellus*, females[34]	VetScan VSPro	28	Whole blood	18.8–25.4	65.0–83.3	
Guinea pig, *C porcellus*, males[34]	VetScan VSPro	28	Whole blood	13.7–29.2	63.3–83.7	

Mean ± SD or population reference interval.

patient. The mixture activates patient factor VII, which then induces fibrin clot formation via common pathway factors, and the time to clot formation is reported. Most commercial PT assays use rabbit-sourced thromboplastin. However, clotting times are shorter and less variable with homologous thromboplastin, even within mammalian species.[22] Reference intervals reported for many species should be applied with caution, since they are dependent on the analyzer, operator and reference population (see **Table 2**).

Activated partial thromboplastin time (APTT): The APTT evaluates the intrinsic and common pathways. A contact activator, consisting of a negatively charged compound such as kaolin, is suspended in calcium and phospholipid and added to platelet-poor plasma from the patient. The negative charges activate factor XII and the enzymatic cascade of the intrinsic (XI, IX, VIII) and common pathways (X, V, II, fibrinogen). Reference intervals for the APTT are available for several exotic companion animal species, but are subject to the same sources of the variability as the PT (see **Table 2**).

Viscoelastic-based tests, such as TEG with the TEG analyzer or rotational thromboelastometry (ROTEM), are global assays of coagulation and fibrinolysis, which evaluate clot formation and lysis over time. Viscoelastic tests can be done in native nonanticoagulated blood if assayed immediately, but in practice are usually performed with citrate-anticoagulated whole blood or plasma.[23] The anticoagulated blood or plasma is recalcified, and typically an activator, such as tissue factor or kaolin, is added; small amounts of tPA can be included to aid evaluation of fibrinolysis.[24,25] With TEG, a torsion pin is inserted into the sample mixture, and the sample cup is rotated; as the sample clots and lyses, forces exerted on the pin alter the torque, which is translated into a fibrin formation and lysis curve. With ROTEM, the cup rotates around a fixed pin; studies have shown that results are not interchangeable between TEG and ROTEM.[26] Commonly reported TEG parameters include time to clot initiation (r), clot formation time (K) and rate of clot formation (alpha angle), maximum clot strength (MA), and percent of clot lysis at 30 minutes (LY30) and 60 minutes (LY60) post maximum amplitude. Use of TEG in veterinary species has been reviewed elsewhere,[27] including publication of reference information, but these data should be applied with caution as results may vary with operator and methodology. Results are affected by storage time and temperature, hemostatic variables (platelet count, fibrinogen concentration), and nonhemostatic variables, such as the hematocrit.[28] Additionally, demonstrated species variation in response to TEG activators requires species-specific method validation.[24] In the absence of reference data, serial monitoring of a patient over time may be useful to monitor disease progression or response to treatment. In rabbits and rodents, the TEG assay has primarily been applied in research settings.[29]

Fibrin(ogen) and crosslinked fibrin degradation products: Plasmin cleaves fibrinogen and fibrin, resulting in fibrin(ogen) degradation products (FDPs), the most commonly used indicator of fibrinolysis. Tests employ monoclonal antibodies that target FDP motifs. In citrated plasma samples, only fibrin-derived FDPs are detected, whereas both fibrin- and fibrinogen-derived products are detected in serum FDP assays. Serum FDPs are not specific for fibrinolysis, and concentrations increase with activated coagulation, increased fibrinogenolysis, or with decreased FDP clearance in cases of liver insufficiency.[30] A more specific indicator of fibrinolytic activity is D-dimer, a degradation product produced by plasmin-mediated cleavage of cross-linked fibrin. Although monoclonal antibodies used in these assays are human-derived, species cross-reactivity allows test validation in several domestic species.[31,32] For exotic species, reactivity likely varies, and test validation would be required prior to assay.

Use of reference intervals or subject-based changes: All hemostatic tests are sensitive to preanalytical factors such as collection technique and storage time and temperature, and reference intervals will vary depending on test methodology and the reference population. Thus, each laboratory should establish in-house reference intervals, and a similar recommendation could be made for clinics using point-of-care analyzers. Reference intervals can be established for exotic species on specific analyzers following published guidelines,[10] ideally with concurrent validation. When developing a reference interval for hemostatic tests, patient age, sex and reproductive status, collection method, and sample handling parameters, such as storage duration and temperature should be recorded and reported. For PT analysis, the source of thromboplastin, and condition (fresh or frozen-thawed) should be stated. For viscoelastic-based testing, the source and concentration of activators (TF, kaolin) and modifiers (tPA) and the timing of analysis is essential to report.

Even with appropriate methodology, the value of population-based reference intervals in coagulation test interpretation is questionable as these intervals may be insufficient to detect clinically significant changes in individual patients for certain analytes.[33] For coagulation tests, the evaluation of reference change values or a percentage or absolute change against the individual patient's baseline may be optimal. However, requiring the PT or APTT to be prolonged by more than 30% above the upper limit of the reference interval, as recommended by some authors,[7] may reduce sensitivity of the assay to detect relevant changes in an individual patient.

Sample Collection and Handling

Appropriate collection procedures are essential for accurate hemostatic testing and this is often an impediment for testing in small exotic mammals. In animals with clinical signs of nontraumatic hemorrhage, using central vessels such as the cranial vena cava, jugular vein, or femoral vein is contraindicated due to the risk of large hematoma formation. All samples for coagulation testing should be collected from the initial puncture with a steady flow into the syringe. Excess pressure or "fishing" can yield hemolysis or tissue contamination which exposes the sample to TF, resulting in coagulation within the collection apparatus and prolongation of certain assays. Needle and syringe size will vary based on patient size and vessel diameter. Selecting a larger gauge needle may decrease shearing of the blood and premature activation of coagulation, and will allow for a faster blood flow into the syringe. Syringe size should be conservative to prevent excess pressure and collapse of the vessel.

Collection directly into citrate anticoagulant within a syringe is recommended, by prefilling the syringe with a specific volume of citrate maintaining the appropriate 1:9 citrate:blood ratio (eg, 0.9 mL of blood into 0.1 ml of 3.2% citrate). Samples need to be redrawn if insufficient blood volume is collected, as underfilling can prolong clotting times due to excess citrate dilution. In guinea pigs evaluated via low-volume sampling, comparable PT and APTT results in paired samples of both 0.5 mL whole blood (added to 55 μL citrate) and 0.1 mL whole blood (added to 11 μL citrate) were reported.[34] Use of a dry syringe to collect samples may be common in exotic clinical practice, as it allows the sample to be split between collection tubes and used for multiple diagnostic tests. However, this method allows for contact activation of the sample within the syringe, and impacts results of PT and APTT tests. Citrated microtainers are available that require as little as 0.5 mL whole blood (Sarstedt Inc, Numbrecht, Germany). The sample should be thoroughly mixed (by gentle inversion) with the anticoagulant, but this will not offset the issue of contact activation when using a dry syringe.

The volume of citrate-anticoagulated whole blood or plasma required for commonly used analyzers varies (**Table 3**). For larger mammals with no volume limitations, samples collected for hemostasis testing should include citrate-anticoagulated plasma for coagulation testing and EDTA-anticoagulated whole blood for a complete blood count, with a blood smear prepared from freshly collected blood (with or without anticoagulant) for optimal assessment of platelet counts and white and red blood cell morphology. Serum or heparinized plasma can be obtained for biochemical profiles for underlying disease, such as renal or hepatic disease, that may result in acquired hemostatic abnormalities. For smaller exotic mammals where sample volume is limited, the minimum database required to evaluate hemostasis would require approximately 0.7 mL for the following tests: (1) freshly prepared whole blood smear for platelet estimation; (2) microhematocrit tube for packed cell volume determination; and (3) one microvolume (0.5 mL) citrate-anticoagulated whole blood tube for coagulation testing. Importantly, use of citrate-anticoagulated whole blood for complete blood cell counts is not ideal, as the anticoagulant can induce platelet clumping and affect platelet morphology.[14]

Access to an in-house coagulation analyzer is optimal, to allow for the use of smaller volumes of whole blood or fresh native blood and immediate results (see **Table 3**). However, most of these analyzers have not been validated for use in exotic mammalian species and significant variation in results based on analyzer type and test procedure are reported.[9,35] For these reasons, results need to be interpreted with comparison to a patient's own baseline, or in-house reference intervals should be established following ASVCP guidelines.[10]

Storage time affects PT and APTT results in veterinary species.[36,37] In rats, the PT was not affected by plasma storage at room temperature or refrigerated temperatures (4°C) for up to 24 h. However, the APTT was prolonged at 24 h of plasma storage regardless of storage temperature.[36] Although observed changes in the PT were relatively small (ie, 8% change in median PT at 48 h of refrigeration in male rats), a marked change in APTT was reported (60% increase in median APTT) at 24 h refrigeration, which could affect clinical decision making.[36] As a general guideline, if point-of-care assays are not available, plasma should be harvested within 30 minutes of sampling and submitted overnight to a laboratory for evaluation within 24 hours of sample collection; for delayed testing, freeze plasma samples and ship on dry ice to ensure more accurate coagulation test results.[38]

Evaluation of Species-specific Hemostatic Disorders

Ferrets: Ferrets have similar causes of coagulopathy as canine and feline patients, but some unique symptoms are also described. Ferrets are sensitive to estrogen-mediated bone marrow toxicity, with aplastic anemia occurring in intact female ferrets or cases of ovarian remnant syndrome in sterilized animals.[39] Thrombocytopenia (<55,000/μL) with subsequent hemorrhage is the most common cause of death associated with this syndrome.[39,40] Increased estrogen concentrations due to hyperadrenocorticism are less commonly associated with bone marrow suppression or clinical hemorrhage.[41]

Genetic, viral and toxic etiologies were considered in 3 cases of an acute hemorrhagic syndrome described in 2010. The syndrome occurred in recently shipped animals <1 year of age and manifested as mucosal and cavitary hemorrhage. Affected animals exhibited a median PT of 77 seconds and a median APTT of 99 seconds versus a median PT and APTT of 10 and 18 seconds in 13 healthy young ferrets, respectively.[42] Lack of further case reports suggest this was a nonrepeatable event.

Table 3 Point-of-care coagulation analyzers with required sample type and volume		
Analyzer	**Sample Type**	**Minimum Sample Volume per Assay**
IDEXX Coag DX Analyzer[a]	Fresh or citrated whole blood	0.2 mL
VetScan VSPro Coagulation Analyzer PT/aPTT[b]	Citrated whole blood	0.1 mL
Zoetis MS QuickVet Coag Analyzer[b]	Citrated whole blood	0.06 mL
Hemoscape 5000 TEG® Analyzer[c]	Fresh or citrated whole blood Citrated plasma	0.36 mL
i-Stat ACT Cartridge[d]	Fresh whole blood	0.04 mL

[a] IDEXX laboratories, Westbrook, ME USA
[b] Zoetis, Parsippany, NJ USA
[c] Haemonetics, Boston, MA USA
[d] Abbott, Chicago, IL USA

Viral infections have been associated with hemostatic disorders of ferrets. Mild to severe thrombocytopenia is occasionally reported in cases of ferret systemic coronavirus. Based on histopathologic review,[43] this thrombocytopenia is attributable to vasculitis and DIC, but one case report describes bone marrow infection, pancytopenia, and diffuse intestinal hemorrhage.[44] In ferrets experimentally inoculated with various strains of influenza, including pandemic H5N1, H1N1, and seasonal H3N2, prolongations in PT and APTT occurred, approximately 30% above baseline, even in mild clinical cases of H3N2 influenza.[45] Frank hemorrhage was not present in these experimental cases. Coagulation time prolongations were more severe in ferrets infected with pandemic H5N1, consistent with the multiorgan hemorrhage described in other species infected with this strain.[46] Increased D-dimer concentrations, fibrin deposition in the lungs, and high von Willebrand factor antigen concentrations suggested coagulation activation and subsequent consumptive coagulopathy in cases of severe influenza.[45]

Recently, ferrets have been used as a model for SARS-Cov-2 infection, as they are susceptible to clinical disease following intranasal inoculation, and can transmit the virus to other ferrets via close direct contact.[47] Although SARS-Cov-2 disease is associated with coagulopathy in human patients, these changes have not been exhibited in model ferrets, who tend to show clinical signs of fever and upper respiratory signs without severe pneumonia, multiorgan infection, or mortality.[47]

As for domestic carnivores, hemostatic testing is indicated in ferrets with clinical signs of hemorrhage or anemia, and as screening tests for animals with severe hepatopathy, cardiovascular disease, sepsis or SIRS. Given their susceptibility to circulating human strains of influenza and coronavirus, evaluating coagulation function in ferrets presenting with serious respiratory disease may also be prudent. The common venipuncture site of the cranial vena cava should be avoided in a ferret with clinical suspicion of coagulopathy, with use of the cephalic or lateral saphenous vein being preferred. Reference intervals for platelet counts and PT and APTT for healthy adult ferrets have been reported using commercial reference laboratories and point-of-care analyzers although these analyzers were not validated for ferrets (see **Table 2**).[8,35] These intervals are only guidelines as intervals will be analyzer dependent. Although reference intervals are not available, the Asserachom D-dimer ELISA (Diagnostica Stago, Inc, Parsippany, NJ, USA) has been used in research settings.[45]

Based on variable utility of D-dimer in dogs[48] and cats,[49] further research is needed on the value of D-dimer for evaluating thrombotic disorders in ferrets. Viscoelastic-based testing has not been described for ferrets.

Rabbits: Primary and secondary hemostasis has been well-studied in the domestic rabbit (*Oryctolagus cuniculus domesticus*) as they are a commonly used biomedical model for human disease. Rabbits have higher endogenous activity of the intrinsic and common pathway components (factors V, VIII, IX, V, and XI); factor VII and TF activities are similar to humans.[7] Platelet responses to most commonly tested agonists, such as thrombin, arachidonic acid and collagen, are similar to human platelets.[7] Rabbits appear to have less fibrinolysis than humans, and are more sensitive to endotoxin-induced DIC.[7] Some rabbit breeds have natural warfarin resistance, with subsequent variability in their susceptibility to anticoagulant rodenticides.[7]

Coagulopathies in companion rabbits are mostly associated with hepatic disorders,[50,51] benzimidazole toxicity and aflatoxicosis,[51,52] and rabbit hemorrhagic disease virus (RHDV) and its variant, RHDV-2.[53] Causes of hepatic injury include hepatic lipidosis, liver lobe torsion, aflatoxicosis, or potentially coccidial hepatitis. In 16 rabbits with liver lobe torsion,[50] 7 animals were mildly to moderately thrombocytopenic (minimum platelet count 46,000/μL [RR 134,000–567,000/μL]), and two animals had prolonged bleeding after venipuncture. Red blood cell fragmentation in 9 animals supported the presence of DIC, although hemostasis testing was not performed.[50] Rabbits are sensitive to aflatoxin-induced hepatic necrosis, with clinical hemorrhage reported in natural cases. In experimental aflatoxicosis of 12 rabbits, prolonged bleeding from venipuncture sites was reported in multiple rabbits, one rabbit exhibited cavitary hemorrhage postmortem, and the mean PT and APTT doubled from baseline during the 3-day period prior to death for all rabbits.[51]

In a review of 13 rabbits with suspected or presumptive benzimidazole toxicosis,[52] clinical signs included epistaxis (*n* = 1) and petechiae and ecchymosis (*n* = 1) in 3 rabbits exhibiting the radiomimetic bone marrow lesions typical of benzimidazole toxicosis; one affected rabbit had no clinical signs of hemorrhage. All three rabbits had abdominal or multiorgan hemorrhage on necropsy.

Rabbit Hemorrhagic Disease Virus and RHDV-2 cause acute hepatic necrosis, with DIC being the most common cause of death. Characteristic necropsy findings include multiorgan congestion and hemorrhage.[53] RHDV-2 may be associated with a subacute clinical course, and these rabbits may present to veterinarians with nonspecific clinical signs, such as lethargy, anorexia, or nonspecific neurologic or respiratory signs.[55] Although rabbits naturally infected with RHDV-2 may not exhibit frank hemorrhage, hemostatic abnormalities are found on testing, including moderate thrombocytopenia (47,000–63,000/μL [RR 134,000–567,000/μL]),[54] hypofibrinogenemia, and prolonged PT and APTT.[55] Pulmonary hemorrhage and a hemorrhagic diathesis, identified on necropsy examination, were attributed to severe hypofibrinogenemia, presumably secondary to hepatic insufficiency from acute hepatocellular necrosis.[55]

Hemostatic testing is indicated in rabbits with clinical signs of hemorrhage, anemia and cases of cardiovascular disease, sepsis or SIRS, hepatitis or liver lobe torsion, or exposure to RHDV, RHDV-2, or benzimidazoles. Based on rabbit stoicism, and the limited antemortem clinical signs in many reported cases, suspicion of disease rather that overt clinical signs is adequate indication to perform hemostasis testing in this species. Reference intervals for PT and APTT in rabbits from 2 point-of-care analyzers (IDEXX Coag Dx and Melet Schloesing Quick Vet Coag Combo) were not interchangeable,[9] emphasizing that reference intervals are analyzer dependent (see **Table 2**). In rabbit models of DIC,[56] FDPs have been measured and D-dimer assays designed for use in rabbits are available (Rabbit D-dimer ELISA kit, Abbexa, UK), but remain unvalidated. Viscoelastic studies of rabbits have provided results for the ROTEM[57] and TEG with native whole blood[58] and citrate-anticoagulated whole blood with variable concentrations of tissue factor.[29] However, no viscoelastic methods have been validated for clinical applications in pet rabbits.

Companion rodents: Coagulopathy is rarely reported in companion rodents. Vitamin C deficiency, or scurvy, can result in bleeding and a prolonged PT in rodent species with a dietary requirement for vitamin C, which includes guinea pigs and likely other hystricomorph rodents.[59] Atrial thrombosis of Syrian hamsters has been associated with DIC, characterized by thrombocytopenia and decreased activity of factors II, VII, VIII and X in affected animals.[60]

Reference data for the PT and APTT are published for several companion rodent species, including rats,[36,61] mice,[62] and guinea pigs,[34] though small sample sizes of <20 animals often preclude calculation of population reference intervals (see **Table 2**). Guinea pigs are biomedical models for leptospirosis[63] and viral hemorrhagic diseases,[64] resulting in some reference information on traditional coagulation[34] and TEG parameters.[64] Thromboelastographic parameters have also been reported for rats [27,65] and mice,[27,62] which provide a basis for developing standard clinical assays in these species. In practice, sample volume requirements and access to peripheral vasculature is a significant limiting factor to coagulation testing in rodents, and likely precludes routine hemostatic evaluation in companion mice, hamsters, and gerbils. Rats, guinea pigs and chinchillas >200 g can be sampled from peripheral vasculature with samples as small as 0.2 mL run directly on point-of-care analyzers.

SUMMARY

Both clinical experience and comparative biomedical research demonstrate that companion exotic mammals are susceptible to the same hemostatic disorders observed in domestic veterinary species, including common causes of thrombocytopenia, prothrombotic disease, factor-deficient coagulopathies, and consumptive coagulopathies, including DIC. In many cases, evaluation of hemostatic tests can detect disorders prior to clinical signs of frank hemorrhage, including cases where significant internal hemorrhage is detected on post-mortem examination. The potential value of these tests is incontrovertible, however logistic constraints and knowledge gaps will continue to limit their application in clinical practice. Further research is needed to validate common analyzers for exotic species; practices using point-of-care analyzers should, at a minimum, establish in-house reference intervals or strive for baseline measurements in patients for use of reference change values. Additionally, further clinical research on the utility of FDP/D-dimer and viscoelastic-based tests to diagnose and monitor hemostatic disorders in companion exotic mammals would be valuable.

CLINICS CARE POINTS

- Frank hemorrhage may not be apparent in patients with a coagulopathy, and a thorough patient history, physical examination and establishment of a differential diagnostic list should be used to determine if hemostatic testing is indicated.

- Platelet counts obtained via smear estimation or automated analyzers can be affected by anticoagulant , storage time, collection procedure, and platelet clumping. Evaluation of a non-anticoagulated or EDTA-anticoagulated whole blood smear made immediately at point of care can allow for a platelet count estimate with evaluation of clumping. Platelet clumping is most often observed along the feathered edge, and will increase with storage time and lower storage temperatures.

- Use of individual patient baselines and subject-based change values may be more clinically useful than population reference intervals for coagulation test interpretation.
- Collection of blood directly into citrate anticoagulant within a syringe is recommended, by prefilling the syringe with a specific volume of citrate to maintain a citrate:blood ratio of 1:9.
- Point-of-care coagulation analyzers can provide PT, APTT, and/or ACT results using as little as 0.1 ml whole blood.
- Coagulation results should always be interpreted in the context of what is known about the patient.

DISCLOSURE

The authors have nothing to disclose.

REFERENCES

1. Gentry P. Comparative aspects of blood coagulation. Vet J 2004;168(3):238–51.
2. Hermida JOS, Montes R, Ramo JAP, et al. Endotoxin-induced disseminated intravascular coagulation in rabbits : Effect of recombinant hirudin on hemostatic parameters, fibrin deposits and mortality. J Lab Clin Med 1998;131(1):77–83.
3. Mackman N. Tissue-specific hemostasis in mice. Arterioscler Thromb Vascu Biol 2005;25:2273–81.
4. Nielsen VG, Elda ES, Redford DT. Characterization of the rabbit as an in vitro and in vivo model to assess the effects of fibrinogenolytic activity of snake venom on coagulation. Basic Clin Pharm Toxicol 2018;122(1):157–64.
5. Holinstat M. Normal platelet function. Cancer Metastasis Rev 2017;36:195–8.
6. Smith SA. The cell-based model of coagulation. J Vet Emerg Crit Care 2009; 19(1):3–10.
7. Dodds W. Rabbits and Ferret hemostasis. In: Fudge A, editor. Laboratory medicine: avian and exotic pets. Philadelphia: WB Saunders; 2000. p. 285–90.
8. Benson KG, Paul-Murphy J, Hart AP, et al. Coagulation values in normal ferrets (Mustela putorius furo) using selected methods and reagents. Vet Clin Path 2008;37(3):286–8.
9. Mentre V, Adeline L, Ronot P. Reference intervals for coagulation times using two point-of-care analysers in healthy pet rabbits (Oryctolagus cuniculus). Vet Rec 2014;174(26):658.
10. Friedrichs KR, Harr KE, Freeman KP, et al. ASVCP reference interval guidelines: Determination of de novo reference intervals in veterinary species and other related topics. Vet Clin Pathol 2012;41(4):441–53.
11. Campbell TW. Peripheral blood of mammals. In: Campbell TW, editor. Exotic animal hematology and cytology. 4th edition. Ames IA: Elsevier Inc; 2014. p. 1–36.
12. George J. Ocular Field Width and Platelet Estimates: To the Editor. Vet Clin Pathol 1999;28:126.
13. Mylonakis ME, Leontides L, Farmaki R, et al. Effect of anticoagulant and storage conditions on platelet size and clumping in healthy dogs. J Vet Diagn Invest 2008; 20(6):774–9.
14. Stokol T, Erb H. A comparison of platelet parameters in EDTA- and citrate-anticoagulated blood in dogs. Vet Clin Pathol 2007;36(2):148–54.
15. Song F, Al-Samkari H. Management of Adult Patients with Immune Thrombocytopenia (ITP): A Review on Current Guidance and Experience from Clinical Practice. J Blood Med 2021;12:653–64.

16. Morowski M, Timo V, Kraft P, et al. Only severe thrombocytopenia results in bleeding and defective thrombus formation in mice. Blood 2013;121(24): 4938–47.
17. Defontis M, Côté S, Stirn M, et al. Optimization of Multiplate® whole blood platelet aggregometry in the Beagle dog and Wistar rat for ex vivo drug toxicity testing. Exp Toxicol Pathol 2013;65(5):637–44.
18. Dugan G, O'Donnell L, Hanbury DB, et al. Assessment of Multiplate® platelet aggregometry using Citrate, Heparin or Hirudin in Rhesus macaques. Platelets 2015;26(8):730–5.
19. Heringer S, Kabelitz L, Kramer M, et al. Platelet function testing in pigs using the Multiplate ® Analyzer. PLoS One 2019;13(8):1–11.
20. Liu Y, Jennings NL, Dart AM, et al. Standardizing a simpler, more sensitive and accurate tail bleeding assay in mice. World J Exp Med 2012;2(2):30–6.
21. Quaknine-Orlando B, Samama CM, Riou B, et al. Role of the hematocrit in a rabbit model of arterial thrombosis and bleeding. Anesthesiology 1999;90(5):1454–61.
22. Kase F. The effect of homo- and heterologous thromboplastins on plasmas of man, several mammalian and two avian species: a comparative study. Comp Biochem Physiol A 1978;61A.
23. Flatland B, Koenigshof AM, Rozanski E, et al. Systematic evaluation of evidence on veterinary viscoelastic testing part 2: Sample acquisition and handling. J Vet Emerg Crit Care (San Antonio) 2014;24(1):30–6.
24. deLaforcade A, Goggs R, Wiinberg B. Systematic evaluation of evidence on veterinary viscoelastic testing part 3: Assay activation and test protocol. J Vet Emerg Crit Care (San Antonio) 2014;24(1):37–46.
25. Kupesiz A, Rajpurkar M, Warrier I, et al. Tissue plasminogen activator induced fibrinolysis: standardization of method using thromboelastography. Blood Coagul Fibrinolysis 2010;21(4):320–4.
26. Goggs R, Brainard B, de Laforcade AM, et al. Partnership on Rotational Visco-Elastic Test Standardization (PROVETS): evidence-based guidelines on rotational viscoelastic assays in veterinary medicine. J Vet Emerg Crit Care (San Antonio) 2014;24(1):1–22.
27. Wiinberg B, Kristensen AT. Thromboelastography in Veterinary Medicine. Semin Thromb Hemost 2010;36(7):747–56.
28. Hanel RM, Chan DL, Conner B, et al. Systematic evaluation of evidence on veterinary viscoelastic testing part 4: Definitions and data reporting. J Vet Emerg Crit Care 2014;24(1):47–56.
29. Nielsen VG, Geary BT, Baird MS. Evaluation of the Contribution of Platelets to Clot Strength by Thromboelastography in Rabbits: The Role of Tissue Factor and Cytochalasin D. Anesth Analg 2000;91:35–9.
30. VanDeWater L, Carr JM, Aronson D, et al. Analysis of Elevated Fibrin(ogen) Degradation Product Levels in Patients With Liver Disease. Blood 1986;67(5): 1468–73.
31. Caldin M, Furlanello T, Lubas G. Validation of an immunoturbidimetric D-dimer assay in canine citrated plasma. Vet Clin Path 2008;29(2):51–4.
32. Martin-Cuervo M, Aguirre CN, Gracia LA, et al. Usefulness of a point-of-care analyzer to measure cardiac troponin i and d-dimer concentrations in critically ill horses with gastrointestinal diseases. J Vet Equine Sci 2020;90.
33. Wiinberg B, Jensen A, Kjelgaard-Hansen, et al. Study on biological variation of haemostatic parameters in clinically healthy dogs. Vet J 2007;174:62–8.
34. Condrey JA, Flietstra T, Nestor KM, et al. Prothrombin Time, Activated Partial Thromboplastin Time , and Fibrinogen Reference Intervals for Inbred Strain 13/

N Guinea Pigs (*Cavia porcellus*) and Validation of Low Volume Sample Analysis. Microorganisms 2020;8:1127.

35. Lichtenberger M., Evaluation of Partial Thromboplastin Time and Prothrombin Time in Ferrets Using Two Different Tests. In: Proceedings Assoc exotic Mamm, Vet, 200, 101–105.

36. Goyal VK, Kakade S, Pandey SK. Determining the effect of storage conditions on prothrombin time, activated partial thromboplastin time and fibrinogen concentration in rat plasma samples. Lab Anim 2015;49(4):311–8.

37. Furlanello T, Caldin M, Stocco A, et al. Stability of stored canine plasma for hemostasis testing. Vet Clin Path 2006;35(2):204–7.

38. Brooks MB. Sampling Instructions: comparative coagulation laboratory. Animal Health Diagnostic Center. Available at: https://www.vet.cornell.edu/animal-health-diagnostic-center/laboratories/comparative-coagulation/sampling-instructions. Accessed November 1, 2021.

39. Kociba GJ, Caputo CA. Aplastic anemia associated with estrus in pet ferrets. J Am Vet Med Assoc 1981;178(12):1293–4.

40. Sherrill A, Gorham J. Bone marrow hypoplasia associated with estrus in ferrets. Lab Anim Sci 1985;35(3):280–6.

41. Bakthavatchalu V, Muthupalani S, Marini RP, et al. Endocrinopathy and Aging in Ferrets. Vet Pathol 2016;53(2):349–65.

42. Johnson-Delaney C. Emerging Ferret Diseases. J Exot Pet Med 2010;19(3): 207–15.

43. Garner MM, Ramsell K, Morera N, et al. Clinicopathologic features of a systemic coronavirus-associated disease resembling feline infectious peritonitis in the domestic ferret (*Mustela putorius*). Vet Pathol 2008;45(2):236–46.

44. Tarbert DK, Bolin LL, Stout AE, et al. Persistent infection and pancytopenia associated with ferret systemic coronaviral disease in a domestic ferret. J Vet Diagn Invest 2020;32(4):616–20.

45. Goeijenbier M, Van Gorp ECM, Van Den Brand J, et al. Activation of coagulation and tissue fibrin deposition in experimental influenza in ferrets. BMC Microbiol 2014;14:134.

46. Maines TR, Lu XH, Erb SM, et al. Avian Influenza (H5N1) Viruses Isolated from Humans in Asia in 2004 Exhibit Increased Virulence in Mammals. J Virol 2005; 79(18):11788–800.

47. Cleary SJ, Pitchford SC, Amison RT, et al. Animal models of mechanisms of SARS-CoV-2 infection and COVID-19 pathology. Br J Pharmacol 2020;177: 4851–65.

48. Stokol T, Brooks MB, Erb HN. D-dimer concentrations in healthy dogs and dogs with disseminated intravascular coagulation. Am J Vet Res 2000;61(4):393–8.

49. Tholen I, Weingart C, Kohn B. Concentration of D-dimers in healthy cats and sick cats with and without disseminated intravascular coagulation (DIC). J Feline Med Surg 2009;11(10):842–6.

50. Graham JE, Orcutt J, Casale SA, et al. Liver lobe torsion in rabbits: 16 cases (2007-2012). J Exot Pet Med 2014;23:258–65.

51. Baker D, Green R. Coagulation Defects of Aflatoxin Intoxicated Rabbits. Vet Pathol 1987;24:62–70.

52. Graham JE, Garner MM, Reavill DR. Benzimidazole toxicosis in rabbits: 13 cases (2003 to 2014). J Exot Pet Med 2014;23:188–95.

53. Abrantes J, van der Loo W, Le Pendu J, et al. Rabbit haemorrhagic disease (RHD) and rabbit haemorrhagic disease virus (RHDV): a review. Vet Res 2012; 43(12):1–19.

54. Gallego M. Laboratory reference intervals for systolic blood pressure , rectal temperature , haematology , biochemistry and venous blood gas and electrolytes in healthy pet rabbits. Open Vet J 2017;7(3):203–7.

55. Bonvehi C, Ardiaca M, Montesinos A, et al. Clinicopathologic findings of naturally occurring Rabbit Hemorrhagic Disease Virus 2 infection in pet rabbits Clinicopathologic findings of naturally occurring Rabbit Hemorrhagic Disease Virus 2 infection in pet rabbits. Vet Clin Pathol 2019;48(1):89–95.

56. Berthelsen LO, Kristensen AT, Wiinberg B, et al. Implementation of the ISTH classification of non-overt DIC in a thromboplastin induced rabbit model. Thromb Res 2009;124(4):490–7.

57. Studer KA, Hanzlicerk A, Di Girolamo N. Effect of rest temperature on rotational thromboelastometry in New Zealand White rabbits. J Vet Diagn Invest 2021; 33(1):47–51.

58. Nielsen VG. The Detection of Changes in Heparin Activity in the Rabbit: A Comparison of Anti-Xa Activity, Thrombelastography ® , Activated Partial Thromboplastin Time, and Activated Coagulation Time. Anesth 2002;95:1503–6.

59. Barkhan P, Howard A. Some blood coagulation studies in normal and scorbutic guinea pigs. Br J Nutr 1959;13:389–400.

60. Mcmartin D, Dodds WJ. Animal model of human disease: atrial thrombosis in aged Syrian hamsters. Am J Pathol 1983;107(2):277–9.

61. Walter GL. Effects of Carbon Dioxide Inhalation on Hematology, Coagulation , and Serum Clinical Chemistry Values in Rats. Toxicol Pathol 1999;27(2):217–25.

62. Kopic A, Benamara K, Schuster M, et al. Coagulation phenotype of wild-type mice on different genetic backgrounds. Lab Anim 2019;53(1):43–52.

63. Yang H, Jiang X, Zhang X, et al. Thrombocytopenia in the experimental leptospirosis of guinea pig is not related to disseminated intravascular coagulation. BMC Infect 2006;6(19):1–9.

64. Slenczka W. Filovirus research: how it began. Curr Top Microbiol Immunol 2017; 411:3–21.

65. Wohlauer M, Moore E, Harr J, et al. A standardized technique for performing thromboelastrography in rodents. Shock 2011;36(5):524–6.

66. Hein J, Spreyer F, Sauter-Louis C, et al. References ranges for laboratory parameters in ferrets. Vet Rec 2012;171:218.

67. He Q, Su G, Liu K, et al. Sex-specific reference intervals of hematologic and biochemical analytes in Sprague-Dawley rats using the nonparametric rank percentile method. PLoS One 2017;12(12):e0189837.

68. O'Connell KE, Mikkola AM, Stepanek AM, et al. Practical Murine Hematopathology : A Comparative Review and Implications for Research. Comp Med 2015; 65(2):96–113.

69. Moore D. Hematology of the Mongolian gerbil (*Meriones unguiculatus*). In: Feldman BF, Zinkl JG, Jain NC, editors. Schalm's veterinary hematology. 5th edition. Philadelphia: Lippincott Williams and Wilkins; 2000. p. 1111–4.

70. Moore D. Hematology of the Syrian (Golden) hamster (*Mesocricetus auratus*). In: Feldman BF, Zinkl JG, Jain NC, editors. Schalm's veterinary hematology. 5th edition. Philadelphia: Lippincott Williams and Wilkins; 2000. p. 1115–9.

71. Spittler AP, Afzali MF, Bork SB, et al. Ag and sex-associated differences in hematology and biochemistry parameters of Dunkin Hartley guinea pigs (*Cavia porcellus*). PLoS One 2021;16(7):e0253794.

72. de Oliveira Silva T, Kreutz LC, Barcellos LJG, et al. Reference values for chinchilla (*Chinchilla laniger*) blood cells and serum biochemical parameters. Ciência Rural St Maria 2005;35(3):602–6.

73. Portilla-de-buen E, Ramos L, Leal C, et al. Activated Clotting Time and Heparin Administration in Sprague – Dawley Rats and Syrian Golden Hamsters. Contemp Top Lab Anim Sci 2004;43(2):21–4.

Endocrine Diagnostics for Exotic Animals

Susan Fielder, DVM, MS, DACVP (Clinical Pathology)[a], João Brandão, LMV, MS, DECZM (Avian)[b],*

KEYWORDS

- Pituitary • Thyroid • Adrenal • Endocrine pancreas • Calcium metabolism

KEY POINTS

- Endocrine diseases are underreported in most exotic species perhaps due to the limited number of validated diagnostic tests and lack of awareness in clinicians.
- Hyperthyroidism is most common in guinea pigs and the measurement of circulating thyroid hormones can be useful in the diagnosis.
- Hypoadrenocorticism (adrenal neoplastic disease) is common in ferrets and ultrasound is considered the gold standard for clinical diagnosis but circulating hormone measurement can also be considered.
- Insulinomas are a common neoplasm in ferrets and clinical diagnosis can be supported by the measurement of glucose using appropriate methods.
- Metabolic bone disease and calcium imbalances are common in captive reptiles but also occur in exotic birds and small mammals, and diagnosis can be made with the determination of total calcium, ionized calcium, and vitamin D.

INTRODUCTION

Endocrinopathies are common in animals. Overall, in exotic animals, endocrinology is not as developed as it is in small companion and large animal species. Nevertheless, many diseases may go under- or undiagnosed due to a lack of clinician awareness, reference intervals for specific hormones, and validated diagnostic tests. This article compiles information about different endocrine organs or groups of organs with endocrine functions, including normal physiological processes, common diseases affecting these organs, and their impact on physiological functions, as well as previously reported cases in exotic animals and diagnostic tests used.

THE HYPOTHALAMUS–PITUITARY AXIS

The hypothalamus is located at the base of the brain and is connected via the infundibulum to the pituitary, which is located just below. In most species, the anterior

[a] Department of Veterinary Pathobiology, College of Veterinary Medicine, Oklahoma State University, 250 McElroy Hall, Stillwater, OK 74078, USA; [b] Department of Veterinary Clinical Sciences, College of Veterinary Medicine, Oklahoma State University, 2065 West Farm Road, Stillwater, OK 74078, USA
* Corresponding author.
E-mail address: jbrandao@okstate.edu

Vet Clin Exot Anim 25 (2022) 631–661
https://doi.org/10.1016/j.cvex.2022.06.003
1094-9194/22/© 2022 Elsevier Inc. All rights reserved.

vetexotic.theclinics.com

pituitary is composed of the pars distalis, pars tuberalis, and the pars intermedia; however, birds and some reptiles lack a pars intermedia.[1–4]

The hypothalamus and pituitary glands control several endocrine systems.[5] The hypothalamus produces many different hormones that either stimulate or inhibit the pituitary to synthesize and secrete hormones that affect a number of systems. Most of these systems will be discussed in further detail later in this article.

DIABETES INSIPIDUS

In mammals, arginine vasopressin (AVP) or antidiuretic hormone (ADH) is produced by the hypothalamus and stored in the posterior pituitary. AVP is released in response to changes in extracellular fluid osmolality and blood pressure and volume. This hormone acts in the kidneys to inhibit diuresis resulting in increased urine osmolality and water retention. Nonmammalian vertebrate species do not produce AVP; instead, these species produce a similar hormone, arginine vasotocin (AVT).[6,7]

Diabetes insipidus (DI) occurs based on the failure to produce, secrete, or respond to AVP. Characterized by the lack of urine concentrating ability in the face of a strong osmotic stimulus, DI results in profound polyuria/polydipsia (PU/PD)[8] and can be classified as central (CDI) or nephrogenic (NDI). In CDI, a lack of AVP due to decreased production or secretion by the hypothalamus or pituitary occurs.[9] In NDI, AVP is present in normal or increased concentrations but the kidneys are unable to respond. NDI can be further classified as primary NDI, a rare congenital defect, or the more common secondary (acquired) NDI that is due to an interference in the normal interaction of AVP and AVP receptors in the kidneys.[10]

Another condition, psychogenic PD, can have a similar presentation to DI and is an important differential. PD is typically seen as a response to PU; however, in psychogenic PD, excessive water intake (behavioral or secondary to another disease) is the primary problem and the PU is a compensatory response to control overhydration.[10]

The most common clinical sign in an animal with DI (CDI or NDI) is PU/PD. As PU/PD is a common clinical sign associated with many diseases, one should first rule out other causes of PU/PD. Both DI and psychogenic polydipsia can present with a markedly dilute urine, and a urine specific gravity (USG) of <1.006 is often seen. Most other causes of PU/PD will not result in marked hyposthenuria.

The most common diagnostic test performed for differentiating DI and psychogenic polydipsia is the water deprivation test. This test determines whether AVP (or vasotocin in nonmammalian species) is released in response to dehydration and the response of the kidneys or a lack thereof to this stimulus. Animals undergoing this test must be closely monitored. An animal with DI may suffer significant complications or death when water is withheld, and this test is contraindicated in an animal that is dehydrated. In this test, water is withheld while body weight and USG (and urine osmolality if possible) are frequently monitored. The test concludes when the patient loses 3% of their body weight or USG exceeds 1.030. Water deprivation of a normal animal or animal with psychogenic polydipsia will result in a release of AVP and concentration of urine specific gravity. Animals with DI are unable to concentrate their urine even in the face of dehydration. In animals that are unable to concentrate, synthetic AVP can be administered at the end of the water deprivation test to differentiate CDI and NDI. In animals with CDI, the administration of AVP should result in the concentration of urine.[10]

Birds

Avian species do not produce AVP but instead produce arginine vasotocin that has similar actions to AVP. DI is rare in birds with reports of CDI in African parrot (*Psittacus erithacus*) and NDI in domestic fowl.[8,11] Polyuria/polydipsia is the major clinical sign for DI, but daily water requirements and renal output can vary based on size and species making evaluation of PU/PD difficult.[12] Because of anatomical characteristics of the bird, urine is often contaminated with fecal material, and this may artificially affect the urine osmolality and USG.[13] Nevertheless, USG has been reported in birds.[14] In addition, USG and urine osmolality were used in cases of DI and psychogenic polydipsia in African gray parrots.[8,15] Measuring AVP concentrations at the beginning of the study and at 72 h of water deprivation has also been suggested.[16]

Mammals

Spontaneous DI has been reported in rats and rabbits.[17–19] The water deprivation test can be used to distinguish between CDI, NDI, and psychogenic polydipsia; however, characteristics specific to some small mammal species must be considered. Gerbils (*Meriones unguiculatus*) will become naturally polydipsic if food is restricted.[20]

THE HYPOTHALAMUS–PITUITARY–THYROID AXIS
Thyroid Hormones

The thyroid gland is well conserved across all vertebrates and produces hormones that are important in growth and metabolism.[21] The follicle is the basic unit of the thyroid and contains colloid, the storage of thyroglobulin. Thyroglobulin is the precursor of thyroid hormone synthesis. Thyroxine (T_4 or 3,5,3′,5′-tetraiodothyronine) is the primary hormone produced and is the storage and transport form of thyroid hormone. Smaller amounts of triiodothyronine (T_3 or 3,5,3′-triiodothyronine) are produced by the thyroid and most T_3 comes from the conversion of T_4 from the tissues. 3,5,3′-triiodothyronine is the more metabolically active form of the thyroid hormone.[22,23]

Production of thyroid hormones requires iodide. Iodide is transported by the follicular cell into the thyroid follicle where it is oxidized and incorporated into the tyrosine residue of thyroglobulin. In the blood, most T_3 and T_4 are bound to plasma proteins, which are called total T_4 (TT_4) and total T_3 (TT_3). A small fraction of each thyroid hormone is not protein bound and is called free hormone, free T_4 (fT_4) and free T_3 (fT_3). Only free hormone is biologically active, entering cells or regulating thyrotropin stimulating hormone (TSH) secretion from the pituitary. Protein-bound thyroid hormones are considered a "reservoir" for free hormone.[24]

Regulation of thyroid activity involves the hypothalamus, pituitary, and thyroid gland (**Fig. 1**). Decreased circulating thyroid hormones and other physiological signals stimulate the release of thyrotropin-releasing hormone (TRH) from the hypothalamus. TRH stimulates the pituitary to release TSH, the primary modulator of thyroid hormone concentration.[24] Increased TSH results in the synthesis and release of T_3 and T_4.[25] This is controlled by a negative feedback loop, and increased thyroid hormones (primarily T_3) result in the decreased release of TSH and, likely, TRH.[26]

Many tests are available to assess thyroid function and more than one test is often necessary for diagnosis. Even with multiple tests, results are often confusing or inconclusive. Measurement of TT_4 is most common and is often used as a screening test in dogs where increased or normal results rule out hypothyroidism.[26] However, in birds, total thyroid hormones are typically low, and this should not be interpreted as indicative of hypothyroidism. The mammal methodology may not be adequate for birds as well as other conditions like nonthyroidal illness syndrome may be involved. Nonthyroidal illnesses such as inflammation, neoplasia, metabolic disease, and other endocrine disorders may result in a low TT_4 in a euthyroid animal (euthyroid sick syndrome or nonthyroidal illness syndrome).[27] This likely results from the

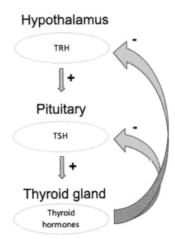

Hypothalamus

TRH

$\Downarrow$ +

Pituitary

TSH

$\Downarrow$ +

Thyroid gland

Thyroid
hormones

Fig. 1. The hypothalamus–pituitary–thyroid axis. Regulation of thyroid activity involves the hypothalamus, pituitary, and thyroid gland. The hypothalamus produces thyrotropin-releasing hormone (TRH), which stimulates the pituitary to produce thyroid-stimulating hormone (TSH). TSH stimulates the thyroid gland to produce thyroid hormones (thyroxine and triiodothyronine). The production of TRH and TSH is stimulated by a negative feedback loop.

inhibition of TSH secretion and T_4 production as well as the decreased concentration or binding affinity of thyroid-binding proteins. Free hormone concentrations are less affected by nonthyroidal illness, and fT_4 may be helpful in differentiating between hypothyroidism and nonthyroidal illness.[27] Recently, euthyroid sick syndrome has been reported in pet rabbits.[28] Measurement of TT_3 and fT_3 was less sensitive than that of TT_4 and fT_4, and most often did not provide additional useful information.[26] Measurement of TSH may be helpful for a diagnosis of hypothyroidism and increased TSH often occurs in hypothyroid dogs; however, it may also be increased in cases of nonthyroidal illness.[26]

Methodology used to determine circulating thyroid hormones concentrations is likely to affect the results. If reference intervals are not available for a specific species using a specific methodology, one should compare other apparently healthy animal(s) of the same species at the same time for comparison. Comparison of thyroid hormones and TSH of captive green-winged macaws (*Ara chloropterus*) using radioimmunoassay (RIA) and chemiluminescent immunoassay (CLIA) revealed that RIA and CLIA were equivalent methods to measure fT_4 and TT_3 levels but not TSH levels.[29] Additionally, CLIA failed to provide valid TT4 concentrations.[29]

Dynamic testing involves the administration of TRH or TSH followed by measurement of TT_4. In a euthyroid patient, an increase in T_3 and T_4 would be expected after administration of TSH or TRH. A lack of response would indicate glandular dysfunction. One report of a Carolina anole (*Anolis carolinensis*) given TRH showed an in vivo increase in plasma T_4 whereas no increase in T_4 occurred after TRH administration in a painted turtle (*Chrysemys picta*).[30,31] TSH stimulation tests are effective in several avian species using bovine, canine, and human TSH.[32–37] TRH and TSH stimulation testing have been reported in rats, mice, ferrets, and guinea pigs (**Table 1**).[38–41] In rats, the TSH stimulation test did not significantly increase the TT_4 values but it did increase that of TT_3. The increase in TT_3 was less substantial as compared with that in mice.[39] TRH stimulation test induced side effects such as hyperventilation, salivation,

Table 1
Thyrotropin-releasing hormone and thyroid-stimulating hormone stimulation testing reported in rats, mice, ferrets, and guinea pigs[38–41]

Species	Dose	Pre-stimulation Value	Post Stimulation Value	Notes
Ferret	Recombinant human thyroid-stimulating hormone or rhTSH (100 µg total dose IM)	TT4 21.3 ± 6.1 nmol/L[a]	TT4 29.9 ± 8.2 nmol/L[a]	Plasma TT4 concentration should be measured 4 h after rhTSH injection
Guinea pig	Recombinant human thyroid-stimulating hormone or rhTSH (100 µg total dose IM)	median, 9.05 (7.39 to 16.99) nmol/L[b]	23.95 ± 4.2 nmol/L[a]	Measurements made at 3 to 4 h
Mice	rhTSH (0.1 µg total dose IP)	TT4 100.4 ± 3.8 nmol/L[a] TT3 1.31 ± 0.03 nmol/L[a] (saline treated [control] animals)	TT4 186.6 ± 5.2 nmol/L[a] TT3 2.83 ± 0.15 nmol/L[a] (rhTSH-treated animals)	Samples collected from euthanized animals at 6 h after treatment
Rat	rhTSH (0.1 µg total dose IP)	TT4 74 ± 1.3 nmol/L[a] TT3 1.23 ± 0.02[a] nmol/L (saline-treated [control] animals)	TT4 77.2 ± 2.6 nmol/L[a] TT3 1.46 ± 0.07 nmol/L[a] (rhTSH-treated animals)	Samples collected from euthanized animals at 6 h after treatment. Changes in TT4 (values extracted from a figure) were not significantly different. TT3 was significantly higher post stimulation

[a] Mean ± SD.
[b] Median (10% to 90% range).

vomiting, and sedation in ferrets.[38] This was not reported with the TSH stimulation test.

Based on the limited knowledge of normal reference values for specific species (**Table 2**), the effect of methodology used to measure circulating hormones, and the potential variable response (e.g., euthyroid sick syndrome), clinicians considering thyroid disease should perform comprehensive panels. These panels should include total and free hormone measurements, and it would be advisable to perform the tests more than once to identify persistent low or high values. In addition, comprehensive health assessments should be performed to identify other conditions that may affect the thyroid function or the circulating thyroid hormone levels.

Table 2
Thyroid related hormones in selected species of exotic mammals

Species[a]	TT4 (nmol/L)	TT3 (nmol/L)	fT4 (pmol/L)	fT3 (pmol/L)	TSH (mIU/L)	Methodology	Target Population
Rabbit	21.88–30.89[b]	1.99–2.2[b]				Unknown	Unknown
	~35 ± 15[c] (n = 10)		26.1 ± 3[c] (n = 5)	7.3 ± 0.2[c] (n = 10)		RIA	Laboratory New Zealand white, 10 weeks old
		~1.3 ± 0.5[c] (n = 10)			~4.3 ± 1.2[c] (n = 10)	RIA	Male laboratory New Zealand white, extrapolated from graph
			22.9 ± 7.0[c] (9–40)[b] (n = 48)			Equilibrium dialysis	Laboratory and breeding population[176]
	35.7 ± 9.6[c] (18–59)[b] (n = 43)	0.46 ± 0.13[c] (0.3–0.7)[b] (n = 36)	50.7 ± 16.1[c] (21–80)[b] (n = 48)	6.8 ± 2.4[c] (1.7–12.4)[b] (n = 42)		RIA	Laboratory and breeding population[176]
Rat	38.61–90.09[b]	0.38–1.54[b]				Unknown	Sprague-Dawley, male
	38.61–90.09[b]	1.23–1.54[b]				Unknown	Sprague-Dawley, female
	32.18–90.09[b]	0.46–1.54[b]				Unknown	Wistar, male
	65.64 ± 5.15[c]	1.01 ± 0.05[c]				Unknown	Long-Evans, male
	63.06 ± 1.29[c]	1.28 ± 0.05[c]				Unknown	Long-Evans, female
	41.18 ± 1.29[c]	0.84 ± 0.05[c]				Unknown	Black hooded/Ztn, male
			28.47 ± 0.71[c]	3.20 ± 0.13[c]		Unknown	Sprague-Dawley, adult
	31.53 ± 2.45[c]	0.76 ± 0.04[c]				TT4 Larsen's method, TT3 RIA	Male Wistar rat
Ferret	18.0 ± 3.6[c] (n = 14)					Solid-phase competitive RIA	Laboratory, 9 females, 5 males
	25.5 ± 6.1[c] (n = 11)					Solid-phase competitive RIA	Pets, 5 females, 6 males
	19.3–38.61[b]					Unknown	Unknown

Value 1	Value 2	Method	Sample
Male 41.7 ± 21.24[c] (n = 31) Female 24.07 ± 10.17[c] (n = 13)	Male 0.89 ± 0.14[c] (n = 31) Female 0.81 ± 0.2[c] (n = 13)	RIA	Commercial vendor, specific pathogen free for Salmonella, Campylobacter, and parasites, 31 males (27 intact, 4 castrated), 13 females (10 intact, 3 spayed)
23.44–37.19[b] (n = 14)	0.98–1.36[b] (n = 14)	RIA	Intact female pets, 9 to 35 months, hospitalized for ovariectomy, either 3–10 days after the beginning of heat (n = 5) or 9–21 days after, with hCG-induced ovulation (n = 6) or out of breeding season (in winter when females were in anoestrus; n = 3)
27 (15.9–42.0)[b] (n = 94)		Chemiluminescence	Clinically healthy pets
22.53 ± 4.63[c] (n = 8)	1.04 ± 0.17[c] (n = 8)	RIA	Adult male, laboratory
24.45 ± 6.44[c] (n = 5)	1.08 ± 0.14[c] (n = 5)	RIA	Adult male, laboratory
32.56 ± 11.97[c] (n = 8)	1.25 ± 0.27[c] (n = 8)	RIA	Adult male, laboratory
37.97 ± 10.17[c] (n = 5)	1.43 ± 0.35[c] (n = 5)	RIA	Adult male, laboratory
45 ± 19[c]	1.08 ± 0.15[c]	Magnetic-antibody immunoassay	Adult female laboratory, extrapolated from graphic

a Values are provided as mean/median values and range/reference interval.
b Values are provided as range.
c Values are provided as mean/median ± standard error/standard deviation of the mean.
Adapted from Brandão et al. unless indicated.[175]

Reptiles

Although the location and anatomy of the thyroid gland varies among reptilian species, the function appears similar to that of mammals. Thyroid dysfunction appears uncommon in reptiles and most cases are thought to be due to changes in light cycles, hibernation, and thermal gradients.[42] Concentrations of TT_4 and fT_4 varied based on species (red-eared sliders [*Trachemys scripta elegans*] and map turtles [*Graptemys* spp.]), season, and sex.[43] Additionally, circulating thyroid hormone concentrations were not always influenced by total protein and albumin.[43]

Goiter has been reported in Galapagos (*Chelonoidis nigra*) and Aldabra tortoises (*Aldabrachelys gigantea*). In one report of a Galapagos tortoise with goiter likely secondary to iodine imbalance, hypothyroidism was diagnosed with a TT_3 of 0.07 nmol/L and a TT_4 of 3.73 nmol/L (compared to 3 apparently euthyroid Galapagos tortoises with a TT_3 of 0.51 to 1.53 nmol/L and a TT_4 of 13.9 to 19.82 nmol/L).[44] Another report of suspected hypothyroidism in an adult sulcata tortoise (*Centrochelys sulcata*) reported a TT_4 of 4.38 nmol/L and clinical improvement with levothyroxine therapy.[45] In a separate study by the same authors, reference values for this species ($n = 12$, median) were TT_4 of 4 nmol/L, fT_4 of 4 pmol/L, TT_4 of 0.15 nmol/L, and fT_3 of 2.9 pmol/L.[45] Proliferative thyroid lesions in a captive population of diplodactylid geckos (*Nephrurus amyae*, *Nephrurus levis*, and *Oedura marmorata*) were reported in 38% of the animals ($n = 8$); no serum thyroid values were provided.[46]

Reports of hyperthyroidism are rare. In one case of a green iguana (*Iguana iguana*), the diagnosis was based on a TT_4 of 30 nmol/L, compared with the reported reference range of 3.81 ± 0.84 nmol/L.[47] Clinical signs in this case included weight loss, polyphagia, hyperactivity, increased aggression, loss of dorsal spines, tachycardia, and a palpable ventral cervical mass. A functional thyroid follicular adenoma was identified and 173 days after surgical removal of the mass, the case TT_4 was within the reference range.[47] In two cases of suspected hyperthyroidism, abnormal shedding was the predominant clinical sign. A geriatric corn snake (*Pantherophis guttatus*) was shedding every 2 weeks and an African helmeted turtle (*Pelomedusa subrufa*) had shed continuously for a 1-year period.[48,49] Both cases responded to treatment with methimazole.

Thyroid neoplasia appears to be rare or underdiagnosed in reptiles with only a few reports of thyroid carcinomas in a Chinese crocodile lizard (*Shinisaurus crocodilurus*), a red-eared slider (*Trachemys scripta elegans*), an Indian black turtle (*Melanochelys trijuga*), a rough knob-tail gecko (*Nephrurus amyae*), and a smooth knob-tailed gecko (*Nephrurus levis*).[46,50–52] Normal ultrasonographic appearance of the thyroid gland of pond turtles (*Trachemys scripta*, $n = 4$).[53]

Birds

The structure of the thyroid gland in avian species is similar to that in mammals; however, the location of the thyroid gland is cranial to or within the thoracic inlet. Differences in size and vascularization occur between species and individuals.[54,55] Control of thyroid hormones in birds has some differences when compared with that in mammals. Corticotrophin-releasing hormone, rather than TRH, stimulates TSH release and T_4 secretion whereas corticosterone exhibits negative feedback on T_4. TRH stimulates growth hormone-releasing hormone resulting in increased T_3 due to the inhibition of degradation of T_3.[56] Release of TSH is also controlled by T_3, and both TSH and growth hormone promote release of T_3 and T_4 from the thyroid.[57] Thyroid-binding globulins are not present in birds, and prealbumin and albumin bind thyroid hormone in the blood. The albumin–T_4 bond is weak and, subsequently, higher fT4 occurs in birds.[57]

Goiter has been reported in many avian species and in one study macaws (specifically blue-and-yellow macaws, *Ara ararauna*) were overrepresented.[58] Iodine deficiency is the most likely cause of goiter in birds.[16,59] Inclusion of broccoli, which is known to have iodine-binding ability, and lack of minerals has been suggested to predispose budgerigars to develop thyroid hyperplasia.[59] Animals with goiter may have normal or abnormal thyroid function and, to the authors' knowledge, reports of assessment of thyroid function in birds with goiter are lacking.[60]

Although hypothyroidism has been reported in birds,[61] diagnosis is difficult. Because of low physiological values in the bird and low sensitivity of current methodologies, TT_3 and TT_4 results are often below reported normal values. Low thyroid hormone values should not be interpreted as diagnostic for hypothyroidism.[62] The authors recommend performing repeated measurement of both free and total hormones. Hyperthyroidism in birds is rarely reported. Hyperthyroidism was diagnosed in a free-ranging male barred owl (*Strix varia*) with a productive thyroid follicular carcinoma diagnosed on necropsy. When compared to controls, thyroid values (TT_4 and fT_4) in this case were increased and supportive of a diagnosis of hyperthyroidism.[63]

Mammals

Among small mammals, thyroid disease most commonly occurs in guinea pigs (*Cavia porcellus*). Hyperthyroidism is most commonly reported, and one pathology service reported thyroid neoplasia as one of the most common neoplasms (3.6%) in the guinea pig.[64] In 40 hyperthyroid guinea pigs, median age 5, no sex predisposition was apparent and clinical signs were weight loss with normal or increase food intake.[65] Most animals treated with thiamazole or carbimazole had decreased TT_4 and clinical improvement occurred in approximately half of the animals.[65] There is only a single report of hypothyroidism in the guinea pig.[66] Reference intervals for thyroid hormones have been reported in several publications, but many different test methodologies were used (**Table 3**).[67–71] One must consider methodology when reviewing reference intervals.

Based on a lack of information for other rodent species, thyroid disease is likely underdiagnosed in rodents. A single case report described concurrent diabetes mellitus and hyperthyroidism in the long-tailed chinchilla (*Chinchilla lanigera*).[72] Most cases are from laboratory animals. Thyroid neoplasia, nonthyroidal illness, hypothyroidism, and hyperthyroidism have been reported in rats.[73,74]

Naturally occurring thyroid dysfunction is rare in rabbits. However, thyroid function can be adversely affected by physiologic stress (nonthyroidal illness).[75] Goiter was reported in rabbits fed a cabbage-based diet for 2 to 3 months.[76] Hyperthyroidism was presumptively diagnosed in two rabbits based on clinical signs, hormone measurement, and scintigraphy.[77] Circulating thyroid hormones were increased (fT_4 28 pmol/L [equilibrium dialysis, $n = 1$] and 50 pmol/L [radioimmunoassay, $n = 1$], and TT_4 46 nmol/L and 36 nmol/L [radioimmunoassay, n = 2]).[77] Thyroid scintigraphy with intravenous technetium 99m pertechnetate revealed an increased thyroid-to-salivary gland ratio.[77,78] Hyperthyroidism was diagnosed and methimazole (1.25 mg total dose PO q12 h) was initiated.[77] Thyroid hormone concentrations decreased after therapy (fT4 13 and 34 pmol/L; TT4 31 and 34 nmol/L), and the animals showed clinical improvement (e.g., weight gain).[77]

Hypothyroidism has been reported in ferrets. In seven ferrets, clinical signs of obesity, lethargy, inactivity, and excessive sleeping were reported. Basal TT_4 was low, and these animals had a limited response in TT_4 to TSH stimulation.[79] Recombinant human TSH has been validated in the ferret for stimulation testing.[40]

Table 3
Normal values of total thyroxine (TT_4), total triiodothyronine (TT_3), free thyroxine (fT_4) and free triiodothyronine (fT_3) of guinea pigs (*Cavia porcellus*)[177]

Population	TT3 (µg/dL)	TT4 (µg/dL)	fT3 (ng/dL)	fT4 (ng/dL)	Data Format
Pet[a,67]		4.17 (3.01–5.33)[d]			Mean (reference interval)
Pet[b,68]		2.1 (1.1–5.2)[d]			Mean (reference interval)
Laboratory[a,67]		4.04 (2.26–5.82)[d]			Mean (reference interval)
Laboratory[c,69]	39–44[e]	2.5–3.2[e]	0.221–0.260[e]	1.26–2.03[e]	Reference interval
Unknown[c,169]	31.7 ± 1.4[f]	4.54 ± 0.443[f]	0.224 ± 0.108[f]	0.67 ± 0.57[f]	Mean ± standard deviation of the mean

[a] Enzyme immunoassay.
[b] Chemiluminescence.
[c] Radioimmunoassay.
[d] Values are provided as mean (reference interval).
[e] Values are provided as reference interval.
[f] Values are provided as mean ± standard error of the mean.

Euthyroid sick syndrome has been recently reported in pet rabbits.[28] Mean TT_4 and fT_4 were significantly lower in sick animals (e.g., fractures and presumed obstructive ileus).[28] However, contrary to dogs, both TT_4 and fT_4 were both similarly decreased in diseased rabbits.[28] Thus for the rabbit at least, TT_4 and fT_4 alone may not provide sufficient evidence of hypothyroidism due to the possibility of nonthyroidal illness syndrome.[28]

THE HYPOTHALAMUS–PITUITARY–ADRENAL AXIS

The adrenal gland is composed of the cortex and the medulla—two histologically and functionally distinct parts. Three zones make up the cortex, the zonae glomerulosa, fasciculata, and reticularis.[80] The main hormones secreted from the adrenal cortex are cortisol, corticosterone, and aldosterone. The zona glomerulosa produces aldosterone. The zona fasciculata and zona reticularis function together, but the zona fasciculata secretes mostly glucocorticoids and the zona reticularis secretes sex hormones. All zones can secrete corticosterone.[80,81] The medulla is composed of a network of chromaffin cells, or pheochromocytes, and produces epinephrin and norepinephrine.[80,82]

Control of the adrenal gland is primarily through ACTH, angiotensin II, and potassium. Released from the pituitary in response to CRH from the hypothalamus, ACTH primarily results in the release of glucocorticoids (cortisol and corticosterone). Glucocorticoids exhibit negative feedback on both CRH and ACTH secretion.[81] In most species, ACTH is secreted constantly in a pulsatile manner but increases secondary to stress. Aldosterone is released in response to angiotensin II and increases in serum potassium concentration.[83]

Adrenal gland structure in exotic species varies. The ferret adrenal gland is anatomically unique and, in addition to the three layers of the cortex seen in most vertebrates, the adrenal cortex also contains two extra less prominent layers—the zonae intermedia and juxtamedullaris.[84] The function of these layers is unclear, but these differences may play a role in the development of adrenal disease in ferrets.[85,86] The adrenal gland of mice contains an extra layer adjacent to the medulla called the X zone.[87] In birds, the cortex and medulla are not distinct from one another.[88] Differences in adrenal gland function in exotic species are seen as well. In birds, rats, and mice, corticosterone is secreted in higher amounts than cortisol.[80] Aldosterone secretion in birds is lower than in other vertebrates.[89]

Hyperadrenocorticism/Hyperandrogenism

Hyperadrenocorticism, increased production of hormones in the adrenal cortex either due to hypertrophy or neoplasia, or both, has been described in exotic mammals. The adrenal gland comprises three layers, each responsible for producing specific hormones. Disease affecting the zona glomerulosa leads to the increased production of mineralocorticoids resulting in hyperaldosteronism or Conn's syndrome whereas disease of the zona fasciculata results in increased production of glucocorticoids causing hypercortisolism or Cushing's syndrome. Increased production of androgens by the zona reticularis results in hyperandrogenism.

Hyperandrogenism, also known as ferret adrenal gland disease, is the most common form of hyperadrenocorticism in pet ferrets. Adrenal gland disease in ferrets should not be confused with Cushing's disease in canines.[90] Although the unique anatomy and physiology of the ferret adrenal gland may play a part in the development of this disease, the removal of gonadal tissue, independent of the age at the time of sterilization, likely influences the development of ferret adrenal disease.[91,92] Several tests are available to diagnose adrenal disease in ferrets. Ultrasound evaluation of the size, shape, and structure of the adrenal gland is considered the gold standard. Adrenal glands may be classified as abnormal when any of the following are present: rounded appearance of the gland, increased size at the cranial or caudal pole, heterogenous structure, increased echogenicity, or signs of mineralization.[93] Increased concentrations of estradiol, androstenedione, and 17a-hydroxyprogetsterone are supportive of adrenal disease but may occur in other conditions and caution is necessary when interpreting these findings.[90] Clinical signs seen with ferret adrenal disease are similar to that seen in ovarian remnant syndrome in female ferrets and the human chorionic gonadotropin (hCG) stimulation test may be helpful in differentiating the two diseases. Clinically however, ovarian remnant syndrome of ferrets is relatively rare in the United States. Hyperandrogenism (commonly hypertestosteronism) secondary to adrenal neoplasia and hyperplasia, with increased sexual and aggressive behavior, has been reported in older neutered, male and female, rabbits.[94–97] Concentrations of adrenal steroids (progesterone, 17-hydroxyprogesterone, androstenedione, testosterone, and cortisol) in 29 neutered rabbits have been reported.[98]

Hyperadrenocorticism has also been reported in other species of exotic mammals. A case of hyperadrenocorticism has been reported in golden hamster (*Mesocricetus auratus*).[99] The patient presented with dermatologic and other clinical signs (PU, PD).[99] Urine cortisol/creatinine ratio was elevated (45.6 although values < 20 were considered normal) and clinical diagnosis of hyperadrenocorticism (presumptive Cushing's disease) was made.[99]

Hyperadrenocorticism (Cushing's syndrome) was suggested to be the third most common endocrinopathy in guinea pigs, and both adrenal- and pituitary-dependent hyperadrenocorticism can be present.[100] In one guinea pig case, hyperadrenocorticism was diagnosed using synthetic ACTH stimulation (5 μg/kg IM, Cosyntropin 0.25 mg/mL; Amphastar Pharmaceuticals Inc., ON, Canada).[101] The ACTH stimulation test revealed markedly elevated pre- and poststimulation cortisol (>1380.0 nmol/L; reference interval for guinea pig serum basal cortisol: 138–828 nmol/L, no reference interval for poststimulation available).[101] In another guinea pig, ACTH stimulation (20 IU total dose IM, Synacthen depot; Novartis Pharma) was used to diagnose Cushing's disease.[102] In this case, radioimmunoassay was used to measure salivary cortisol.[102] Hypercortisolism and adrenal gland hyperreactivity was identified after ACTH stimulation in the affected guinea pig (721 ng/mL).[102] This value was shown to be elevated when compared with that of poststimulation controls (pet guinea pigs 125 ng/mL; laboratory guinea pigs 6.6 ± 3.4 ng/mL [n = 100] and 157 ± 53 ng/mL [n = 8]).[102]

ENDOCRINE PANCREAS

The pancreas is composed of both exocrine and endocrine components. The exocrine component is made up of acinar cells and is involved in digestion. The endocrine component consists of nests of cells known as the islets of Langerhans.[80] In mammals, the islets of Langerhans are composed of several cell types including glucagon-secreting alpha cells, insulin-secreting beta cells, somatostatin-secreting delta cells, pancreatic polypeptide cells, and ghrelin-producing epsilon cells.[103–105] Hormones produced by these cells are primarily responsible for glucose homeostasis.[104] Glucagon is produced in much lower concentration than insulin and has opposing effects on glucose homeostasis leading to an increase in blood glucose.[106] Somatostatin inhibits the release of both insulin and glucagon.[106]

NEOPLASIA

Functional neoplasms are one of the most common diseases to affect the endocrine pancreas. Insulinomas are functional beta cell tumors that secrete insulin typically resulting in hypoglycemia.[107,108]

Mammals

Insulinomas are one of the two most common neoplasms in ferrets and make up about 25% of all neoplasms diagnosed in this species.[90] Spontaneous insulinomas have been reported in guinea pigs, rats, and in a rabbit.[109–113]

Hypoglycemia is a common finding in animals with insulinoma, but hypoglycemia alone is not diagnostic as many other conditions can result in hypoglycemia (sepsis, neoplasia, lab delay in assay based on shipment). In general, glucose levels below 70 mg/dL (3.9 mmol/L) prior to any treatment are suggestive of hypoglycemia, levels between 80 to 90 mg/dL (4.4 to 5 mmol/L) are borderline low and should be monitored, and values above 100 mg/dL (5.6 mmol/L) are not concerning. Diagnosis requires the presence of a hypoglycemia with concurrent hyperinsulinemia. Owing to the high prevalence of disease in the ferrets, hypoglycemia alone is highly indicative of insulinoma, but not pathognomonic. Although insulin can be measured and normal insulin levels have been reported in ferrets,[114] interpretation can be challenging as the influence of the time period since the last food ingestion has not been well defined. Measurement of fructosamine, a glycated protein used to assess glucose concentrations over the previous 1 to 3 weeks, has been diagnostically useful for dogs.[115,116] However, in ferrets, no significant differences between the healthy and hypoglycemic ferrets was noted.[117] Therefore, the fructosamine concentration and fructosamine–albumin ratio do not appear useful to assess insulinoma-associated chronic hypoglycemia in ferrets.[117]

Diabetes Mellitus

Diabetes mellitus (DM) is the most common disease associated with the endocrine pancreas in dogs and cats. DM is the result of insulin deficiency (absolute or relative). In type I DM there is a lack of insulin secretion. In type II DM there is a lack of receptor response to insulin (insulin resistance).[118] Both types result in decreased tissue utilization of glucose, accelerated hepatic glycogenolysis and gluconeogenesis, and accumulation of glucose in the circulation.

Reptiles

Despite numerous anecdotal reports of DM in reptiles, a lack of evidence in peer reviewed literature exists. Hyperglycemia may occur in reptiles for several reasons including metabolic conditions, systemic diseases, and physiologic variability; however, a persistent, marked hyperglycemia of >200 mg/dL is considered suggestive of DM.[119] Diabetes mellitus has been reported in red-eared sliders (*Trachemys scripta elegans*), desert tortoises (*Gopherus agassizii*), Chinese water dragons (*Physignathus cocincinus*), western pond turtles (*Actinemys marmorata*), Exuma Island iguanas (*Cyclura cychlura figginsi*), inland bearded dragons, and the green iguana.[119,120]

Another condition in reptiles that results in a persistent, severe hyperglycemia (>900 mg/dL) has been reported in inland bearded dragons. Gastric neuroendocrine carcinomas are a highly malignant neoplasm that arise from the mucosa and submucosa of the gastric wall. The neoplastic cells overproduce somatostatin resulting in decreased secretion of insulin and subsequent hyperglycemia.[121,122] Diagnosis is typically based on a persistent and severe hyperglycemia. Other useful diagnostics include diagnostic imaging for the assessment of gastric masses and presence of metastasis, and fine needle aspiration and cytological assessment. One case report described the diagnosis of this tumor based on cytology. Cytological characteristics of gastric neuroendocrine carcinomas are similar to those of other mammalian neuroendocrine tumors (**Fig. 2**).[123]

Birds

Glucose metabolism in birds is poorly understood and differs from mammals in several ways. Birds have lower concentrations of insulin and higher concentrations of glucagon within the pancreas and plasma concentrations of glucagon are 10 to 50 times higher when compared with mammals.[16] Birds appear more sensitive to glucagon than insulin, and in some bird species (granivores) glucagon is likely a more effective regulator of glucose than insulin.[16,124] Birds also maintain higher concentrations of blood glucose, and chickens normally have glucose concentrations twice that of mammals.[125]

In birds, DM has been reported in Psittaciformes, Ramphatidae, Accipitriformes, and Sphenisciformes.[126–133] Diagnosis of DM may be made based on a persistent hyperglycemia and glucosuria. The marked hyperglycemia is typically above 1000 mg/dL.[134] Pancreatic biopsies may be helpful but are rarely performed.[134]

Mammals

Although DM has been reported in exotic mammals, the disease is uncommon. Animals in the suborder Hystricomorpha (guinea pigs and degus) have physiologic differences associated with DM, and degus may be one of the most common exotic small

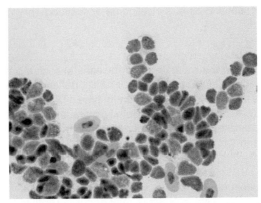

Fig. 2. Fine needle aspiration biopsy of liver mass from an inland bearded dragon (*Pogona vitticeps*) diagnosed with a gastric neuroendocrine carcinoma. Intact neoplastic cells are small, cuboidal with a high nuclear:cytoplasmic ratio and scant basophilic cytoplasm. Nuclei are generally round with stippled chromatin and lack visible nucleoli. (Aqueous Romanowsky stain. 1,000 × original magnification). (Image courtesy J. Meinkoth, Stillwater, OK.)

mammals to develop DM.[135] In degus, insulin has less than 10% of the biological activity found in other species.[136,137] To counter this, degus have increased numbers of insulin receptors and higher insulin concentrations.[136] DM in degus is related to a high-starch diet and obesity making it similar to type II (adult-onset nontinsulin-dependent) in humans.[138] In f chinchillas, DM, most likely type II, has been reported. These animals had marked hyperglycemia (4 times the upper reference limit, specific values not reported) with glucosuria and ketonuria.[139] DM has also been reported in guinea pigs and these animals had hyperglycemia.[140–143] Spontaneous DM has rarely been reported in New Zealand white rabbits.[144]

In ferrets, most DM cases were iatrogenic because of surgical removal of an insulinoma. The hyperglycemia in these cases is usually transient, and insulin and glucose levels typically normalize over time. Reports of spontaneous DM in the ferret are comparatively rare.[145,146]

Glucose Measurement

Measurement of blood glucose is important for diagnosis and management of DM. Point-of-care units for testing blood glucose are commonly used in exotic small mammal patients due to the small sample size required and the rapid results. Although the use of a glucometer (as is used in humans) is common in rabbits, ferrets require a veterinary-specific blood glucose unit set to "canine."[147,148] Recently, a study of the effect of hematocrit on the glucose measurements with human portable point-of-care glucometer in rabbits, showed that blood glucose concentrations were falsely low with hematocrits < 31% and falsely high if hematocrit > 43%.[149] A correction formula improved accuracy for human glucometers but not for veterinary glucometers.[149] Although not scientifically validated in ferrets, similar effects may occur. Accurate glucose measurement requires laboratory units to be accurate.

CALCIUM METABOLISM

Calcium is an essential element with two primary functions. Calcium provides structural strength and support for bones within hydroxyapatite but is also critical for numerous cellular functions.[80,150] Calcium can be found both intracellularly and extracellularly. Most calcium (99%) is bound in skeletal bone and serves as a storage pool for regulating plasma calcium concentrations. About half of extracellular calcium is protein bound (primarily albumin) or complexed (citrate or sulfate) and only the remaining half, ionized (iCa) or free calcium, is biologically active. The calcium measured on a typical biochemistry profile, "total" calcium concentration, consists of all fractions (protein bound, complexed, and iCa).[151]

In most mammals, the parathyroid glands are responsible for calcium, magnesium, and phosphorus homeostasis. Plasma calcium levels are maintained within a narrow range despite fluctuations in dietary calcium intake, bone resorption and remodeling, renal excretion, and changing demands.[80] Chief cells from the parathyroid glands synthesize and release PTH in response to low plasma calcium levels. By increasing calcium resorption from bone, by increasing calcium reabsorption in the proximal tubules of the kidneys, and by stimulating the hydroxylation of 25-hydroxycholecalciferol (vitamin D_3) to its active form, 1,25-dihydroxycholecalciferol (calcitriol) PTH mobilizes calcium.[152] Effects of vitamin D include increasing intestinal absorption of calcium, magnesium, and phosphorus, increasing renal reabsorption of calcium and phosphorus, and increasing bone resorption.[80]

Calcitonin is produced by the parafollicular cells in the thyroid and plays a minor role in calcium homeostasis. The primary role of calcitonin is to reduce hypercalcemia following dietary intake. Calcitonin is secreted in response to hypercalcemia and decreases bone resorption. Calcitonin does not affect the kidneys or intestines.[151] Glucocorticoids also likely decrease plasma calcium levels by reducing intestinal calcium absorption and reducing PTH-stimulated renal calcium reabsorption.[80]

There are many forms of vitamin D. Two naturally occurring forms are cholecalciferol (vitamin D3) and ergocalciferol (vitamin D2).[153] Vitamin D can also be synthesized in the skin with sun exposure (ultraviolet B [UVB] radiation) and must be activated in the kidneys to form 1,25-dihydroxyvitamin D_3 or calcitriol.[153] Active vitamin D_3 stimulates calcium, phosphorus, and magnesium absorption in the intestines; calcium and phosphate reabsorption in the kidneys; and bone resorption.[80]

Reptiles

Calcium imbalance is a common problem in reptiles and is often referred to in the broad term of metabolic bone disease (MBD). Diseases included in MBD are due to abnormal levels and function of minerals such as calcium, phosphorus, and magnesium or vitamin D and PTH. Low plasma calcium concentrations based on nutritional and environmental factors are the initial problem and hypocalcemia stimulates the release of PTH from the parathyroid glands resulting in bone resorption and reduced bone density.[154]

Nutritional secondary hyperparathyroidism is the most common form of MBD in captive reptiles.[155] Although it varies between species, most lizards and chelonians are unable to obtain vitamin D solely from dietary sources.[156] These species rely on light exposure and adequate temperature for subsequent endogenous vitamin D production and maintenance of appropriate levels.[157] Animals in captivity may not have adequate exposure to UVB light resulting in low levels of vitamin D.[158]

As clinical signs of MBD are variable and nonspecific, numerous tests are recommended for diagnosis. Radiographic imaging allows for detection of potential pathologic fractures and evaluation of bone density. Radiographic evidence is often present in chronic disease, but radiographic images may appear normal in early disease. Serum or plasma calcium evaluation is necessary for diagnosis and evaluation of both total calcium and iCa are recommended for interpretation. The evaluation of

1,25-dihydroxyvitamin D_3 is also recommended and is available through several commercial labs. Species-dependent reference intervals are available in the current literature (**Table 4**), and seasonal variations and effect of sex have also been reported.[159–162] Reference intervals for PTH have not been well established in reptiles. Renal disease is often a secondary and life-threatening condition associated with MBD and assessment of renal function is recommended.

Birds

Although hypocalcemia is not seen as frequently in birds as it is in reptiles, it should still be considered. Control of calcium is similar to that of mammals, but there are several differences. Like mammals, in birds the calcium homeostasis is controlled primarily by PTH, calcitonin, and vitamin D, but estrogens and prostaglandins are also involved. Mammalian assays can be used to evaluate PTH levels in birds, but average PTH concentrations in birds are lower than in mammals.[150] Calcitonin concentrations are typically much higher in birds than in mammals, and calcitonin is produced by the ultimobranchial glands in birds, which is a separate structure from the thyroid gland[163]; however, the function of calcitonin in calcium regulation in birds is unclear based on contradictory reports. Birds can also utilize a form of vitamin D, 24,25-dihydroxxholecalciferol that mammals cannot.

Hypocalcemia syndrome in African gray parrots has been well described. Although several theories have been advanced, the etiology of the condition remains unknown. A recent report described a case of a hypocalcemic African gray parrot that was nonresponsive to calcium supplementation. Plasma magnesium concentrations in this bird were low and upon magnesium supplementation, both calcium and magnesium concentrations normalized, and clinical signs improved.[164] In humans, evidence suggests that magnesium is necessary for proper parathyroid gland function.[165,166] Therefore, the measurement of total calcium, ionized calcium, and magnesium should be measured in cases of suspected hypocalcemia. Reference intervals for Mg, Ca, and D_3 have been reported for African gray and Hispaniolan Amazon parrots (**Table 5**).[167]

During egg laying, there are increased demands for calcium. A marked increase in plasma protein occurs concomitantly leading to a significant increase in total available calcium. As in mammals, only about 40% of calcium is protein bound in birds.[16,80] In laying hens, a sigmoidal pattern occurs for concentrations of iCa that peaks within 3 to 6 h of oviposition and then falls to low levels until next oviposition.[168] Thus, high circulating concentrations of total calcium are expected in laying female birds. Total calcium can reach values as high as 40 mg/dL without clinical complications.[150]

Mammals

Information regarding the influence of UVB on the production of endogenous vitamin D is limited, but studies in guinea pigs, chinchillas, rats, and rabbits demonstrate their ability to produce endogenous vitamin D following exposure to artificial UVB light (**Table 6**).[169–172] Calcium metabolism appears independent of vitamin D in domestic rabbits. Rabbits passively absorb calcium from the intestine and maintain total serum calcium concentrations that can be up to 50% higher than what is reported in other mammals.[171] Among mammals, MBD is likely to occur in sugar gliders (*Petaurus breviceps*), tamarins, and marmosets.[173,174] These animals should be assessed similarly to reptiles; Diagnostics should include ionized calcium and diagnostic imaging.

Table 4
Calcium metabolism hormones other related molecules in selected species of exotic reptiles

Species	25-Hydroxycholecalciferol (nmol/L)	1,25-Dihydroxychole-Calciferol (pmol/L)	Total Calcium (mg/dL)	Ionized Calcium (mmol/L)	Methodology	Information
Green iguana				Males 1.32[a,b] (n = 29); Gravid females 1.21[a] (n = 21); Nongravid females 1.30[a] (n = 17)	iCa i-stat	Captive, 2 to 4 years old
Ball python	No UVB exposure 197 ± 35[d] (n = 8); 70-day UVB exposure 203.5 ± 13.8[d] (n = 6)			No UVB exposure 1.84 ± 0.05[d] (n = 8); 70-day UVB exposure 1.78 ± 0.07[d] (n = 6)	Unknown	Captive, >4 years old; exposed to UVB (n = 6 females); not exposed to UVB (n = 3 females and 5 males)
Inland bearded dragon			With UVB supplementation 17.72 ± 4[d] (n = 8); 83 days without UVB 13.88 ± 0.36[d] (n = 10)	With UVB supplementation 1.3 ± 0.1[d] (n = 4); 83 days without UVB 1.48 ± 0.1[d] (n = 10)	TCAutomation clinical analyzer, iCa clinical analyzer	Captive adult female
Inland bearded dragon	UVB exposure 178.4 ± 9[d], No UVB exposure 9.9 ± 1.3[d]	UVB exposure 1.205 ± 0.100[d]; No UVB exposure 0.229 ± 0.025[d]			RIA	Captive raised, 6 months old, (n = 40 males and 44 females)

(continued on next page)

Table 4
(continued)

Species	25-Hydroxycholecalciferol (nmol/L)	1,25-Dihydroxychole-Calciferol (pmol/L)	Total Calcium (mg/dL)	Ionized Calcium (mmol/L)	Methodology	Information
Veiled chameleon	UVB exposure 142[a]; With Ca and vitamin A 160[a]; With Ca, vitamin A, cholecalciferol, and UVB >250[a]; With Ca, vitamin A, and cholecalciferol 102[a]		UVB exposure 8.8[a]. No UVB exposure 8[a] With Ca, vitamin A, and UVB 11.2[a]. With Ca and vitamin A 12.4[a]. With Ca, vitamin A, cholecalciferol, and UVB 12.4[a]. With Ca, vitamin A, and cholecalciferol) 18.4[a]		TCAutomation clinical analyzer, 25(OH)D3 HPLC	6 months old, captive reared (n = 29 males, 27 females)
Corn snake	No UVB supplementation 57.33 ± 45.59[d] (0–132)[c] (n = 12); With 28-day UVB supplementation 196.0 ± 16.73[d] (121–232)[c] (n = 12)				RIA	Captive, not fed during the study
Red-eared slider	No UVB supplementation 10.7 ± 3.4[d] (5–14)[c] (n = 6); 30-day UVB supplementation 71.7 ± 46.9[d] (34–155)[c] (n = 6)				Unknown	Yearlings, captive

[a] Values reported as mean/median.
[b] Values are provided as mean/median values and range/reference interval.
[c] Values are provided as range.
[d] Values are provided as mean/median ± standard error/standard deviation of the mean.

Table 5
Calcium metabolism hormones and other related molecules in selected species of exotic mammals

Species[a]	PTH (pmol/L)	25-Hydroxycholecalciferol (nmol/L)	1,25-Dihydroxycholecalciferol (pmol/L)	Total Calcium (mg/dL)	Ionized Calcium (mmol/L)	Magnesium (mg/dL)	Methodology	Information
Rabbit							Unknown	Unknown
		No UVB supplementation at day 0 (D0) 29.7 ± 14.9[c] (n = 4) No UVB supplementation D14 31.7 ± 9.9[c] (n = 4) D0 prior to UVB exposure 38.8 ± 21.4[c] (n = 5) D14 after UVB exposure 66.4 ± 14.3[c] (n = 5)	88.8 ± 12[c]				Unknown	6 weeks old, dwarf mixed breed
			125.8 ± 9.8[c] (n = 19)				Unknown	6 week old, dwarf mixed breed
	2.83 ± 0.34[c] (n = 9)				1.71 ± 0.02[c] (n = 9)		Immuno-radiometric	New Zealand white of both sexes, aged 9–15 months
	3.31 ± 0.64[c] (n = 10)				1.69 ± 0.02[c] (n = 10)		Immuno-radiometric	New Zealand white of both sexes, aged 9–15 months
					1.67–1.85[b] (n = 44)		i-stat	Unknown
						2.11 ± 0.28[c] (n = 110);	Clinical analyzer	Male, New Zealand

(continued on next page)

Table 5
(continued)

Species[a]	PTH (pmol/L)	25-Hydroxycholecalciferol (nmol/L)	1,25-Dihydroxychole-Calciferol (pmol/L)	Total Calcium (mg/dL)	Ionized Calcium (mmol/L)	Magnesium (mg/dL)	Methodology	Information
Chinchilla		Pre-UVB exposure 110.7 ± 39.5[c] (63–158)[b] (n = 5) D16 UVB exposure 189 ± 102.7[c] (91–319)[b] (n = 5) No UVB exposure at D0 92.2 ± 52[c] (31–166)[b] (n = 5) No UVB exposure at D16 87.8 ± 34.4[c] (53–126)[b] (n = 5)		9.0 ± 1.47[c] (6.1–10.8)[b] (n = 10)				white, 4–7 months
				9.0 ± 1.47[c] (6.1–10.8)[b] (n = 10)			RIA	8-week-old
							RIA	8-week-old
				9.5 ± 0.9[c] (7.4–11.5)[b] (n = 16)		3.8 ± 0.2[c] (3.3–4.2)[b] mg/dL (n = 16)	Colorimetric	Commercial purpose (fur), adult males
				9.28 ± 1.52[c] (n = 20)		2.9 ± 0.41[c] mg/dL (n = 20)	Spectrometry	Commercial purpose, 2–4-year-old female
Guinea pig (Cavia porcellus)		36.33 ± 24.42[c] (10–114)[b] (n = 6)			1.52 ± 0.07[c] (1.35–1.65)[b] (n = 6)		RIA	14- to 16-week-old, female intact Hartley, no UVB supplementation

101.49 ± 21.81[c] (67–165)[b] (n = 6)	1.58 ± 0.09[c] (1.29–1.74)[b] (n = 6)	RIA		14- to 16-week-old, female intact Hartley, UVB supplemented for 6 months
10.32–12.64[b] (n = 58)	1.73–3.84[b] mg/dL (n = 58)	Clinical analyzer		Healthy pets, 24 males, 34 females, ranging from 8 weeks to 5 years old

[a] Values are provided as mean/median values and range/reference interval.
[b] Values are provided as range.
[c] Values are provided as mean/median ± standard error/standard deviation of the mean.
Adapted from Brandão et al.[175]

Table 6
Plasma values of total calcium, phosphorus, magnesium, and calcium:phosphorus ratio for captive African gray parrots (*Psittacus erithacus*) and Hispaniolan Amazon parrots (*Amazona ventralis*)[167]

Test	Males and Females		Non-egg Laying Females	
	African gray parrots (n = 24)	Hispaniolan Amazon parrots (n = 26)	African gray parrots (n = 19)	Hispaniolan Amazon parrots (n = 25)
Calcium mg/dL (mmol/L)				
Mean ± SD	10.77 ± 3.72 (2.69 ± 0.93)	10.03 ± 2.3 (2.51 ± 0.58)	9.02 ± 0.65 (2.26 ± 0.16)	9.6 ± 0.54 (2.4 ± 0.14)
Reference interval	8.20–20.20 (2.05–5.05)	8.80–10.40 (2.20–2.60)	8.10–10.80 (2.03–2.70)	8.80–10.30 (2.20–2.58)
Phosphorus mg/dL (mmol/L)				
Mean ± SD	4.09 ± 2.42 (1.32 ± 0.78)	2.96 ± 1.02 (0.96 ± 0.33)	3.72 ± 0.9 (1.2 ± 0.29)	2.8 ± 0.66 (0.9 ± 0.21)
Reference interval	2.50–5.90 (0.81–1.91)	1.80–4.40 (0.58–1.42)	2.40–5.30 (0.78–1.71)	1.80–3.80 (0.58–1.23)
Magnesium mg/dL (mmol/L)				
Mean ± SD	2.48 ± 0.38 (1.02 ± 0.16)	2.43 ± 0.32 (1.0 ± 0.13)	2.32 ± 0.16 (0.95 ± 0.07)	2.4 ± 0.3 (0.99 ± 0.12)
Reference interval	2.10–3.40 (0.86–1.40)	1.90–3.10 (0.78–1.27)	2.00–2.60 (0.82–1.07)	1.90–3.00 (0.78–1.23)
Calcium:phosphorus ratio				
Mean ± SD	2.7 ± 0.65	3.57 ± 0.81	2.55 ± 0.6	3.6 ± 0.82
Reference interval	1.81–3.77	2.62–5.39	1.67–3.50	2.62–5.39

African gray parrots were housed in an open aviary with exposure to sunlight in Mississippi (USA) while the Hispaniolan Amazon parrots were housed in an indoor close aviary in Louisiana (USA).[167] Results represent all tested animal (males and females) and only non-egg laying animals (i.e., males and non-laying females).[167]

DISCLOSURE

No conflict of interest to disclose.

REFERENCES

1. Norris D. Vertebrate endocrinology. 4th edition. San Diego (CA): Academic Press; 2007.
2. Ball JN, Baker BI. 1 - The pituitary gland: anatomy and histophysiology.. In: Hoar WS, Randall DJ, editors. Fish Physiology. In: Hoar W, Randall D, editors. The endocrine system, vol. 2. New York, NY: Academic Press; 1969. p. 1–110.
3. Goodman H. Pituitary gland. In: Goodman H, editor. Basic medical endocrinology. Boston, MA: Academic Press -Elsevier; 2010. p. 29–42.
4. Herring P. Further observations upon the comparative anatomy and physiology of the pituitary body. Exp Physiol 1913;6:73–108.
5. Welbourn R. The history of endocrine surgery. New York: Praeger Publishers; 1990.
6. Heller H, Pickering B. Neurohypophysial hormones of non-mammalian vertebrates. J Physiol 1961;155:98.
7. Rice G. Plasma arginine vasotocin concentrations in the lizard Varanus gouldii (Gray) following water loading, salt loading, and dehydration. Gen Comp Endocrinol 1982;47:1–6.
8. Starkey SR, Wood C, de Matos R, et al. Central diabetes insipidus in an African Grey parrot. J Am Vet Med Assoc 2010;237:415–9.
9. Bichet DG. Nephrogenic diabetes insipidus. Am J Med 1998;105:431–42.
10. Nelson R. Water metabolism and diabetes insipidus. In: Feldman E, Nelson R, Reusch C, et al, editors. Canine and feline endocrinology. St Louis, (MO): Elsevier; 2015. p. 1–22.
11. Braun EJ, Stallone JN. The occurrence of nephrogenic diabetes insipidus in domestic fowl. Am J Physiol 1989;256:F639–45.
12. Bartholomew GA, Cade TJ. The water economy of land birds. Auk 1963;80:504–39.
13. Kurien BT, Everds NE, Scofield RH. Experimental animal urine collection: a review. Lab Anim 2004;38:333–61.
14. Tschopp R, Bailey T, Di Somma A, et al. Urinalysis as a noninvasive health screening procedure in Falconidae. J Avian Med Surg 2007;21:8–12.
15. Lumeij J, Westerhof I. The use of the water deprivation test for the diagnosis of apparent psychogenic polydipsia in a socially deprived African grey parrot (Psittacus erithacus erithacus). Avian Pathol 1988;17:875–8.
16. Lumeij J. Endocrinology. In: Ritchie B, Harrison G, Harrison L, editors. Avian medicine: principles and application. Lake Worth (FL): Wingers Pub.; 1994. p. 582–606.
17. Cheng K, Friesen H, Martin J. Neurophysin in rats with hereditary hypothalamic diabetes insipidus (Brattleboro strain). Endocrinology 1972;90:1055–63.
18. Boorman G. Diabetes insipidus syndrome in a rabbit. J Am Vet Med Assoc 1969;155:1218–20.
19. Kalimo H, Rinne UK. Ultrastructural studies on the hypothalamic neurosecretory neurons of the rat. Z für Zellforschung Mikroskopische Anatomie 1972;134:205–25.
20. Kutscher CL, Stillman RD, Weiss IP. Food-deprivation polydipsia in gerbils (Meriones unguiculatus). Physiol Behav 1968;3:667–71.

21. Zhang J, Lazar MA. The mechanism of action of thyroid hormones. Annu Rev Physiol 2000;62.

22. Yen PM. Physiological and molecular basis of thyroid hormone action. Physiol Rev 2001;81:1097–142.

23. Westgren U, Melander A, Wåhlin E, et al. Divergent effects of 6-propylthiouracil on 3, 5, 3′-triiodothyronine (T3) and 3, 3′, 5′-triiodothyronine (RT3) serum levels in man. Eur J Endocrinol 1977;85:345–50.

24. Scott-Moncrieff J. Hypothryoidism. In: Feldman E, Nelson R, Reusch C, et al, editors. Canine and feline endocrinology. St Louis(MO): Elsevier; 2015. p. 78–9.

25. Little JW. Thyroid disorders. Part I: hyperthyroidism. Oral Surg Oral Med Oral Pathol Oral Radiol Endod 2006;101:276–84.

26. Ferguson DC. Testing for hypothyroidism in dogs. Vet Clin North Am Small Anim Pract 2007;37:647–69.

27. Warner MH, Beckett GJ. Mechanisms behind the non-thyroidal illness syndrome: an update. J Endocrinol 2009;205:1–13.

28. Thöle M, Brezina T, Fehr M, et al. Presumptive nonthyroidal illness syndrome in pet rabbits (Oryctolagus cuniculus). J Exot Pet Med 2019;31:100–3.

29. Vieira KR, Faillace AC, Oliva LR, et al. Comparison of Serum Thyroid Hormone Levels in Green-winged Macaws (Ara chloropterus) Using Radio and Chemiluminescent Immunoassays. J Avian Med Surg 2021;35:187–95.

30. Licht P, Denver RJ. Effects of TRH on hormone release from pituitaries of the lizard, Anolis carolinensis. Gen Comp Endocrinol 1988;70:355–62.

31. Sawin CT, Bacharach P, Lance V. Thyrotropin-releasing hormone and thyrotropin in the control of thyroid function in the turtle, Chrysemys picta. Gen Comp Endocrinol 1981;45:7–11.

32. Lothrop C Jr, Loomis M, Olsen J. Thyrotropin stimulation test for evaluation of thyroid function in psittacine birds. J Am Vet Med Assoc 1985;186:47–8.

33. Lumeij J, Westerhof I. Clinical evaluation of thyroid function in racing pigeons (Columba livia domestica). Avian Pathol 1988;17:63–70.

34. Williamson R, Davison T. The effect of a single injection of thyrotrophin on serum concentrations of thyroxine, triiodothyronine, and reverse triiodothyronine in the immature chicken (Gallus domesticus). Gen Comp Endocrinol 1985;58:109–13.

35. Zenoble R, Kemppainen R, Young D, et al. Endocrine responses of healthy parrots to ACTH and thyroid stimulating hormone. J Am Vet Med Assoc 1985;187:1116–8.

36. Harms C, Hoskinson J, Bruyette D, et al. Development of an experimental model of hypothyroidism in cockatiels (Nymphicus hollandicus). Am J Vet Res 1994;55:399–404.

37. Greenacre C, Jaques J. TSH testing in birds using canine, bovine, or human TSH. WA: Proceedings Association Avian Veterinarians Seattle; 2011. p. 49.

38. Heard D, Collins B, Chen D, et al. Thyroid and adrenal function tests in adult male ferrets. Am J Vet Res 1990;51:32–5.

39. Colzani RM, Alex S, Fang S-I, et al. The effect of recombinant human thyrotropin (rhTSH) on thyroid function in mice and rats. Thyroid 1998;8:797–801.

40. Mayer J, Wagner R, Mitchell MA, et al. Use of recombinant human thyroid-stimulating hormone for thyrotropin stimulation testing in euthyroid ferrets. J Am Vet Med Assoc 2013;243:1432–5.

41. Mayer J, Wagner R, Mitchell MA, et al. Use of recombinant human thyroid-stimulating hormone for evaluation of thyroid function in guinea pigs (Cavia porcellus). J Am Vet Med Assoc 2013;242:346–9.

42. Rivera S, Lock B. The reptilian thyroid and parathyroid glands. Veterinary Clin North Am Exot Anim Pract 2008;11:163–75.

43. Leineweber C, Öfner S, Stöhr AC, et al. A comparison of thyroid hormone levels and plasma capillary zone electrophoresis in red-eared sliders (Trachemys script a elegans) and map turtles (Graptemys spp.) depending on season and sex. Vet Clin Pathol 2020;49:78–90.

44. Norton TM, Jacobson ER, Caligiuri R, et al. Medical management of a Galapagos tortoise (Geochelone elephantopus) with hypothyroidism. J Zoo Wildl Med 1989;20(2):212–6.

45. Franco KH, Hoover JP. Levothyroxine as a treatment for presumed hypothyroidism in an adult male African spurred tortoise (Centrochelys [formerly Geochelone] sulcata). J Herpetological Med Surg 2009;19:42–4.

46. Hadfield CA, Clayton LA, Clancy MM, et al. Proliferative thyroid lesions in three diplodactylid geckos: Nephrurus amyae, Nephrurus levis, and Oedura marmorata. J Zoo Wildl Med 2012;43:131–40.

47. Hernandez-Divers SJ, Knott CD, MacDonald J. Diagnosis and surgical treatment of thyroid adenoma-induced hyperthyroidism in a green iguana (Iguana iguana). J zoo Wildl Med 2001;32:465–75.

48. Frye F. Biomedical and surgical aspects of captive reptile husbandry. Malabar, FL: Krieger Pub Co; 1981. April 18-23.

49. Kubiak M. Hyperthyroidism Diagnosis and Treatment in an African Helmeted Turtle. Proceedings of the 2nd International Conference on Avian, Herpetological, and Exotic Mammal Medicine Paris, France, 2015;421.

50. Cowan DF. Diseases of captive reptiles. J Am Vet Med Assoc 1968;153:848–59.

51. Gál J, Csikó G, Pásztor I, et al. First description of papillary carcinoma in the thyroid gland of a red-eared slider (Trachemys scripta elegans). Acta Vet Hung 2010;58:69–73.

52. Whiteside DP, Gamer MM. Thyroid adenocarcinoma in a crocodile lizard, Shinisaurus crocodilurus. J Herpetological Med Surg 2001;11:13–6.

53. Pajdak-Czaus J, Terech-Majewska E, Będzłowicz D, et al. Applicability of thyroxine measurements and ultrasound imaging in evaluations of thyroid function in turtles. J Vet Res 2019;63:267.

54. Radek T, Piasecki T. Topography and arterial supply of the thyroid and the parathyroid glands in selected species of Falconiformes. Anat Histol Embryol 2007;36:241–9.

55. Radek T, Piasecki T. The topographical anatomy and arterial supply of the thyroid and parathyroid glands in the budgerigar (Melopsittacus undulatus). Folia Morphol 2004;63:163–71.

56. McNabb F. Thyroids. In: Scanes C, editor. Sturkie's Avian physiology. San Diego: Academic Press; 2015. p. 535–47.

57. Merryman JI, Buckles EL. The avian thyroid gland. Part one: a review of the anatomy and physiology. J Avian Med Surg 1998;12(4):234–7.

58. Schmidt RE, Reavill DR. Thyroid hyperplasia in birds. J Avian Med Surg 2002;16:111 4.

59. Loukopoulos P, Bautista AC, Puschner B, et al. An outbreak of thyroid hyperplasia (goiter) with high mortality in budgerigars (Melopsittacus undulatus). J Vet Diagn Invest 2015;27:18–24.

60. Chen AY, Bernet VJ, Carty SE, et al. American Thyroid Association statement on optimal surgical management of goiter. Thyroid 2014;24:181–9.

61. Oglesbee BL. Hypothyroidism in a scarlet macaw. J Am Vet Med Assoc 1992;201:1599–601.

62. Fudge A, Speer B. Selected controversial topics in avian diagnostic testing. Semin Avian Exot Pet Med 2001;10(2):96–101.

63. Brandão J, Manickam B, Blas-Machado U, et al. Productive thyroid follicular carcinoma in a wild barred owl (Strix varia). J Vet Diagn Invest 2012;24:1145–50.

64. Gibbons PM, Garner MM, Kiupel M. Morphological and immunohistochemical characterization of spontaneous thyroid gland neoplasms in guinea pigs (Cavia porcellus). Vet Pathol 2013;50:334–42.

65. Girod-Rüffer C, Müller E, Marschang R, et al. Retrospective study on hyperthyroidism in guinea pigs in veterinary practices in Germany. J Exot Pet Med 2019; 29:87–97.

66. Mayer J, Wagner R, Taeymans O. Advanced diagnostic approaches and current management of thyroid pathologies in Guinea pigs. Veterinary Clin North Am Exot Anim Pract 2010;13:509–23.

67. Fredholm D, Cagle L, Johnston M. Evaluation of precision and establishment of reference ranges for plasma thyroxine using a point-of-care analyzer in healthy guinea pigs (Cavia porcellus). J Exot Pet Med 2012;21:87–93.

68. Müller K, Müller E, Klein R, et al. Serum thyroxine concentrations in clinically healthy pet guinea pigs (Cavia porcellus). Vet Clin Pathol 2009;38:507–10.

69. Castro MI, Alex S, Young RA, et al. Total and free serum thyroid hormone concentrations in fetal and adult pregnant and nonpregnant guinea pigs. Endocrinology 1986;118:533–7.

70. Anderson R, Nixon D, Akasha M. Total and free thyroxine and triiodothyronine in blood serum of mammals. Comp Biochem Physiol A, Comp Physiol 1988;89: 401–4.

71. Quimby F. The clinical chemistry of laboratory animals. 2nd ed. Philadelphia: Taylor & Francis; 1999.

72. Fritsche R, Simova-Curd S, Clauss M, et al. Hyperthyroidism in connection with suspected diabetes mellitus in a chinchilla (Chinchilla laniger). Vet Rec 2008; 163:454–6.

73. Thorson L. Thyroid diseases in rodent species. Veterinary Clin North Am Exot Anim Pract 2014;17:51–67.

74. Bray GA, York DA. Thyroid function of genetically obese rats. Endocrinology 1971;88:1095–9.

75. Mebis L, Debaveye Y, Ellger B, et al. Changes in the central component of the hypothalamus-pituitary-thyroid axis in a rabbit model of prolonged critical illness. Crit Care 2009;13:R147.

76. Chesney AMCT, Webster B. Endemic Goitre in Rabbits. I. Incidence and Characteristics. Bull Johns Hopkins Hosp 1928;43:261–77.

77. Brandão J, Higbie C, Rick M, et al. Naturally occurring idiopathic hyperthyroidism in two pet rabbits. St. Antonio, TX: 1st ExoticsCon; 2015. p. 341–2.

78. Brandão J, Ellison M, Beaufrère H, et al. Quantitative 99m Technetium Pertechnetate Thyroid Scintigraphy in Euthyroid New Zealand Rabbits (Oryctolagus cuniculus). American College of Veterinary Radiology Annual Scientific Conference St. Louis, MO, October 21-24, 2014;62.

79. Wagner R. Hypothyroidism in Ferrets. Proceedings of the Association of Exotic Mammal Veterinary Conference Oakland, CA, October 23-26, 2012;29-31.

80. Engelking L, Rebar A. Metabolic and endocrine physiology. Jackson, WY: Tenton NewMedia; 2012.

81. Behrend E. Canine hyperadrenocorticism. In: Feldman E, Nelson R, Reusch C, et al, editors. Canine and feline endocrinology. St Louis, MO: Elsevier; 2015. p. 377–80.

82. Hartman F, Brownell K. The hormone of the adrenal cortex. Exp Biol Med 1930; 27:938–9.
83. Scott-Moncrieff J. Hypoadrenocorticism. In: Feldman E, Nelson R, Reusch C, et al, editors. Canine and feline endocrinology. St Louis, MO: Elsevier; 2015. p. 377–80.
84. Bielinska M, Parviainen H, Kiiveri S, et al. Review paper: origin and molecular pathology of adrenocortical neoplasms. Vet Pathol 2009;46:194–210.
85. Miller C, Marini R, Fox J. Diseases of the endocrine system. In: Fox J, Marini R, editors. Biology and diseases of the ferret. 3rd ed. Ames, Iowa: Wiley-Blackwell; 2014. p. 377–400.
86. Holmes RL. The adrenal glands of the ferret, Mustela putorius. J Anat 1961;95: 325–36.
87. Deacon CF, Mosley W, Jones IC. The X zone of the mouse adrenal cortex of the Swiss albino strain. Gen Comp Endocrinol 1986;61:87–99.
88. Carsia R, Harvey S. Adrenals. In: Whittow G, editor. Sturkie's avian physiology. San Diego, CA: Academic Press; 2000. p. 489–538.
89. de Matos R. Adrenal steroid metabolism in birds: anatomy, physiology, and clinical considerations. Veterinary Clin North Am Exot Anim Pract 2008;11:35–57, vi.
90. Chen S. Advanced diagnostic approaches and current medical management of insulinomas and adrenocortical disease in ferrets (Mustela putorius furo). Veterinary Clin North Am Exot Anim Pract 2010;13:439–52.
91. Vinke C, van Deijk R, Houx B, et al. The effects of surgical and chemical castration on intermale aggression, sexual behaviour and play behaviour in the male ferret (Mustela putorius furo). Appl Anim Behav Sci 2008;115:104–21.
92. Shoemaker NJ, Schuurmans M, Moorman H, et al. Correlation between age at neutering and age at onset of hyperadrenocorticism in ferrets. J Am Vet Med Assoc 2000;216:195–7.
93. Kuijten AM, Schoemaker NJ, Voorhout G. Ultrasonographic visualization of the adrenal glands of healthy ferrets and ferrets with hyperadrenocorticism. J Am Anim Hosp Assoc 2007;43:78–84.
94. Lennox A, Chitty J. Adrenal Neoplasia and Hyperplasia as a Cause of Hypertestosteronism in Two Rabbits. J Exot Pet Med 2006;15:56–8.
95. Baine K, Newkirk K, Fecteau K, et al. Elevated testosterone and progestin concentrations in a spayed female rabbit with an adrenal cortical adenoma. Case Rep Vet Med 2014.
96. Wright T, Eshar D, Rooney T, et al. Use of a deslorelin implant for management of hyperandrogenism associated with excessive sex hormone production in a female spayed pet rabbit (Oryctolagus cuniculus). J Exot Pet Med 2022;40:12–5.
97. Rose JB, Vergneau-Grosset C, Steffey MA, et al. Adrenalectomy and Nephrectomy in a Rabbit (Oryctolagus cuniculus) With Adrenocortical Carcinoma and Renal and Ureteral Transitional Cell Carcinoma. J Exot Pet Med 2016;25:332–41.
98. Fecteau KA, Deeb BJ, Rickel JM, et al. Diagnostic Endocrinology: Blood Steroid Concentrations in Neutered Male and Female Rabbits. J Exot Pet Med 2007;16. 256–9.
99. Martinho F. Suspected case of hyperadrenocorticism in a golden hamster (Mesocricetus auratus). Veterinary Clin North Am Exot Anim Pract 2006;9:717–21.
100. Jekl V, Hauptman K, Knotek Z. Evidence-Based Advances in Rodent Medicine. Veterinary Clin North Am Exot Anim Pract 2017;20:805–16.
101. Zaheer OA, Beaufrère H. Treatment of hyperadrenocorticism in a guinea pig (Cavia porcellus). J Exot Pet Med 2020;34:57–61.

102. Zeugswetter F, Fenske M, Hassan J, et al. Cushing's syndrome in a guinea pig. Vet Rec 2007;160:878–80.
103. Elayat AA, el-Naggar MM, Tahir M. An immunocytochemical and morphometric study of the rat pancreatic islets. J Anat 1995;186(Pt 3):629–37.
104. Andralojc KM, Mercalli A, Nowak KW, et al. Ghrelin-producing epsilon cells in the developing and adult human pancreas. Diabetologia 2009;52:486–93.
105. Wierup N, Svensson H, Mulder H, et al. The ghrelin cell: a novel developmentally regulated islet cell in the human pancreas. Regul Peptides 2002;107:63–9.
106. Nussey S, Whitehead S. Endocrinology: an integrated approach. Oxford: CRC Press; 2013.
107. Lester NV, Newell SM, Hill RC, et al. Scintigraphic diagnosis of insulinoma in a dog. Vet Radiol Ultrasound 1999;40:174–8.
108. Goutal CM, Brugmann BL, Ryan KA. Insulinoma in dogs: a review. J Am Anim Hosp Assoc 2012;48:151–63.
109. Hess LR, Ravich ML, Reavill DR. Diagnosis and treatment of an insulinoma in a guinea pig (Cavia porcellus). J Am Vet Med Assoc 2013;242:522–6.
110. Harcourt-Brown FM, Harcourt-Brown SF. Clinical value of blood glucose measurement in pet rabbits. Vet Rec 2012;170:674.
111. Agúndez MG, Velasco CI. Case report of a guinea pig (Cavia porcellus) with a surgically treated insulinoma. J Exot Pet Med 2020;33:50–3.
112. Adissu HA, Turner PV. Insulinoma and squamous cell carcinoma with peripheral polyneuropathy in an aged Sprague–Dawley rat. J Am Assoc Lab Anim Sci 2010;49:856–9.
113. Robertson J, Brandão J, Blas-Machado U, et al. Spontaneous pancreatic islet cell adenoma with peripheral neuropathy in a pet rat (Rattus norvegicus). J Exot Pet Med 2019;28:166–72.
114. Mann F, Stockham S, Freeman M, et al. Reference intervals for insulin concentrations and insulin: glucose ratios in the serum of ferrets. Scientifur 1995; 19:289.
115. Mellanby RJ, Herrtage ME. Insulinoma in a normoglycaemic dog with low serum fructosamine. J Small Anim Pract 2002;43:506–8.
116. Thoresen SI, Aleksandersen M, Lønaas L, et al. Pancreatic insulin-secreting carcinoma in a dog: fructosamine for determining persistent hypoglycaemia. J Small Anim Pract 1995;36:282–6.
117. Duhamelle A, Vlaemynck F, Loeuillet E, et al. Clinical value of fructosamine measurements and fructosamine-albumin ratio in hypoglycemic ferrets (Mustela Putorius Furo). J Exot Pet Med 2018;27:103–7.
118. Nelson R. Canine diabetes mellitus. In: Feldman E, Nelson R, Reusch C, et al, editors. Canine and feline endocrinology. St Louis, MO: Elsevier; 2015. p. 213–7.
119. Stahl S. Hyperglycemia in reptiles. In: Mader D, editor. Reptile medicine and surgery. 2nd edition. St. Louis, Missouri: Saunders Elsevier; 2006. p. 822–30.
120. Barten S. Lizards. In: Mader D, editor. Reptile medicine and surgery. 2nd edition. St. Louis, Missouri: Saunders Elsevier; 2006. p. 683-605.
121. Ritter JM, Garner MM, Chilton JA, et al. Gastric neuroendocrine carcinomas in bearded dragons (Pogona vitticeps). Vet Pathol 2009;46:1109–16.
122. Mans C. Clinical update on diagnosis and management of disorders of the digestive system of reptiles. J Exot Pet Med 2013;22:141–62.
123. Anderson KB, Meinkoth J, Hallman M, et al. Cytological diagnosis of gastric neuroendocrine carcinoma in a pet inland bearded dragon (Pogona Vitticeps). J Exot Pet Med 2019;29:188–93.

124. Braun EJ, Sweazea KL. Glucose regulation in birds. Comp Biochem Physiol B, Biochem Mol Biol 2008;151:1–9.
125. Akiba Y, Chida Y, Takahashi T, et al. Persistent hypoglycemia induced by continuous insulin infusion in broiler chickens. Br Poult Sci 1999;40:701–5.
126. Desmarchelier M, Langlois I. Diabetes mellitus in a nanday conure (Nandayus nenday). J Avian Med Surg 2008;22:246–54.
127. Pilny AA, Luong R. Diabetes Mellitus in a Chestnut-fronted Macaw (Ara severa). J Avian Med Surg 2005;19:297–302, 296.
128. Appleby RC. Diabetes mellitus in a budgerigar (Melopsittacus undulatus). Vet Rec 1984;115:652–3.
129. Altman R, Kirmayer A. Diabetes mellitus in the avian species [Parakeets]. J Am Anim Hosp Assoc 1976;531–7.
130. Ryan C, Walder E, Howard E. Diabetes-mellitus and islet cell-carcinoma in a parakeet. J Am Anim Hosp Assoc 1982;18:139–42.
131. Douglass E. Diabetes mellitus in a toco toucan. Mod Vet Pract 1981;62:293–5.
132. Candeletta SC, Homer BL, Garner MM, et al. Diabetes mellitus associated with chronic lymphocytic pancreatitis in an African grey parrot (Psittacus erithacus erithacus). J Assoc Avian Veterinarians 1993;7(1):39–43.
133. Wallner-Pendleton EA, Rogers D, Epple A. Diabetes mellitus in a red-tailed hawk (Buteo jamaicensis). Avian Pathol 1993;22:631–5.
134. Pilny AA. The avian pancreas in health and disease. Veterinary Clin North Am Exot Anim Pract 2008;11:25–34.
135. Spear G, Caple M, Sutherland L. The pancreas in the degu. Exp Mol Pathol 1984;40:295–310.
136. Edwards MS. Nutrition and behavior of degus (Octodon degus). Veterinary Clin North Am Exot Anim Pract 2009;12:237–53.
137. Opazo JC, Soto-Gamboa M, Bozinovic F. Blood glucose concentration in caviomorph rodents. Comp Biochem Physiol A: Mol Integr Physiol 2004;137:57–64.
138. Campbell-Ward M, Rand J. Diabetes mellitus in other species. In: Rand J, Behrend E, Gunn-Moore D, editors. Clinical endocrinology of companion animals. 1st edition. Ames, IA: John Wiley & Sons; 2013. p. 191–200.
139. Mans C, Donnelly T. Disease Problems of Chinchillas. In: Quesenberry K, Carpenter J, editors. Ferrets, rabbits, and rodents: clinical medicine and surgery. 3rd edition. St. Louis, MO: Elsevier/Saunders; 2012. p. 311–25.
140. Vannevel J. Diabetes mellitus in a 3-year-old, intact, female guinea pig. Can Vet J 1998;39:503.
141. Belis JA, Curley RM, Lang M. Bladder dysfunction in the spontaneously diabetic male Abyssinian-Hartley guinea pig. Pharmacology 1996;53:66–70.
142. Ewringmann A, Göbel T. Diabetes mellitus bei Kaninchen, Meerschweinchen und Chinchilla. Kleintierpraxis 1998;43:337–48.
143. Glage S, Kamino K, Jörns A, et al. Hereditary hyperglycaemia and pancreatic degeneration in Guinea pigs. J Exp Anim Sci 2007;43:309–17.
144. Roth S, Conaway H. Animal model of human disease. Spontaneous diabetes mellitus in the New Zealand white rabbit. Am J Pathol 1982;109:359.
145. Benoit-Biancamano M-O, Morin M, Langlois I. Histopathologic lesions of diabetes mellitus in a domestic ferret. Can Vet J 2005;46:895.
146. Boari A, Papa V, Di Silverio F, et al. Type 1 diabetes mellitus and hyperadrenocorticism in a ferret. Vet Res Commun 2010;34:107–10.
147. Petritz OA, Antinoff N, Chen S, et al. Evaluation of portable blood glucose meters for measurement of blood glucose concentration in ferrets (Mustela putorius furo). J Am Vet Med Assoc 2013;242:350–4.

148. Selleri P, Di Girolamo N, Novari G. Performance of two portable meters and a benchtop analyzer for blood glucose concentration measurement in rabbits. J Am Vet Med Assoc 2014;245:87–98.

149. Cutler DC, Koenig A, Di Girolamo N, et al. Investigation for correction formulas on the basis of packed cell volume for blood glucose concentration measurements obtained with portable glucometers when used in rabbits. Am J Vet Res 2020;81:642–50.

150. de Matos R. Calcium metabolism in birds. Veterinary Clin North Am Exot Anim Pract 2008;11:59–82.

151. Feldman E. Hypercalcemia and primary hyperparathyroidism. In: Feldman E, Nelson R, Reusch C, et al, editors. Canine and feline endocrinology. St Louis, MO: Elsevier; 2015. p. 580–3.

152. Åkerström G, Hellman P, Hessman O, et al. Parathyroid glands in calcium regulation and human disease. Ann N Y Acad Sci 2005;1040:53–8.

153. Cui Y, Rohan TE. Vitamin D, calcium, and breast cancer risk: a review. Cancer Epidemiol Prev Biomarkers 2006;15:1427–37.

154. McWilliams D. Nutrition research on calcium homeostasis. I. Lizards (with recommendations). Int Zoo Yearb 2005;39:69–77.

155. Mader D. Metabolic bone disease. In: Mader D, editor. Reptile medicine and surgery. 2nd edition. St. Louis, Missouri: Saunders Elsevier; 2006. p. 841–51.

156. Hedley J. Metabolic bone disease in reptiles: part 1. UK Vet Companion Anim 2012;17:52–4.

157. Ferguson GW, Gehrmann WH, Karsten KB, et al. Do panther chameleons bask to regulate endogenous vitamin D3 production? Physiol Biochem Zool 2003; 76:52–9.

158. Dittmer K, Thompson K. Vitamin D metabolism and rickets in domestic animals: a review. Vet Pathol 2011;48:389–407.

159. Eatwell K. Variations in the concentration of ionised calcium in the plasma of captive tortoises (Testudo species). Vet Rec 2009;165:82–4.

160. Eatwell K. Plasma concentrations of 25-hydroxycholecalciferol in 22 captive tortoises (Testudo species). Vet Rec 2008;162:342–5.

161. Selleri P, Di Girolamo N. Plasma 25-hydroxyvitamin D3 concentrations in Hermann's tortoises (Testudo hermanni) exposed to natural sunlight and two artificial ultraviolet radiation sources. Am J Vet Res 2012;73:1781–6.

162. Stringer EM, Harms CA, Beasley JF, et al. Comparison of ionized calcium, parathyroid hormone, and 25-hydroxyvitamin D in rehabilitating and healthy wild green sea turtles (Chelonia mydas). J Herpetological Med Surg 2010;20:122–7.

163. Johnston MS, Ivey ES. Parathyroid and ultimobranchial glands: calcium metabolism in birds. Semin Avian Exot Pet Med 2002;11(2):84–93.

164. Kirchgessner MS, Tully TN Jr, Nevarez J, et al. Magnesium therapy in a hypocalcemic African grey parrot (Psittacus erithacus). J Avian Med Surg 2012;26: 17–21.

165. Anast CS, Mohs JM, Kaplan SL, et al. Evidence for parathyroid failure in magnesium deficiency. Science 1972;177:606–8.

166. Anast CS, Winnacker JL, Forte LR, et al. Impaired release of parathyroid hormone in magnesium deficiency. J Clin Endocrinol Metab 1976;42:707–17.

167. de Carvalho FM, Gaunt SD, Kearney MT, et al. Reference intervals of plasma calcium, phosphorus, and magnesium for African grey parrots (Psittacus erithacus) and Hispaniolan parrots (Amazona ventralis). J Zoo Wildl Med 2009;40: 675–9.

168. Luck M, Scanes C. Plasma levels of ionized calcium in the laying hen (Gallus domesticus). Comp Biochem Physiol A Physiol 1979;63:177–81.
169. Watson MK, Stern AW, Labelle AL, et al. Evaluating the clinical and physiological effects of long term ultraviolet B radiation on guinea pigs (Cavia porcellus). PLoS One 2014;9:e114413.
170. Rivas AE, Mitchell MA, Flower J, et al. Effects of ultraviolet radiation on serum 25-hydroxyvitamin D concentrations in captive chinchillas (Chinchilla laniger). J Exot Pet Med 2014;23:270–6.
171. Emerson JA, Whittington JK, Allender MC, et al. Effects of ultraviolet radiation produced from artificial lights on serum 25-hydroxyvitamin D concentration in captive domestic rabbits (Oryctolagus cuniculi). Am J Vet Res 2014;75:380–4.
172. Abulmeaty MMA. Sunlight exposure vs. vitamin D supplementation on bone homeostasis of vitamin D deficient rats. Clin Nutr Exp 2017;11:1–9.
173. Power M, Koutsos L. Marmoset nutrition and dietary husbandry. London, UK: The common marmoset in captivity and biomedical research Academic Press; 2019. p. 63–76.
174. Hatt JM, Sainsbury AW. Unusual case of metabolic bone disease in a common marmoset (Callithrix jacchus). Vet Rec 1998;143:78–80.
175. Brandão J, Rick M, Mayer J. Endocrine system. In: Mitchell M, Tully T, editors. Current therapy in exotic pet practice. Oxford (UK): Elsevier; 2016. p. 277–351.
176. Brandão J, Rick M, Tully Jr TN. Measurement of Serum Free and Total Thyroxine and Triiodothyronine Concentrations in Rabbits Exoticscon. Proceedings of the Exoticscon, Portland, OR, August 27 - September 1, 2016;485-486.
177. Brandão J, Vergneau-Grosset C, Mayer J. Hyperthyroidism and hyperparathyroidism in guinea pigs (Cavia porcellus). Veterinary Clin North Am Exot Anim Pract 2013;16:407–20.

Digital Cytology in Exotic Practice

Tips to Optimize Diagnosis

Richard Dulli, DVM[a], Sabrina D. Clark, DVM, PhD, DACVP, MRCVS[b],*

KEYWORDS

- Digital microscopy • Exotic animals • Images • Scanner • Static • Telecytology

KEY POINTS

- Recognizing the advantages and limitations of digital cytology are important to maximize this techniques' clinical usefulness.
- Sample preparation techniques can improve the likelihood of obtaining a cytologic diagnosis/interpretation for digital submissions.
- To acquire the best images for static digital cytology submission, microscope settings must be properly optimized via Köhler illumination.
- While standard pathologist slide review or biopsy with histopathologic evaluation may still be required for definitive interpretation and diagnosis, we provide specific examples to highlight the benefits of incorporating digital cytology into exotic animal clinical practice.

INTRODUCTION

Digital cytology refers to microscopic images of a cytologic preparation converted to a digital format. This can be as elaborate as whole slide imaging (WSI) via scanners designed to digitize a whole slide to allow evaluation at various magnifications or as simple as an image capture from a single field of view through a microscope's ocular using a camera or smartphone. Digital cytology has fundamentally changed the involvement of the clinical pathologist in patient care, particularly as a point-of-care diagnostic service that can now be incorporated into real-time case management. However, to maximize the usefulness of this service, the clinician must understand both the advantages and limitations of digital cytology. Additionally, based on the incorporation of digital cytology, digital sample preparation and capture often becomes the responsibility of the practice staff. Thus, all individuals involved should feel comfortable with sample acquisition and preparation, and have optimized

[a] Department of Veterinary Pathobiology, College of Veterinary Medicine & Biomedical Sciences, Texas A&M University, 4467 TAMU, College Station, TX 77840, USA; [b] Zoetis, Inc., 10 Sylvan Way, Parsippany, NJ 07054, USA
* Corresponding author. 10 Sylvan Way, Parsippany, NJ 07054.
E-mail address: sdclarkdvm@gmail.com

Vet Clin Exot Anim 25 (2022) 663–678
https://doi.org/10.1016/j.cvex.2022.06.004
1094-9194/22/© 2022 Elsevier Inc. All rights reserved.
vetexotic.theclinics.com

microscopy skills to achieve high-quality diagnostic and digitally decipherable samples. Furthermore, through viewing highlighted features of real digital cases, one may better gauge the benefits of digital cytology as a diagnostic tool to incorporate into daily practice.

Several advantages of digital cytology over traditional microscopy make it desirable for various applications, including as a point-of-care diagnostic tool in a practice setting. One of the greatest advantages of incorporating digital cytology into general practice use is the rapid turnaround times allowed with digital evaluation. Submission of cytology samples with conventional send-out services can take more than 24 to 48 hours to receive a cytopathologist's interpretation. However, with digital imaging, digital cytology companies can provide turnaround times of 2 hours or less. This decreased time to results translates to more immediate therapeutic planning and better patient outcomes in exotic animal practice. A rapid turnaround time also allows for the acquisition of additional samples, if needed, before the patient has left the clinic, should the original sample prove inconclusive, thus reducing the need for multiple hospital visits before diagnosis. Furthermore, static cytology images or WSI are more easily shared and viewed by multiple pathologists simultaneously and digital cytology files can be transmitted almost instantaneously, without risk of loss or damage to slides, which allows for rapid second opinion evaluation. This is particularly advantageous for exotic hematology and cytology samples, for which some pathologists may have limited diagnostic experience, allowing for prompt consultation with those more experienced. Additionally, during the evaluation of the digital sample, pathologists can capture images of multiple areas of interest. These images can then be incorporated into the cytologic report and inserted directly into the patient's record. The clinician then has a specific image to share with owners to both improve the explanation of a diagnosis and allow for the monitoring of response to therapy or progression of the disease.

With the growing adoption of WSI for primary diagnosis, awareness of this technique's limitations is crucial for the best results. Cytologic preparations have an inherent three-dimensionality for cell clusters or piles, making fine focus an essential tool in the cytopathologist's repertoire. However, WSI scanners generally scan slides at a single depth, resulting in the loss of fine focus and a subsequent reduction in the ability to evaluate some important cellular details. This limitation can be partially overcome by Z-stacking, a technique that scans the slide at multiple depths and overlays the scans to allow depth evaluation in the viewing software. Unfortunately, Z-stacking also causes multiple-fold increases in scanning and transfer time, along with file size, which makes its use impractical for most applications, particularly point-of-care services. Differences in color and brightness associated with WSI may also affect the appearance and description of cytologic features.[1] Finally, many commercial WSI scanners do not scan at more than 400X magnification to reduce file size and scan time. While this magnification is suitable for many cytologic samples, observation of very small features such as bacteria or intracellular granules may be more challenging. In the authors' experience, bacteria can be identified on digital cytology, but the diagnostic sensitivity may be lower compared with traditional microscopy. To overcome these limitations and improve diagnostic sensitivity, several digital cytology services offer an additional service (often at no additional charge) to allow for the submission of the glass slide in specific cases to confirm the presence or absence of bacteria or other organisms, if suspected. Despite these limitations, the growing application of WSI in general practice for primary diagnosis suggests that both practitioners and cytopathologists who use this technology deem its diagnostic accuracy acceptable and valuable for clinical application. Validation studies of WSI digital cytology for primary diagnosis in veterinary medicine are limited but also support this notion.[2,3]

Other applications of digital cytology include scanning only portions of a slide selected by the submitter (region of interest or ROI cytology) and the capturing individual static microscope images using a camera or smartphone, both of which can then be submitted for pathologist review. With both techniques, the experience of the individual choosing the fields and capturing the images is critical to ensure high-quality representative images for evaluation. Additionally, capturing several regions or images increases the chance that all important features of the sample are represented.[4] With low numbers of images or an inexperienced capturer, the risk of focusing on nonrepresentative features increases and could lead to a nondiagnostic sample, or worse, a misdiagnosis.[5] For example, capturing images of a reactive mesenchymal population without the inclusion of inflammatory cells could lead to a misdiagnosis of sarcoma, which could have a severe negative impact on patient outcome. Nonetheless, static image digital cytology can be useful in clinical practice and is suited for a quick preliminary diagnosis, and second opinion cytology (eg, what is this weird parasite?).

GETTING THE MOST OUT OF DIGITAL CYTOLOGY

To take digital images of a cytologic sample from a glass slide, capturing the highest quality image possible is essential. Obtaining high-quality, representative images depend on multiple factors including sample acquisition and preparation, microscopy skills, cytology evaluation skills, and image capturing skills. This section is meant to help the reader optimize all these elements to maximize the diagnostic quality of samples when using digital cytology. Additionally, this section will discuss when extra effort is required for certain sample types to complete the analysis beyond the cytologic evaluation.

Sample Acquisition and Preparation

For solid tissues and masses, little adjustment is required to typical sample preparation when using digital cytology instead of standard sample shipment. The following general advice for obtaining good quality cytologic smears is not specific to digital cytology unless specified. For sample acquisition, the technique of fine-needle aspiration biopsy (FNAB) is most commonly used (**Box 1**).

While other techniques have been described for preparing smears, the pull-apart method (sometimes referred to as a slide-over-slide smear) is generally the best for spreading cells, and optimal for digital cytology in which excess three-dimensionality can limit interpretation. A hair dryer without heat can be used instead of air drying the sample. Do not use heat to dry the sample to avoid altering cellular morphology.[6]

The technique of fine-needle biopsy without aspiration is similar to FNAB but can be conducted with or without a syringe attached and without any negative pressure applied. This technique relies on capillary action for the exfoliation of tissue cells into the needle and is generally preferred for highly vascularized masses and tissues to limit blood contamination. Once the sample is in the needle, cells are ejected onto the slide and smeared as for FNAB.

In contrast to solid tissues and masses, body fluid analysis requires extra effort from the practitioner when using digital cytology relative to the ease of simply sending off the sample to a reference laboratory. We estimate the time required between 30 minutes to an hour; therefore, sample shipment should be carefully considered for body fluid analysis. The additional time and equipment required to occur because, in addition to the cytologic evaluation, body fluid analysis generally includes the assessment of the fluid including physical characteristics of the fluid, total protein

---

Box 1
Preparing a fine-needle-aspirate biopsy and pull-apart smear

1. Prepare all supplies - a 20 ga to 25 ga needle attached to a 3 mL to 12 mL syringe with the plunger seal broken and properly labeled glass slides.

2. Insert the needle into the mass and apply light, constant negative aspirational pressure via the syringe plunger.

3. Redirect the needle along multiple planes to sample different areas of the mass, being careful to withdraw the needle most of the way out of the mass before redirecting to avoid tissue laceration.

4. When the sample is visible within the needle's hub, release the suction and withdraw the needle.

5. Disconnect the needle from the syringe and pull back the plunger, then reattach the needle.

6. Place the needle over a glass slide and eject the contents onto the slide.

7. Place a second (spreader) slide over the sample perpendicular to the base slide without forcefully squashing the sample as the weight of the second slide by itself is sufficient.

8. Pull slides apart along the base slide to create 2 viable smears (**Fig. 1**).

9. Allow slides to air dry before staining.

---

concentration, pack cell volume (PCV), and total nucleated cell count, and may also include specific biochemical and microbiological tests. The physical characteristics including color (eg, red, yellow, colorless) and clarity (eg, clear, cloudy, flocculent) should be directly observed and recorded. The fluid's PCV should be evaluated and recorded, if the fluid has redness. The total protein concentration should be assessed by refractometry. A fluid cell count (excluding erythrocytes and thrombocytes) may not be possible in your clinic, but, can be performed similarly to a leukocyte count in peripheral blood by using a reagent to lyse erythrocytes and then counting nucleated

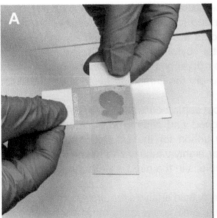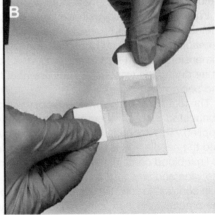

Fig. 1. Pull apart preparation. (*A*) A spreader slide (second glass slide) is gently placed on top of the material collected from the fine-needle aspiration biopsy (FNAB) without downward pressure, to avoid cell lysis. The weight of the spreader slide is typically enough to smear the sample. (*B*) The spreader slide is then pulled forward in one smooth motion across the bottom slide to spread the sample in an even thin layer.

cells in a hemocytometer. In some instances, the total nucleated cell count can be obtained using certain hematology instruments; however, these methods are yet to be validated for use in exotic species. When using digital cytology for the evaluation of a body fluid, as much of this analysis as possible should be performed in house, recorded, and reported to the consulting pathologist to help ensure the most accurate interpretation possible.

In addition to the noncytologic components of fluid analysis, for digital cytology, the submitting hospital should prepare a concentrated smear along with a direct smear. A direct smear is prepared similarly to that of a blood film and is used to estimate the cellularity of the fluid sample. Concentrating techniques are a routine part of fluid analysis as low cellularity is a common feature of nonexudative effusions. The simplest concentrating technique is a thick line preparation (also referred to as a line prep). For this technique, a drop of the fluid is placed on one end of the slide and is smeared relatively slowly with a spreader slide, as preparation for a blood smear. However, instead of following through to the end with the smear, the spreader slide is abruptly lifted midway through the slide to deposit larger cells in a thick line at the point whereby the spreader slide was lifted. Centrifugation of the fluid is an alternative technique to creating a concentrated sample. After centrifugation, the cells are concentrated in a pellet at the bottom of the tube, and the remaining supernatant is discarded. The cell-rich pellet is then resuspended in the remaining fluid and a drop of this fluid is smeared in the same technique as a blood film. Combining the above 2 techniques will further concentrate the sample. Two additional techniques for concentrating samples, cytocentrifugation and cytosedimentation, require specialized equipment and are unavailable in most veterinary practices. These techniques concentrate cells into a small circular area either quickly through centrifugation, or slowly through sedimentation, and are sometimes required for the evaluation of extremely low cellularity fluids including cerebrospinal fluid.

Staining

With routine send-out cytology, unstained slides are generally submitted to allow the laboratory to use their own associated equipment and specialized stains (Modified Giemsa or Wrights stains). For digital cytology, aqueous Romanowsky staining procedures (sold under a variety of trade names including Diff-Quik) are commonly used in most veterinary practices and are acceptable for routine cytologic evaluation. The staining procedure takes minutes and involves sequential dipping through first the cyan (light blue) methanol fixative, then the pink/orange acidic stain or solution II (attracted to basic molecules such as most proteins), and finally the purple basic stain or solution III (attracted to acid molecules such as nucleic acids). The slide can then be rinsed in tap water and air dried. While the manufacturer's recommended protocol for staining is a good place to start, it is generally based on use for blood smears. In the authors' experience, 20 one-second dips in the fixative with 10 one-second dips each in solutions II & III, followed by a water rinse is the optimum protocol for most cytologic samples submitted for digital evaluation. In some instances, overstaining can be corrected when using those "forgiving" aqueous stain kits by dipping the slide in the methanol fixative a few times to reduce both purple and pink stains. In rare situations, should highly cellular samples be under-stained, additional dips in the pink and/or purple stain can be performed. It is also important to dip the slides rather than pool the stain on the glass slide laying on a flat surface as this causes discoloration within various areas of the slide hindering interpretation.

Reliance on in-house staining requires routine care and maintenance of the stain station and its components. Stains must be changed routinely, approximately every

1 to 2 weeks depending on how often they are used. Otherwise, the dyes in the solution will become progressively depleted leading to under-staining of samples and/or build-up of stain precipitate or contamination of stain with microorganisms. Stain precipitates can mimic bacterial organisms hindering the interpretability of the sample and prompting a request for additional sample submission and delaying interpretation. It is highly recommended that a busy practice maintain 2 separate stain stations, one for contaminated sites such as ears, fecals, choanae, cloacae, and the oral cavity, and another for the evaluation of cytologic aspirates to avoid contamination and thus misinterpretation of infectious agents. If excess stain debris or extracellular bacteria that may not have originated from the patient site are noted in the sample, the stain should be changed immediately. Finally, it is critical that unstained samples intended for cytologic evaluation are NEVER placed close to formalin. Formalin fumes permanently alter the affinity of cells to Romanowsky stains and ruin the ability to interpret any cellular aspects of the cytologic sample. All slides submitted for digital cytology should be carefully stored (preferable in a slide box, at a controlled room temperature) until a final report is obtained from the pathologist in case rescans or additional diagnostic testing is requested and to allow for clinician review and education.

Köhler Illumination

Köhler illumination is the first critical microscopy skill to be mastered for obtaining optimal digital cytology static images. Köhler Illumination provides optimum contrast and resolution by focusing and centering the light path from the light source and spreading the light evenly over the field of view to best evaluate fixed and stained specimens. For a microscope to be set up for Köhler illumination, it must have 2 adjustable iris diaphragms: the aperture iris diaphragm at the substage condenser (A) and the field iris diaphragm (B) nearer to the light source (**Fig. 2**).

The aperture iris diaphragm controls the angular aperture of the cone of light from the condenser, while the field iris diaphragm controls the circle of light illuminating the specimen. The substage condenser must be capable of focusing up and down and must be fitted with an aperture iris diaphragm that can be opened and closed by a lever or knob. The light path must be fitted with a condensing lens, a collector lens, and a field iris diaphragm that can also be opened and closed. The procedure to perform proper Köhler illumination is described in **Box 2**.

Choosing Areas of Image Capture

Experience helps to avoid the pitfalls of misleading or nondiagnostic images. However, becoming an expert in cytopathology before taking pictures would obviate the need for consultation. Therefore, here are a few tips to assist in the selection of the best areas to fully represent the cytologic sample.

Low power is your friend

First, grossly evaluate the slide, via the so-called "1X view," to identify the focal blue/purple areas which may represent high cellularity aggregates. These areas are worth looking at immediately when assessing the glass slide. Regardless of what you see grossly, it is still recommended that you scan the entire slide at 100X magnification (10X objective) to observe the best and most cellular areas of the slide. Capturing at least one image at lower power is helpful to represent the overall cellularity of the sample. Once you have a good idea of whereby the best areas of the smear are, you can then increase magnification for further evaluation and capture multiple images with confidence that you're best representing the entirety of the smear.

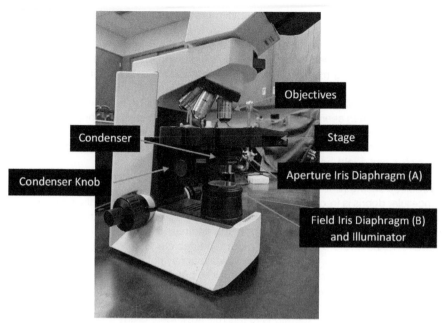

Fig. 2. Major control parts of the microscope. To allow a microscope to be set up for Köhler illumination, it must have two adjustable iris diaphragms: the aperture iris diaphragm at the substage condenser (A) and the field iris diaphragm (B) nearer to the light source.

Recognizing intact cells

Cytologic preparations often have variable numbers of lysed or disrupted cells as an artifact of smear preparation. In lysed cells, the "naked" nucleus is the component most commonly recognized and mistaken for a significant finding. Lysed cell nuclei range in appearance from minimally disrupted, appearing as just a normal free nucleus

---

Box 2
Obtaining Köhler illumination for the sample

1. Turn on the microscope and open entirely both the field diaphragm (see **Fig. 2**A) and the substage condenser diaphragm (see **Fig. 2**B).

2. Place a clean stained slide on the stage and, while on the 10X objective, focus on the sample on the slide.

3. Close the field diaphragm at the base of the microscope about 90% to observe a small polygon-shaped light field.

4. If the polygon is not centered in the field of view, use the cantering or centering screws on the condenser to center it.

5. Using the condenser knob, raise or lower the condenser until the polygons' outline has sharp, crisp edges.

6. Refocus on the specimen on the slide.

7. Once the slide is in focus and the polygon has sharp edges, the condenser is properly adjusted and optimized. Open the field diaphragm until the edges of the polygon disappear from view.

8. Congratulations, you are now using Kohler illumination to achieve the best view and image capture of your sample

without any cytoplasm, to completely obliterated with chromatin strewn across multiple fields resulting in nuclear streaming (**Fig. 3**). Unfortunately, even with minimally disrupted nuclei, cytologic features of the disrupted cell are not reliable for diagnostic purposes; little to no useful information can be gleaned from a disrupted cell. Therefore, when evaluating microscopic fields to capture, make sure cells of interest are intact. Intact cells have both a nucleus and cytoplasm. The sole exception to this rule is the high fragility and lysis that are consistent features of neuroendocrine tumors. These tumors often seem cytologically as free nuclei in a sea of cytoplasm (see **Fig. 8** for an example of this pattern).[7] Thus, if lysed cells are a highly repeatable feature in your sample, particularly despite good sampling and preparation techniques, take a few pictures; it might be important.

If you keep seeing it, it might be important
Noncellular debris is frequently observed in cytologic preparations. This debris may be an artifact of sample preparation and handling or may be representative of the lesion. Although differentiating between debris and findings important to the lesion can be challenging, as a rule of thumb, the more repeatable a feature is in your smear, the more likely it is to be significant. For example, you may not recognize the blue globular material present in an avian coelomic effusion, but when you see a lot of them and conclude they are a significant feature of your sample, you'll be one step closer to identifying them as egg lipoprotein consistent with egg yolk coelomitis. Of course, there are nearly endless exceptions to this rule so, if there is any doubt, take a picture.

Take more pictures
In a recent study evaluating static image digital cytology, better diagnostic accuracy occurred when 5 images were examined compared with 2, especially with an inexperienced cytologist obtaining images.[4] The optimal number of pictures to maximize accuracy is unknown but likely varies widely based on the sample type and quality. Luckily, modern smartphones can store a myriad of pictures. So, if there's ever any doubt, keep shooting!

Capture every cell population
A common mistake in cytologic evaluation is to focus on only the largest (both in size and frequency) cell population to the exclusion of other important features. In some cases, the recognition of a second cell population, for example, an inflammatory

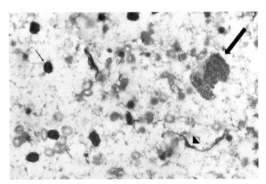

Fig. 3. Ruptured cell nuclei can range in appearance from minimally disrupted, appearing as just a normal free nucleus without any cytoplasm (*thin arrow*) to completely obliterated (*thick arrow*) to strewn nuclear streaming (*arrowhead*) material. All images: quick type Romanowsky stain.

population (eg, heterophils, macrophages, lymphocytes, plasma cells), can dramatically change the overall interpretation. Identification of a second cell population is often complicated by blood contamination (an unavoidable consequence of stabbing a tissue with a needle) which naturally includes low numbers of leukocytes in numbers and proportions that correlate with the amount of erythrocytes present. Thus, a true second population from the tissue would include inflammatory cells in greater frequency than expected from the degree of peripheral blood contamination. Most neoplastic lesions lack a significant second cell population, so if you don't appreciate one, that's fine. Remember to look for more subtle features and don't fixate on the most obvious ones, and this will help you minimize the risk of omitting important cytologic features.

Provide a frame of reference
The size of cytologic structures is important for accurate interpretation of both inflammatory and neoplastic lesions, identification of etiologic agents, and assessing criteria of malignancy, respectively. Unfortunately, accurately assessing the size of cells or objects in static images can be difficult. To address this, all submitted images should include the objective magnification at which they were captured (ie, 10X, 40X, 100X, and so forth). Additionally, capturing a tissue cell population and including a cell of known size, such as erythrocytes and/or heterophils/neutrophils can serve as size markers for the evaluation of cell size and further facilitate interpretation.

Capturing Static Digital Images

Capturing good quality images with a microscope used to require expensive specialized mounted cameras. Today, thanks to incredible advancements in smartphone technology, almost everyone has a high-quality, high-resolution digital camera in their pocket. These days, taking digital cytology images is as easy as lining up a smartphone camera with the microscope ocular and snapping a picture. To obtain the best quality images possible, a few things you should focus on (pun intended) are described in **Box 3**. Taking pictures via a smartphone camera can be frustrating but becomes easier with practice. Alternatively, many products now on the market are designed to mount a smartphone camera in line with the ocular lens to increase stability. These products vary widely in their compatibility and ease of use, so do your research to find the amount that works best for you, your smartphone, and your microscope.

CLINICS CARE POINTS

- Following sample aspiration, the pull-apart technique for film preparation is best at producing a monolayer of cells for digital cytology submission.

- Quick Romanowsky stains are suitable for digital cytology evaluation, but routine cleaning and maintenance of the stain is imperative. Fresh clean stain enhances stain quality and minimizes stain debris and bacterial mimics. If you don't know the last time your stain station was refreshed, have it conducted before staining cytologic samples.

- Your microscope must be clean and well maintained and have proper Köhler illumination performed to obtain the highest diagnostic quality possible, particularly when submitting static images for digital cytologic evaluation.

CLINICAL RELEVANCE

In this section, the advantages of incorporating digital cytology into exotic animal practice are highlighted. These examples are taken from actual cases submitted for

---

Box 3
Tips for static images capture from the microscope ocular via smartphone

- Holding your smartphone horizontally allows for better camera stabilization (**Fig. 4**).
- Stabilize your hand by holding onto the microscope ocular.
- Zoom in with your camera to fill the camera field with your image.
- Tap the screen once before taking the picture to allow the camera to auto-focus.
- Take multiple images

---

the digital evaluation and clinical usefulness of digital submission is emphasized whereby applicable.

Case 1: Blood smear from a 12-year-old woman red-eared slider (*Trachemys scripta elegans*) (**Fig. 5**). Evaluation of the digital blood smear confirmed hematopoietic neoplasia consistent with leukemia that is likely of lymphocytic origin.

Case 2: Aspirate from swelling on the tail of an 11-year-old man intact bearded dragon (*P vitticeps*) (**Fig. 6**). While the sample has a large amount of blood contamination, heterophils are collectively increased throughout the entirety of the sample. Although an underlying neoplastic cell population cannot be excluded, the increased proportion of heterophils suggests an inflammatory lesion and bacterial culture with susceptibility testing is warranted for the evaluation of an infectious agent.

Case 3: Aspirate from a small, raised, round, flesh-colored mass at the right commissure of the beak in between the feathers of a 3-year-old woman Cockatiel (*N. hollandicus*) (**Fig. 7**). The sample is moderately cellular with a large amount of blood and necrotic debris. There are moderate numbers of macrophages including multinucleated giant macrophages with fewer heterophils supporting a predominant granulomatous inflammatory response. Additionally, numerous septate fungal hyphae of various lengths that are approximately 4 to 5 μm in width with clear, mostly parallel-sided cell walls and an occasional ball-shaped terminal end are noted throughout the sample. These structures vary from nonstaining to light to dark blue and occasionally exhibit 45° degree branching angles. These cytomorphologic features are most supportive of *Aspergillus* sp.; however, definitive diagnosis should be based on fungal culture.

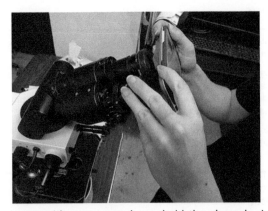

Fig. 4. To take an image with your smartphone, hold the phone horizontally with both hands and then steady the phone by placing your fingers on one eyepiece while holding the camera's lens over the other eyepiece to see the image through the ocular.

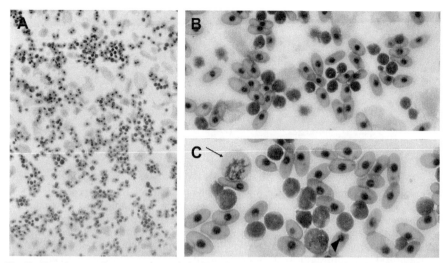

Fig. 5. Blood smear from a red-ear slider (*Trachemys scripta elegans*). (*A*) At lower magnification (10X), a significant leukocytosis is appreciated. (*B*) At 65X, the leukocyte population is predominated by an increased proportion of mononuclear cells most consistent with lymphocytes. (*C*) At higher magnification (100X), increased atypical mitotic figures (*arrow*) are appreciated along with increased lymphocytes and rare mature heterophils (*arrowhead*). All images: quick type Romanowsky stain.

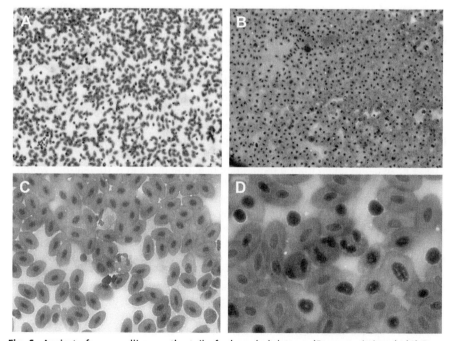

Fig. 6. Aspirate from swelling on the tail of a bearded dragon (*Pogona vitticeps*). (*A*) From lower magnification (10X), the sample is heavily hemodiluted. (*B*) An increased proportion of heterophils is appreciated (22X), especially considering a normal white cell count. (*C*) The sample is predominated by nondegenerate heterophils (50X) to suggest an inflammatory component, (*D*) and heterophils do not display overt phagocytosis (107X). All images: quick type Romanowsky stain.

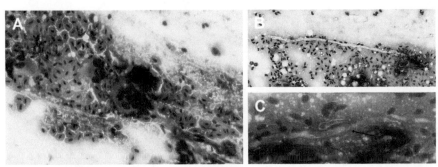

Fig. 7. Aspirate of a small firm mass at the right commissure of the beak in a Cockatiel (*Nymphicus hollandicus*). (*A*) The sample is predominated by granulomatous inflammation including multinucleated giant macrophages (40X). (*B*) Numerous fungal hyphae are noted throughout the sample (40X). (*C*) These septate hyphae vary from nonstaining (*arrow*) to dark blue and have clear, thin, parallel cell walls often with a bulbous terminal end, which are features most consistent with *Aspergillus* sp. (100X), supporting a diagnosis of aspergillosis.

Case 4: Aspirate from a subcutaneous mass on the back of a 2-year-old woman spayed Flemish giant rabbit (*Oryctolagus cuniculus domesticus*) (**Fig. 8**). While the sample contains a moderate amount of blood, it is highly cellular and composed predominantly of lymphocytes. Within the lymphocyte population, there is some occasional heterogeneity with a collective marked expansion of intermediate to large lymphocytes and a discordant increase in plasma cells. These findings are highly concerning for lymphoma with highest consideration given to a T cell-rich B cell lymphoma.

Case 5: Aspirate taken from a ventral, highly mobile, firm, large, round neck mass in a 3-year-old woman intact guinea pig (*C porcellus*) (**Fig. 9**). Clinically, the mass was suspected to be an abscessed lymph node. However, digital cytologic evaluation reveals a population of cells that display a "neuroendocrine" pattern and a lack of an inflammatory infiltrate. Given the cytologic appearance of the sample in conjunction with the location of the mass, a thyroid tumor is considered most likely.

Case 6: Aspirate taken from a hard, immobile, oral mass in a 10-year-old woman intact rabbit (*Oryctolagus cuniculus domesticus*), unspecified breed (**Fig. 10**). Clinical findings included apparent gingival hyperplasia and gingivitis. The digital cytologic evaluation reveals a sample predominated by an epithelial cell population that displays mild atypia with a concurrent mild inflammatory infiltrate and evidence of necrosis. Based on the cytologic findings, highest consideration is given to an epithelial neoplasm, particularly a mixed or complex odontoma. A biopsy sample of the mass was submitted, and histopathologic evaluation confirmed an epithelial tumor likely of odontogenic origin. Unfortunately, the tissue sample taken for biopsy was too small to evaluate tumor margins and thus it could not be determined if the mass was benign or malignant.

Case 7: Aspirate taken from a firm dermal mass on the right lateral chest at the margin of the spines and haired skin in a 4-year-old man intact hedgehog (*A albiventris*) (**Fig. 11**). The sample is markedly cellular consisting of mesenchymal cells displaying marked atypia including marked anisocytosis, anisokaryosis, multinucleation, anisonucleoliosis (variation in nucleolar size), nuclear molding, and bizarre mitotic figures, supporting a diagnosis of a sarcoma.

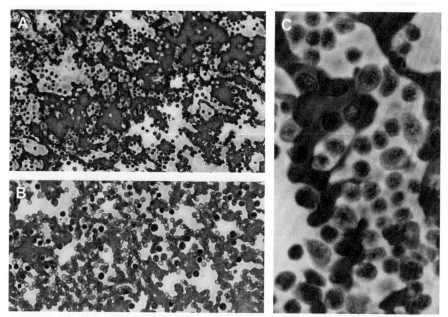

Fig. 8. Aspirate from a subcutaneous mass on the back of a rabbit (*Oryctolagus cuniculus domesticus*). (*A*) The sample is highly cellular although hemodiluted (20X). (*B*) At 43X, it is evident that the sample is comprised predominantly of lymphocytes. (*C*) Collectively, there is a marked expansion of intermediate to large lymphocytes that display atypia, raising concern for a T-cell-rich B-cell lymphoma (108X). All images: quick type Romanowsky stain.

Case 8: Aspirate from the liver in a 7-year-old woman spayed ferret (*M furo*) (**Fig. 12**). The sample is highly cellular and while discernible hepatocytes are not identified, there is a marked proliferation of intermediate to large lymphocytes that range from approximately 9 to 15 µm with small but increased amounts of light blue cytoplasm and a single, round to ovoid nucleus that displays an open chromatin pattern, variably prominent nucleoli, and rare mitotic figures supporting a diagnosis of lymphoma.

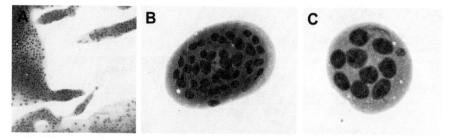

Fig. 9. Aspirate from a ventral neck mass in a guinea pig (*Cavia porcellus*). (*A*) At low magnification (10X), a neuroendocrine pattern, often described as "nuclei floating in a sea of cytoplasm," is appreciated. The sample was not smeared following aspiration, so cells remain in thick droplets. (*B*) Atypical features including anisokaryosis and prominent nucleoli occur within the cell population (60X). (*C*) Due to the thickness of the preparation, cellular features are challenging to evaluate, but variation in nucleolar size, shape, and number is appreciable in cell nuclei at higher magnification (100X). All images: quick type Romanowsky stain.

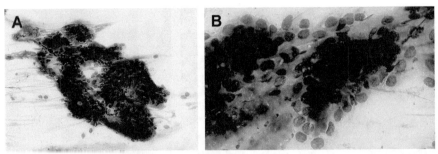

Fig. 10. Aspirate from an oral mass in a rabbit (*Oryctolagus cuniculus domesticus*). (*A*) On digital cytology, the sample is highly cellular, and cells appear of epithelial origin (10X). (*B*) Collectively, cells display some mild atypia raising concern for an epithelial neoplasm (40X), particularly a mixed or complex odontoma. Histopathologic evaluation confirmed a tumor of odontogenic origin, although it was unclear from the biopsy sample if it was benign or malignant. All images: quick type Romanowsky stain. (*Courtesy of* Heska Corporation, Loveland, CO; with permission.)

The patient also had a clinical history of enlarged hepatic lymph nodes, but those were not aspirated.

Case 9: Aspirate of a firm but moveable subcutaneous mass in the right axillary region of a 5 1/2 -year-old woman intact hedgehog (*A albiventris*) (**Fig. 13**). The sample is highly cellular consisting of mostly variably granulated mast cells that exhibit moderate anisocytosis and anisokaryosis along with rare binucleation. Occasional small to intermediate-sized lymphocytes in addition to a moderate proliferation of eosinophils and scattered reactive fibroblasts are also noted, the latter 2 of which are commonly noted as secondary features in mast cell tumors. Based on the location and increased prevalence of lymphocytes, there was a concern that the mass could represent an

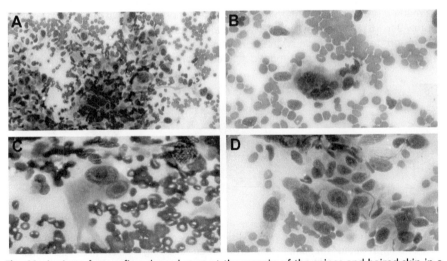

Fig. 11. Aspirate from a firm dermal mass at the margin of the spines and haired skin in a hedgehog (*Atelerix albiventris*). (*A*) At 25X, the sample is highly cellular consisting of markedly atypical mesenchymal cells. (*B*), (*C*), and (*D*) At higher magnification (50X, 40X, and 60X, respectively), cells display marked criteria of malignancy such as multinucleation (*B, D*) and macronucleoli (*C*). All images: quick type Romanowsky stain.

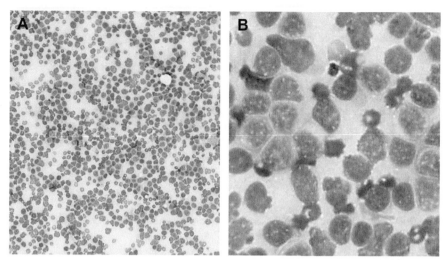

Fig. 12. Liver aspirate from a ferret (*Mustela furo*). (*A*) At 20X, the sample seems highly cellular. (*B*) At 100X, the liver is infiltrated by a marked proliferation of intermediate to large lymphocytes supporting a diagnosis of lymphoma. All images: quick type Romanowsky stain.

axillary lymph node to which the mast cell tumor had metastasized, but histopathologic confirmation was not pursued. It is important to note that in some instances the aqueous-based Romanowsky quick stains will wash out mast cell granules, making them appear colorless to faintly granular. Thus, when using these stains, care must be taken when assessing granularity, which can be an indication of a high-grade tumor, and cells must not be confused for other discrete cell tumors, both of which can influence treatment and prognostic considerations.

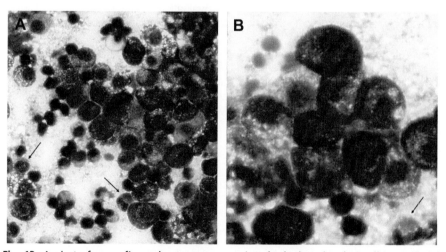

Fig. 13. Aspirate from a firm subcutaneous mass in a hedgehog (*Atelerix albiventris*). (*A*) The sample is comprised of densely packed mast cells which support a diagnosis of mast cell tumor along with increased numbers of eosinophils (*arrows*) (50X). (*B*) At 100X magnification, mast cells are variably granulated and display mild to moderate anisocytosis and anisokaryosis. All images: quick type Romanowsky stain.

SUMMARY

As technology continues to advance, the importance of digital cytology in veterinary medicine, including exotic animal practice, will likely continue to grow. Whether it is used for primary diagnosis, second opinion consultation, or educational purposes, the speed and convenience of transmitting digital images allow for the implementation of cytology in ways that were impossible 20 years ago. Current limitations of digital cytology, specifically with static image cytology, include reliance on microscopy and image capturing the experience of individuals submitting samples. However, with either practice or the addition of whole slide scanners into practice use, veterinarians and their support staff can use digital cytology to enhance their veterinary services and provide high-quality care to all patients.

DISCLOSURE

Dr R. Dulli has no relevant financial or nonfinancial interests to disclose. Dr S.D. Clark is affiliated with and receives a salary from Zoetis, Inc.

REFERENCES

1. Bonsembiante F, Martini V, Bonfanti U, et al. Cytomorphological description and intra-observer agreement in whole slide imaging for canine lymphoma. Vet J 2018;236:96–101.
2. Bonsembiante F, Bonfanti U, Cian F, et al. Diagnostic Validation of a Whole-Slide Imaging Scanner in Cytological Samples: Diagnostic Accuracy and Comparison With Light Microscopy. Vet Pathol 2019;56(3):429–34.
3. Bertram CA, Gurtner C, Dettwiler M, et al. Validation of Digital Microscopy Compared with Light Microscopy for the Diagnosis of Canine Cutaneous Tumors. Vet Pathol 2018;55(4):490–500.
4. Brooker AJ, Krimer PM, Meichner K, et al. Impact of photographer experience and number of images on telecytology accuracy. Vet Clin Pathol 2019;48(3):419–24.
5. Blanchet CJK, Fish EJ, Miller AG, et al. Evaluation of Region of Interest Digital Cytology Compared to Light Microscopy for Veterinary Medicine. Vet Pathol 2019;56(5):725–31.
6. De Witte FG, Hebrard A, Grimes CN, et al. Effects of different drying methods on smears of canine blood and effusion fluid. PeerJ 2020;8:e10092.
7. Raskin RE. Chapter 2 - General categories of cytologic interpretation. In: Raskin RE, Meyer DJ, editors. Canine and feline cytology: a color atlas and interpretation guide. 3rd edition. St. Louis, Missouri: Elsevier; 2016. p. 16–33.

II. Select Avian Diagnostic Analytes

Avian Inflammatory Markers

Raquel M. Walton, VMD, MS, PhD, Diplomate ACVP (Clinical Pathology)[a,*],
Andrea Siegel, DVM, Diplomate ACVP (Clinical Pathology)[b]

KEYWORDS

- Inflammatory biomarkers • Inflammation • Avian • Acute phase proteins
- Acute phase response • Protein electrophoresis

KEY POINTS

- Inflammatory biomarkers can be useful in identifying subclinical disease in avian species and may serve as bioindicators of population and individual health.
- Hematologic indicators of inflammation include the complete blood count, white blood cell count (WBC), heterophil to lymphocyte ratio, WBC morphology, hematocrit, and mean cell volume.
- Iron and iron-associated proteins (unsaturated iron-binding capacity) are implicated in inflammation in birds as in other species.
- Primary acute phase protein biomarkers studied in avian species include ovotransferrin/transferrin, ceruloplasmin, haptoglobin (PIT54), hemopexin, fibrinogen, serum amyloid A, α1-acid glycoprotein, and mannan-binding lectin.

INTRODUCTION

Clinical inflammation was first characterized in the first century AD by the Roman scholar Celsus as comprising 4 principle features: heat (calor), pain (dolor), redness (rubor), and swelling (tumor). Our knowledge of inflammation has progressed to the cellular and even molecular level since this simplest 4-word definition nearly 2 millennia ago. Inflammation is a fundamental response to diverse diseases ranging from trauma and infection to immune-mediated disease and neoplasia. As such, inflammation can be a nonspecific finding but remains a valuable indicator of pathology that can itself lead to disease if left unchecked.[1] This article focuses on inflammatory biomarkers that are currently available and clinically useful in avian species and others under investigation.

Inflammatory biomarkers are identified via evaluation of whole blood and plasma and can be divided into acute and chronic, with varying degrees of specificity and sensitivity. The tests used to elucidate inflammatory disease in avian species

[a] IDEXX Laboratories, Inc., 216 Delmar Street, Philadelphia, PA 19128, USA; [b] IDEXX Laboratories, Inc., 510 E. 62nd Street, New York, NY 10065, USA
* Corresponding author.
E-mail address: Raquel-Walton@idexx.com

Vet Clin Exot Anim 25 (2022) 679–695
https://doi.org/10.1016/j.cvex.2022.05.002

predominantly comprise hematologic and protein evaluation (**Box 1**). Changes in the peripheral blood associated with inflammation reflect responses that have occurred over days to a week or more, whereas changes in select plasma proteins may occur within hours following a systemic inflammatory stimulus. Inflammatory biomarkers are not uniformly affected in inflammatory disease states; thus, evaluation of multiple markers is likely to increase the sensitivity of detection. For example, toxic change in heterophils may be evident in the absence of abnormalities in the leukocyte count; evaluation of both a blood smear and the quantitative data may identify an inflammatory stimulus missed by a complete blood count (CBC) alone. If a CBC fails to identify evidence of inflammation, expanding testing to include protein evaluation may be indicated. Because the CBC and protein evaluation assess different aspects of the inflammatory/immune response, both types of tests are recommended in birds to identify inflammation. Proteins may be evaluated generally via plasma protein electrophoresis and some can be measured individually. Although clinicians are reminded that clinical pathology should confirm a diagnosis rather than create one, the stoic, yet fragile nature of many avian species makes the finding of occult inflammation of critical importance.

THE ACUTE PHASE RESPONSE

The acute phase response (APR) is an evolutionarily conserved innate defense activated at the beginning of tissue injury in vertebrates. The response is mediated by proinflammatory cytokines, such as interleukin-1, interleukin-6, and tumor necrosis factor alpha, which produce a neurophysiological cascade of immunologic recruitment and inflammation, iron sequestration, alterations in lipids, fever, muscle

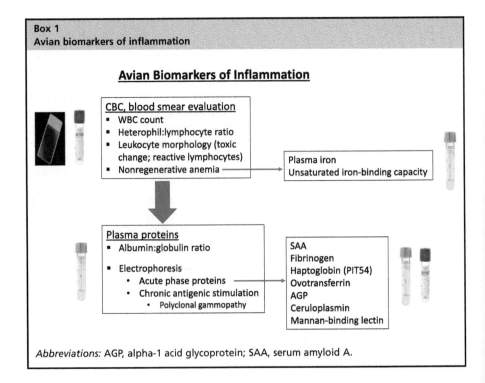

Box 1
Avian biomarkers of inflammation

Avian Biomarkers of Inflammation

CBC, blood smear evaluation
- WBC count
- Heterophil:lymphocyte ratio
- Leukocyte morphology (toxic change; reactive lymphocytes)
- Nonregenerative anemia → Plasma iron / Unsaturated iron-binding capacity

Plasma proteins
- Albumin:globulin ratio
- Electrophoresis
  - Acute phase proteins → SAA / Fibrinogen / Haptoglobin (PIT54) / Ovotransferrin / AGP / Ceruloplasmin / Mannan-binding lectin
  - Chronic antigenic stimulation
    - Polyclonal gammopathy

Abbreviations: AGP, alpha-1 acid glycoprotein; SAA, serum amyloid A.

catabolism, and release of glucocorticoids via modulation of the hypothalamic-pituitary-adrenal axis.[2,3] Proinflammatory cytokines initiate and mediate the APR directly and via proteins referred to as acute phase proteins (APPs). The effects downstream of this cascade are appreciated to varying degree in peripheral blood cell counts, changes in iron and iron-associated proteins, and alterations in APPs, most of which are produced by the liver. As implied by the name, APPs are involved in the first line of defense against microorganisms (innate immunity), yet also play a role in chronic inflammation.[4] Cytokine release and the APR subsequent to tissue injury are conserved mechanisms in vertebrates; however, the molecules involved differ among species.[3,5]

Whereas specific biological functions of APP have been extensively studied, they remain incompletely elucidated. These proteins play an important role in the APR via direct antiviral and antibacterial activity, uptake of extracellular hemoglobin, iron and free radicals, and modulation of the inflammatory response.[6,7] In response to inflammation, APPs rapidly increase or decrease and are accordingly characterized as either positive or negative. In all species, including birds, albumin functions as a negative APP.[5] Positive APPs identified in avian species include serum amyloid A (SAA), haptoglobin (PIT54), hemopexin, fibrinogen, α1-acid glycoprotein, ceruloplasmin, mannan-binding lectin, and transferrin/ovotransferrin.[5,7–9] Transferrin is a negative APP in mammals but acts as a positive APP in chickens (*Gallus domesticus*).[8,10] Positive APPs variably increase in response to inflammation and are grouped as minor ($\leq$2-fold increase), moderate (5- to 10- fold), or major (10- to 1000-fold increase) depending on the magnitude of increase. Major APPs tend to increase markedly within the first 48 hours of the stimulus and decline rapidly due to a short half-life. Moderate and minor proteins tend to increase more slowly and have a more prolonged duration. As expected, chronic inflammatory processes are usually associated with minor and moderate APPs.[7,8] Chickens are the best studied of the avian species, and for them, SAA is characterized as a major APP; PIT54, hemopexin, fibrinogen, α1-acid glycoprotein, ceruloplasmin, mannan-binding lectin, and transferrin/ovotransferrin are characterized as moderate and minor APPs.[7] In birds, most of the published studies on APPs are on chickens, raptors, and parrots, but more species, including pigeons, are being investigated.[7,11–14] In plasma electrophoresis, the APPs migrate within the alpha- and beta-globulin fractions and immunoglobulins within the beta- and gamma-globulins, but there are significant differences between species, even within the same phylogenetic order.

PLASMA PROTEINS: ACUTE PHASE PROTEINS AND IMMUNOGLOBULINS
Protein Electrophoresis

APPs may be measured indirectly through protein electrophoresis or individually for those APPs with available, validated assays. Expert opinion currently holds that the sensitivity of protein electrophoresis for APPs may be higher than that of using individual APP assays in some avian species, as has been reported for penguins.[15] Plasma protein electrophoresis (PPE) provides quantitative data that may have a subjective component as the data are derived from where the technician (or clinical pathologist) chooses to divide the densitometer tracing. Although there are established guidelines for delineating protein fractions to mitigate subjectivity, techniques vary between laboratories. Moreover, interspecies differences in migration distances and fraction concentrations are well documented, which can complicate the choice of fraction separation.[11–13] Different laboratories may also use different electrophoresis analyzers. Because of variation in technique and analyzers, results between laboratories may not be comparable. Thus, veterinary clinicians, biologists, and scientists should only compare patient data generated from the same laboratory.[16] As for any laboratory data, PPE interpretation requires species and method-specific reference intervals, which may not be available. In the absence of an appropriate reference interval, comparison of results from other, apparently unaffected or healthy individuals of the same species, sex and age group, or from a previous sample of the same patient may be necessary for a meaningful interpretation. For best results, samples should be shipped immediately to the reference laboratory and assayed promptly. Significant differences occur in globulin migration after 2 days of refrigeration.[11] Sample conditions such as lipemia and hemolysis affect interpretation, as they may produce peaks in the beta- and gamma-globulin fractions, respectively.[11]

Birds generally have 5 protein fractions that resolve on protein electrophoresis: albumin, alpha1-globulin, alpha2-globulin, beta-globulins, and gamma-globulins (**Fig. 1**). In birds, as in all species evaluated, albumin constitutes the largest protein fraction in health and has a high negative charge and low molecular weight so that it migrates to the anode and conventionally to the left of the densitometer tracing followed by the alpha1-, alpha-2, beta-, and gamma-globulins. Some species, such as the African gray parrot (*Psittacus erithacus*), may have 2 distinct beta-globin fractions, but the fractions are generally combined and reported as a single value by convention.[11] Many avian species have an additional detectable protein that is more negatively charged than albumin that migrates closer to the anode, to the left of albumin, and is therefore referred to as prealbumin (see **Fig. 1**).[17]

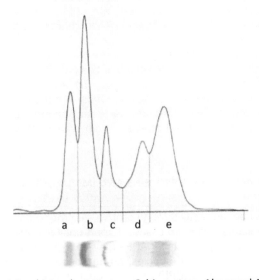

Fig. 1. Plasma protein electrophoretogram, Sebia system. Abnormal PPE from a cockatiel (*Nymphicus hollandicus*) with a history of fungal infection and evidence of macrophagic inflammation on choanal cytology. There is a prominent prealbumin fraction (a) in this species. Gamma-globulins are increased, but the alpha- and beta-globulin concentrations are within reference intervals for this species (using the Sebia methodology). a, prealbumin; b, albumin; c, alpha-globulin; d, beta-globulin; e, gamma-globulins Sebia system methodology.

Prealbumin

Prealbumin binds thyroid hormones and retinol and in humans is termed transthyretin.[17] Similar to albumin, prealbumin likely functions as a negative APP in birds with aspergillosis, and decreases may indicate inflammation.[18] Established species-specific reference intervals are essential in the interpretation of prealbumin, as it varies significantly between avian species. Large prealbumin fractions are reported in cockatiels (*Nymphicus hollandicus*), budgies (*Melopsittacus undulatus*), and Quaker parakeets (*Myiopsitta monachus*), whereas prealbumin may be absent or very minimal in African Gray parrots or chickens (see **Fig. 1**; **Fig. 2**).[11] Prealbumin also varies with the electrophoretic methodology used and is significantly lower in the same individual when measured with the Sebia system compared with the Helena or Beckman systems.[16] Because molting is under the control of thyroid hormones, increases in prealbumin have been reported during molting season, and molt status may affect interpretation.[19,20]

Albumin

Albumin, as a negative APP, can be valuable as a biomarker of inflammation and decreases up to 75% are reported in chickens.[7] In captive flamingos (*Phoenicopterus ruber*) with pododermatitis, decreased albumin concentration was the sole inflammatory biomarker correlated with clinical pododermatitis scores.[12] Similarly, decreases in albumin and total albumin (albumin and prealbumin) were the only abnormal electrophoretic findings in falcons (*Falco peregrinus, Falco rusticolus, Falco cherrug, and Falco pelegrinoides bablyonicus*) with confirmed aspergillosis.[18] Total albumin concentration proved a prognostic indicator in Gentoo penguins (*Pygoscelis papua papua*) with aspergillosis.[21] Albumin does not consistently decrease in all inflammatory conditions as has been noted in some reports of avian mycobacteriosis in which albumin concentrations (determined by electrophoresis) were not different from healthy controls.[14]

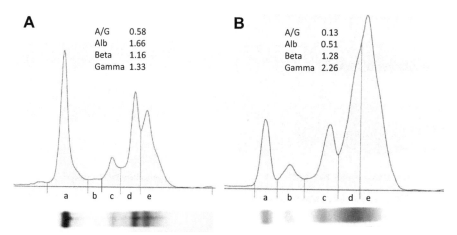

Fig. 2. Plasma protein electrophoretogram, Sebia system. Abnormal PPE from 2 chickens (*Gallus domesticus*) with unknown history. Similar to African gray parrots (*Psittacus erithacus*), prealbumin is barely discernible in chickens. (*A*) There are elevations in the beta- and gamma globulin peaks and albumin is within reference limits; the decreased A/G ratio reflects hyperglobulinemia. (*B*) There is marked hypoalbuminemia and elevations in the beta- and globulins with a corresponding marked decrease in A/G ratio. a, albumin; b, alpha1-globulin; c, alpha2-globlulin; d, beta-globulin; e, gamma-globulins Sebia system methodology.

Alpha-globulins

The alpha-globulin fractions contain APPs such as alpha1-acid glycoprotein (alpha1-globulin fraction) and haptoglobin/PIT54 (alpha2-globulin fraction). The alpha-globulins represent the lowest percentage of electrophoretic plasma proteins in psittacine birds and can be difficult to accurately quantitate due to the low concentration.[11] Alpha-globulin concentrations are higher and better defined in raptors, the domestic chicken, and penguins (*Pygoscelis papua papua* and *Spheniscus demersus*).[13,22] Several raptor species (*Haliaeetus leucocephalus; Parabuteo unicinctus; Strix varia; Tyto alba; Bubo virginianus*) may have an alpha1-globulin peak that arises as a right shoulder off the albumin peak that should not be misinterpreted as bisalbuminemia (Fig. 3).[10] Alpha2-globulins frequently increase in acute inflammation as reported in penguins with aspergillosis. Although changes in protein fractions associated with inflammation are nonspecific, alpha2-globulins were increased in penguins with aspergillosis and not in those with non-*Aspergillus* inflammatory conditions; alpha2-globulins showed aspergillosis specificity of 92% with a positive cutoff of 1.16 g/dL in *S demersus*.[22]

Beta-globulins

Fibrinogen, SAA, transferrin/ovotransferrin, and complement migrate within the beta-globulin fraction, and increases are associated with the APR and inflammation. Because the beta-globulin fraction includes SAA, a major APP in many species, the largest changes in electrophoretic patterns attributed to inflammation often occur in this fraction. However, vitellogenin and beta-lipoproteins associated with egg production also migrate within this fraction. Thus increases in beta-globulins can also be noted with oviparous females.[17,23] Moderate to marked lipemia also produces significant increases in the beta-globin peak.[11] One of the largest differences between serum and plasma electrophoresis samples manifests in the beta-globulin peak due to the absence of fibrinogen in serum. The importance of sample type (plasma vs serum) in the interpretation of electrophoresis data cannot be overemphasized. Increases in beta-globulins occur frequently in aspergillosis, sarcocystosis, and mycobacteriosis, and in noninfectious inflammatory conditions such as arthritis and metastatic carcinoma.[13,14,21,22,24–26]

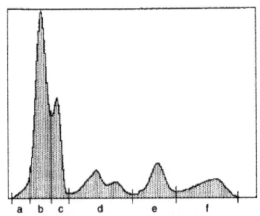

Fig. 3. Plasma protein electrophoretogram, Normal PPE from a clinically healthy bald eagle (*Haliaeetus leucocephalus*). Note the prominent alpha1-globulin shoulder (c) that should not be misinterpreted as bisalbuminemia. a, prealbumin; b, albumin; c, alpha1-globulin; d, alpha2-globulin; e, beta-globulin; f, gamma-globulins *Beckman system methodology*.

Gamma-globulins

Immunoglobulins and degraded complement migrate within this far right region of the electrophoretogram. Increases in immunoglobulins reflect chronic antigenic stimulation, as the humoral response is delayed relative to the innate immune response. Thus, marked increases in gamma-globulin tend to occur with diseases such as chlamydiosis (acute form), sarcocystosis (nonperacute), or mycobacteriosis. Gamma-globulin expression in aspergillosis and chlamydiosis is variable as the humoral response may be suppressed with chronicity.[27,28] The variable gamma-globulin expression in chronic infection has been attributed to immune evasion in chlamydiosis and immune suppression in aspergillosis.[29,30] In psittacine birds, hemolysis produces a spike in the gamma fraction, and interpretation of hemolyzed samples should be avoided.[11]

Albumin:Globulin Ratio

Total protein measurement comprises albumin and globulins. The A/G ratio is conventionally calculated using combined PPE concentrations of prealbumin and albumin as "A" and all globulin fractions as "G," although prealbumin is not universally used in the calculation.[12,17] Albumin concentration measured by the usual bromocresol green methodology in automated analyzers is inaccurate for most avian species and should not be used for calculations.[31] Acute or chronic inflammation may increase total protein due to elevations in globulin fractions. However, because albumin is a negative APP in most species, albumin concentration may decrease with inflammation, bringing the total protein concentration within the reference limits. In contrast, these changes will typically result in a decrease in the albumin/globulin ratio (A:G). Thus, in birds A:G is of greater clinical utility than the total protein concentration as an inflammatory indicator. However, loss of albumin in glomerular and intestinal diseases and decreased production in liver failure and starvation will also result in decreased A:G, thus a decreased A:G is not pathognomonic for inflammation. Similarly, decreased A:G in oviparous females should be interpreted with caution, as there may be a physiologic decrease in A:G due to an estrogen-induced hyperglobulinemia attributable to proteins involved in egg formation.[17] Sample quality affects PPE results, and decreases in A:G may occur due to hemolysis, lipemia, and refrigerated storage for more than 2 days.[11]

As a biomarker of inflammation, A:G may prove useful as a prognostic indicator in some diseases. Optimized test cutoffs determined using receiver operating characteristic curves showed total albumin concentration and A:G were of greatest prognostic use in discriminating survival and death in Gentoo penguins (*Pygoscelis papua papua*) with aspergillosis.[21] Decreased A:G is a common finding across many avian species for many inflammatory diseases.[13,21,22,25,26]

Acute Phase Proteins

With the exception of fibrinogen, testing for most APPs in birds is not readily available at most diagnostic laboratories in the United States, and most evaluations are performed for research studies. Haptoglobin testing is not species-specific, as the assay relies on hemoglobin binding,[32] but many APP assays require species-specific antibodies and need to be validated across species. The most widely commercially available APP tests are SAA, haptoglobin, and fibrinogen, most of which have been validated for chickens. APPs may be sensitive for disease diagnosis, treatment monitoring, and health screening, but lack specificity. Given that the concentration of the acute phase protein is proportional to the severity of the disease process, quantification of acute phase proteins may provide diagnostic and prognostic information. In addition, because the APP response is subject to the nature of the pathologic process, stage, and severity, simultaneous measurement of several APPs may be more useful for the clinical interpretation than determination of a sole APP.[33]

Alpha-1 acid glycoprotein

Kits for alpha1-acid glycoprotein (AGP) are commercially available and validated for chickens, thus AGP is one of the most widely measured APPs in this species. As a binding protein with antiinflammatory activity, AGP may bind lipopolysaccharide (LPS).[4,7] Studies in bacterial and viral infections indicate AGP is a moderate APP that peaks within 24 hours after *Escherichia coli* lipopolysaccharide injections. The magnitude of increase correlates with disease severity in infectious bursal disease infection (IBDV). In the study, a highly virulent strain with extensive and severe lesions increased AGP concentrations 6-fold versus a 3-fold increase for a virulent reference strain without lesions.[7] As a nonspecific marker of inflammation, AGP has also been used to assess overall flock health in chickens.[34]

Fibrinogen

Fibrinogen (FB) is a glycoprotein synthetized by the liver involved in the coagulation cascade and immune response (innate and T-cell mediated).[4] During the APR, FB increases after vascular disruption and provides a substrate for fibrin formation, tissue repair, and migration of inflammatory cells among other actions.[35] A plasma sample is essential when measuring fibrinogen, as serum does not contain the clotting proteins. In chickens FB is a positive APP increasing up to 4-fold in response to *E coli* and other gram-negative bacteria.[7,36] In 77% of birds with confirmed bacterial infection, representing 20 bacterial species, FB increased.[37] However, significant increases in FB were not found in chicks infected with IBDV.[38]

Mannan-binding lectin

Mannan-binding lectin is a minor APP, and peak increases are documented in chickens with various viral infections 3 to 7 days postinfection. With a carbohydrate recognition domain capable of binding bacteria, viruses, fungi, and parasites, mannan-binding lectin decreases can occur with binding despite its role as a positive APP. Decreases in mannan-binding lectin occur in *Pasteurella multocida* infection in chickens and ducks following LPS treatment.[7,39]

Serum amyloid A

SAA, an apolipoprotein of high-density lipoproteins, is a moderate to major APP in most species.[8,40] Physiologic functions of SAA include chemotaxis of neutrophils and monocytes, phagocytic activity enhancement, bacterial toxin inactivation, opsonization, and inhibition of viral infectivity.[41] In addition, SAA plays a role in leukocyte-mediated inflammatory response modulation and in downregulating the inflammatory process.[8,41] Lastly, as an apolipoprotein, SAA modulates cholesterol transport necessary for cell membrane repair and removal of lipid debris from damaged tissue. In chickens, SAA is a major APP peaking 12 to 24 hours postchallenge.[7] Thus, SAA has been used to screen health status in many avian species. Concentrations of SAA were significantly increased in several falcon species (including *Falco rusticola*) with inflammatory disease compared with healthy and noninflammatory disease groups.[42] In another study evaluating diagnosis of premortem aspergillosis, most adults and all the juvenile falcons (*Falco rusticola x Falco cherrug* hybrid) with *Aspergillus* granulomas had significantly increased SAA concentrations.[40] However, greater than 50% of juvenile falcons without granulomas also had increased SAA concentrations, elucidating the need for more APP research in birds.

Several studies have investigated the magnitude of SAA increase with different inflammatory stimuli. In chickens, SAA increased 100- to 1000-fold 12 hours after turpentine and *Staphylococcus aureus* injection using a chicken-specific SAA antibody enzyme-linked immunoassay.[7] In contrast, SAA only increased 1.5- to 2-fold in more recent studies in birds infected with IBDV and infectious bronchitis virus using murine antibody.[38] This wide variation in SAA response may result from the etiologic agent or the methods used. A study comparing APP concentrations in historical and modern broiler breeding lines showed age-related differences. However, a lack of significant changes between broiler breeder lines revealed fluctuations in APP during this period of life. Thus, determination of normal values of APP over the life span of broiler chickens is warranted in order to best use APP diagnostically.[43]

Although the mechanism is not completely understood, persistently increased SSA concentrations along with continued inflammatory stimulus results in AA amyloid formation and pathologic deposition of amyloid in tissues.[4,7] Amyloidosis (AA type) is common in waterfowl, Galliformes, and occasionally reported in turkeys.[7] Concentrations of SAA are significantly increased in brown layer chickens with amyloid arthropathy compared with healthy controls.[41]

Heme-binding proteins: haptoglobin (PIT54)

Heme-binding proteins, including haptoglobin, form complexes with hemoglobin to scavenge free hemoglobin preventing oxidative damage and limiting iron availability for bacterial growth. In addition, haptoglobin also has antiinflammatory properties through prostaglandin synthesis modulation and granulocyte chemotaxis inhibition.[4,7] In chickens, a hemoglobin-binding protein was detected by electrophoresis after turpentine-induced inflammation. Despite a lack of a haptoglobin encoding gene in chickens, a heme-binding protein with a similar function (PIT54) has evolved to replace the function of haptoglobin in this species and other birds including geese, ostriches, and emus.[44,45] Interestingly, haptoglobin along with PIT54 has been conserved in primitive Palaeognathae birds (ostriches and emus) and more recently found in cormorants.[46] Several publications in chickens have studied the PIT54 response to different pathogens, finding a significant increase after infectious bronchitis virus infection, parenteral administration of *Salmonella typhimurium* LPS, and intracrop inoculation of *Salmonella gallinarum*, and following experimental infection with *E coli* alone and combined with *Eimeria tenella*.[36,38,47] Contrarily, no change or decrease of PIT54 occurs with some fungal infections in birds.[48] Thus, evaluating a panel of APP in birds may be more helpful for the diagnosis of aspergillosis, given the variable haptoglobin response depending on the type of infection. *Hemopexin* (HX) is another heme-binding protein and positive APP in chickens that increases rapidly after infection.[7] Increased concentrations ranging from 1.5- to 3-fold in HX have been demonstrated using *E coli* and *S typhimurium* LPS and intracrop administered *S gallinarum*.[47,49]

Ceruloplasmin

Ceruloplasmin is a copper-storage and transport protein with antioxidant activity that functions as a minor to moderate APP in birds; peak concentrations occur within 1 to 5 days of insult, depending on the inflammatory stimulus. Increases in ceruloplasmin occur with bacterial and parasitic (*Eimeria*) infections in chickens and following LPS treatment of ducks.[39] However, ceruloplasmin decreased in IBDV infection. It is uncertain whether the negative APP response for ceruloplasmin is unique to IBDV infection or occurs in all viral infections.[7,38]

Transferrin/ovotransferrin

Transferrin and ovotransferrin (conalbumin) are identical iron-binding proteins with some glycosylation differences that act as an APP in chickens.[9,10] Ovotransferrin has direct antimicrobial effects via permeation of the outer membrane of *E coli*, and documented immunomodulatory effects include induction of the respiratory burst activity and degranulation of heterophils and macrophages.[7] In contrast to mammals in which transferrin is downregulated in the APR, ovotransferrin is a positive APP in infectious and noninfectious inflammatory conditions in birds.[8–10]

Unsaturated iron-binding capacity

Unsaturated iron binding capacity (UIBC) measures the portion of transferrin that has yet to be saturated with iron and reflects reserve capacity of transferrin. Total iron-binding capacity (TIBC) is the sum of UIBC and iron and represents transferrin levels. During the APR, serum transferrin, as an iron-binding protein, sequesters iron, rendering it unavailable for bacterial growth.[50] Because transferrin is a positive APP in avian species, UIBC and TIBC are expected to increase during the APR in birds. However, TIBC and UIBC were similar in sick and healthy red-tailed hawks (*Buteo jamaicensis*), elucidating the differences in APP response among different species.[51] In addition, the type of inflammation and the timing of sampling during the APR could have effects on UIBC. For instance, fuel oil exposure in mallard ducks caused decreased plasma UIBC and plasma iron compared with the control group, whereas ducks treated with bacterial LPS had increased UIBC.[39] In quail (*Coturnix japonica*) with aspergillosis, UIBC and TIBC increased and positively correlated with disease severity CFU numbers of Aspergillus cultured.[48]

Plasma iron

Plasma iron is a negative acute phase reactant in both mammals and birds. Decreased iron during the APR occurs as a result of hepatic sequestration, decreased intestinal absorption, and increased iron binding.[50] Decreased plasma iron occurs in poultry with viral and bacterial diseases as well as in sick and injured hawks (*B jamaicensis*) compared with normal populations.[51] In contrast, increased iron was found in a study evaluating inflammatory markers in Japanese quail (*C japonica*) experimentally infected with *Aspergillus fumigatus*. Aspergillus-induced impaired cellular iron uptake leading to increased iron levels in plasma has been proposed as an explanation for this unexpected finding.[48]

HEMATOLOGIC INDICATORS OF INFLAMMATION
The Leukon

Of the current available tests that may identify inflammation, the CBC is the most common diagnostic test ordered. Although both the erythron and leukon may serve as indicators of inflammation, some quantitative and qualitative leukocyte data are more specific than red blood cell data (**Boxes 2** and **3**). Although some older studies suggest that up to 30% of birds may have inflammation not evident on evaluation of the CBC, some recent studies have shown that clinically ill psittacine birds were more likely to have abnormal quantitative CBC results than PPE.[52] However, as species-specific PPE reference intervals are generated and PPE becomes more standardized, identification of abnormal results will improve.

The most specific leukon changes indicating inflammation are heterophilia with a left-shift, eosinophilia, and monocytosis, which are compatible with acute inflammation, eosinophilic inflammation, and macrophagic inflammation, respectively. Although inflammation is nonspecific, patterns of leukocytosis may suggest specific

---

Box 2
Inflammatory indicators in the leukon

Heterophilia with left-shifting: acute inflammation

Heteropenia ± left-shifting: severe, acute inflammation (rule out other causes of heteropenia)

Lymphocytosis: chronic antigenic stimulation (rule out other causes of lymphocytosis)

Eosinophilia: eosinophilic inflammation

Monocytosis: inflammation with a macrophagic component (acute or chronic inflammation)

Inverted heterophil:lymphocyte ratio (in lymphocyte-predominant species): acute inflammation (rule out stress)

Toxic change: severe inflammation

Reactive lymphocytes: chronic antigenic stimulation

---

diseases. Heterophilia, eosinophilia, and monocytosis with lymphopenia is supportive of a diagnosis of mycobacteriosis in raptors (*Haliaeetus leucocephalus*; *Buteo jamaicensis; Buteo lineatus; B virginianus*) with appropriate clinical signs and/or radiographic features of mycobacterial infection.[25,53]

Similarly, morphologic changes in leukocytes such as toxic change in heterophils is specific for severe inflammation, and reactive change in lymphocytes indicates antigenic stimulation (**Figs. 4–7**). Lymphocytosis, inverted heterophil:lymphocyte ratios (H:L), and heteropenia may also be indicators of inflammation but are less specific, as they may have noninflammatory causes. In avian species such as Amazon parrots (*Amazona* spp.) and some passerines (canaries, *Serinus canaria forma domestica*) with lymphocytes as the predominant leukocyte, inversion of the H:L in absence of absolute heterophilia can indicate acute, heterophilic inflammation. However, lymphopenia due to noninflammatory processes such as the corticosteroid response, certain viral infections, or damage to the bursa can also result in inversion of the H:L.[27]

Although the leukon can be a valuable indicator of inflammation, it can take days to weeks for some changes to manifest. The bone marrow response to proinflammatory cytokines resulting in leukocytosis is not immediate. Studies in dogs, likely applicable to many species, demonstrate that leukocytosis due to a systemic inflammatory stimulus occurs up to 4 to 7 days following the initial stimulus.[54] Moreover, localized inflammation, or compartmentalized inflammation such as that within the gut or brain, may not result in changes in leukocyte concentrations.

The Erythron

The presence of nonregenerative anemia may indicate chronic inflammation; however, nonregenerative anemia is not specific for inflammation and noninflammatory causes must be considered. Nonregenerative anemia due to inflammatory disease (previously known as "anemia of chronic disease") is common in many species, including birds.

Box 3
Inflammatory indicators in the erythron

Nonregenerative anemia: chronic inflammation (rule out other causes of nonregenerative anemia)

Microcytosis, hypochromia: chronic inflammation (rule out iron deficiency anemia)

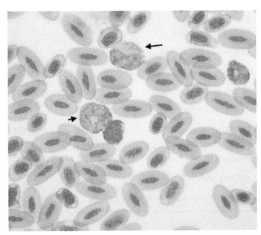

Fig. 4. Blood smear (100x), Wright-Giemsa stain, red-tailed hawk (*Buteo jamaicensis*). Toxic change in heterophils characterized by loss of secondary granules (*long arrow*), increased cytoplasmic basophilia, and presence of primary granules (*short arrow*).

The pathogenesis of inflammatory anemia stems from a relative iron deficiency due to the effects of proinflammatory cytokines on iron metabolism as well as direct inhibition of erythropoiesis. Inflammatory cytokines cause upregulation of the APP hepcidin in the liver, which causes decreased intestinal iron absorption. Inflammatory cytokines also stimulate increased transferrin iron binding and increased production of ferritin (the storage form of iron) effectively sequestering iron.[50] In addition to direct inhibition of erythropoiesis by inflammatory cytokines, this reduced iron availability also suppresses erythropoiesis and contributes to anemia. The effects of these changes appear after a week or more rather than hours to days in most species but have not been specifically investigated for avian species.

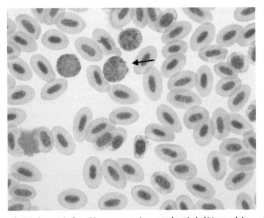

Fig. 5. Blood smear (100x), Wright-Giemsa stain, cockatiel (*Nymphicus hollandicus*). Toxic change in heterophils characterized by presence of purple primary granules (*arrow*) with loss of secondary granules. Note the reactive lymphocyte with deeply basophilic cytoplasm above the toxic heterophil.

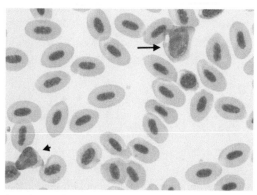

Fig. 6. Blood smear (100x), Wright-Giemsa stain, cockatiel (*Nymphicus hollandicus*). Reactive lymphocyte (*long arrow*) characterized by intermediate size and deeply basophilic cytoplasm. A normal lymphocyte (*short arrow*) is present in the lower left corner.

Because of decreased iron availability due to iron sequestration, anemia of inflammatory disease may be microcytic and hypochromic, although it is typically normocytic and normochromic. If absolute iron deficiency is ruled out, microcytic/hypochromic or normocytic/normochromic nonregenerative anemia may indicate chronic inflammation in birds.[55] Microcytosis and hypochromia are typically assessed on blood film evaluation (**Fig. 8**), as mean cell volume and mean cell hemoglobin concentration are not usually reported in birds. Microcytic anemia is characterized by greater than 5% microcytic erythrocytes.[56]

DISCLOSURE

R.M. Walton and A. Siegel declare they have nothing to disclose.

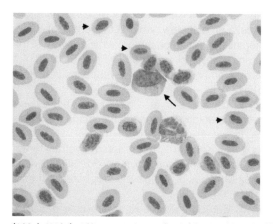

Fig. 7. Blood smear (100x), Wright-Giemsa stain, cockatiel (*Nymphicus hollandicus*). Reactive lymphocyte (*long arrow*) with deeply basophilic cytoplasm enhancing the paranuclear Golgi clearing. The bird was anemic (23%) with increased numbers of microcytic RBCs (*arrowheads*). RBC, red blood cell.

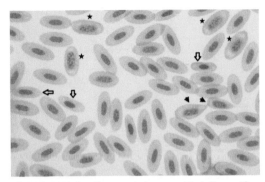

Fig. 8. Blood smear (100x), Wright-Giemsa stain, songbird (Passeriformes, species not reported). Anemia with hypochromic (*stars*) and microcytic (*open arrows*) erythrocytes and keratocytes (*arrowheads*). Hypochromia and microcytosis may be present with anemia of inflammatory disease and with iron deficiency anemia. Keratocytes are often associated with fragmentation injury due to microvascular disease (eg, thrombosis) or increased erythrocyte fragility due to iron deficiency.

REFERENCES

1. Liu CH, Abrams ND, Carrick DM, et al. Biomarkers of chronic inflammation in disease development and prevention: challenges and opportunities. Nat Immunol 2017;18(11):1175–80.
2. Owen-Ashley NT, Wingfield JC. Acute phase responses of passerine birds: characterization and seasonal variation. J Ornithol 2007;148(Suppl 2):583–91.
3. Cray C. Acute Phase Proteins in Animals. In: Michael CP, editor. Animal models of molecular pathology. Vol 105. (Progress in molecular biology and translational science). St Louis (MO): Academic Press; 2012. p. 113–50.
4. Cerón JJ, Eckersall PD, Martínez-Subiela S. Acute phase proteins in dogs and cats: current knowledge and future perspectives. Vet Clin Path 2005;34(2):85–99.
5. Romo MR, Pérez-Martínez D, Ferrer CC. Innate immunity in vertebrates: an overview. Immunology 2016;148(2):125–39.
6. Murata H, Shimada N, Yoshioka M. Current research on acute phase proteins in veterinary diagnosis: an overview. Vet J 2004;168(1):28–40.
7. O'Reilly EL, Eckersall PD. Acute phase proteins: a review of their function, behaviour and measurement in chickens. World's Poult Sci J 2014;70(1):27–44.
8. Cray C, Zaias J, Altman NH. Acute phase response in animals: a review. Comp Med 2009;59(6):517–26.
9. Xie H, Newberry L, Clark FD, et al. Changes in serum ovotransferrin levels in chickens with experimentally induced inflammation and diseases. Avian Dis 2002;46(1):122–31.
10. Rath NC, Anthony NB, Kannan L, et al. Serum ovotransferrin as a biomarker of inflammatory diseases in chickens. Poult Sci 2009;88(10):2069–74.
11. Cray C, Rodriguez M, Zaias J. Protein electrophoresis of psittacine plasma. Vet Clin Path 2007;36(1):64–72.
12. Delk KW, Wack RF, Burgdorf-Moisuk A, et al. Acute phase protein and electrophoresis protein fraction values for captive american flamingos (*Phoenicopterus ruber*). J Zoo Wildl Med 2015;46(4):929–33.
13. Tatum LM, Zaias J, Mealey BK, et al. Protein electrophoresis as a diagnostic and prognostic tool in raptor medicine. J Zoo Wildl Med 2000;31(4):497–502.

14. Mayahi M, Khajeh G, Mosavari N, et al. Serum protein profiles in domestic pigeons naturally infected with *Mycobacterium avium* subsp. avium. Vet Clin Path 2013;42(2):212–5.
15. Cray C. Biomarkers of inflammation in exotic pets. J Exot Pet Med 2013;22(3): 245–50.
16. Cray C, King E, Rodriguez M, et al. Differences in protein fractions of avian plasma among three commercial electrophoresis systems. J Avian Med Surg 2011;25(2):102–10.
17. Lumeij JT. Avian Clinical Biochemistry. In: Kaneko JJ, Harvey JW, Bruss ML, editors. Clinical biochemistry of domestic animals. 6th edition. St Louis (MO): Academic Press; 2008. p. 839–72.
18. Kummrow M, Silvanose C, Somma AD, et al. Serum protein electrophoresis by using high-resolution agarose gel in clinically healthy and *aspergillus* species-infected falcons. J Avian Med Surg 2012;26(4):213–20.
19. Cookson EJ, Hall MR, Glover J. The transport of plasma thyroxine in White storks (*Ciconia ciconia*) and the association of high levels of plasma transthyretin (thyroxine-binding prealbumin) with moult. J Endocrinol 1988;117(1):75–84.
20. Spagnolo V, Crippa V, Marzia A, et al. Reference intervals for hematologic and biochemical constituents and protein electrophoretic fractions in captive common buzzards (*Buteo buteo*). Vet Clin Path 2006;35(1):82–7.
21. Naylor AD, Girling SJ, Brown D, et al. Plasma protein electrophoresis as a prognostic indicator in Aspergillus species-infected Gentoo penguins (*Pygoscelis papua papua*). Vet Clin Path 2017;46(4):605–14.
22. Desoubeaux G, Rodriguez M, Bronson E, et al. Application of 3-hydroxybutyrate measurement and plasma protein electrophoresis in the diagnosis of aspergillosis in African penguins (*Spheniscus demersus*). J Zoo Wildl Med 2018;49(3): 696–703.
23. Harr KE. Clinical chemistry of companion avian species: a review. Vet Clin Pathol 2002;31(3):140–51.
24. Cray C, Watson T, Rodriguez M, et al. Application of galactomannan analysis and protein electrophoresis in the diagnosis of aspergillosis in avian species. J Zoo Wildl Med 2009;40(1):64–70.
25. Tell LA, Ferrell ST, Gibbons PM. Avian mycobacteriosis in free-living raptors in california: 6 Cases (19972001). J Avian Med Surg 2004;18(1):30–40.
26. Cray C, Zielezienski-Roberts K, Bonda M, et al. Serologic diagnosis of sarcocystosis in psittacine birds: 16 Cases. J Avian Med Surg 2005;19(3):208–15.
27. Melillo A. Applications of serum protein electrophoresis in exotic pet medicine. Vet Clin North Am Exot Anim Pract 2013;16(1):211–25.
28. Werner LL, Reavill DR. The diagnostic utility of serum protein electrophoresis. Vet Clin North Am Exot Anim Pract 1999;2(3):651–62.
29. Cramer RA, Rivera A, Hohl TM. Immune responses against *Aspergillus fumigatus*: what have we learned? Curr Opin Infect Dis 2011;24(4):315–22.
30. Radomski N, Einenkel R, Müller A, et al. Chlamydia–host cell interaction not only from a bird's eye view: some lessons from *Chlamydia psittaci*. Febs Lett 2016; 590(21):3920–40.
31. Cray C, Wack A, Arheart KL. Invalid measurement of plasma albumin using bromocresol green methodology in penguins (*Spheniscus* species). J Avian Med Surg 2011;25(1):14–22.
32. Eckersall PD, Duthie S, Safi S, et al. An automated biochemical assay for haptoglobin: Prevention of interference from albumin. Comp Haematol Int 1999;9(3): 117–24.

33. Eckersall PD, Bell R. Acute phase proteins: Biomarkers of infection and inflammation in veterinary medicine. Vet J 2010;185(1):23–7.

34. Tuyttens F, Heyndrickx M, Boeck MD, et al. Broiler chicken health, welfare and fluctuating asymmetry in organic versus conventional production systems. Livest Sci 2008;113(2–3):123–32.

35. Davalos D, Akassoglou K. Fibrinogen as a key regulator of inflammation in disease. Semin Immunopathol 2012;34(1):43–62.

36. Georgieva TM, Koinarski V, Urumova V, et al. Effects of *Escherichia coli* infection and *Eimeria tenella* invasion on blood concentrations of some positive acute phase proteins (haptoglobin (PIT 54), fibrinogen and ceruloplasmin) in chickens. Revue De Medecine Veterinaire 2010;161:84–9.

37. Hawkey C, Hart MG. An analysis of the incidence of hyperfibrinogenaemia in birds with bacterial infections. Avian Pathol 1988;17(2):427–32.

38. Nazifi S, Dadras H, Hoseinian SA, et al. Measuring acute phase proteins (haptoglobin, ceruloplasmin, serum amyloid A, and fibrinogen) in healthy and infectious bursal disease virus-infected chicks. Comp Clin Pathol 2010;19(3):283–6.

39. Lee KA, Tell LA, Mohr FC. Inflammatory markers following acute fuel oil exposure or bacterial lipopolysaccharide in mallard ducks (*Anas platyrhynchos*). Avian Dis 2012;56(4):704–10.

40. Fischer D, Waeyenberghe LV, Cray C, et al. Comparison of diagnostic tools for the detection of aspergillosis in blood samples of experimentally infected falcons. Avian Dis 2014;58(4):587–98.

41. Salama SA, Gouwy M, Damme JV, et al. The turning away of serum amyloid A biological activities and receptor usage. Immunology 2021;163(2):115–27.

42. Caliendo V, McKinney P, Bailey T, et al. Serum amyloid a as an indicator of health status in falcons. J Avian Med Surg 2013;27(2):83–9.

43. O'Reilly EL, Bailey RA, Eckersall PD. A comparative study of acute-phase protein concentrations in historical and modern broiler breeding lines. Poult Sci 2018; 97(11):3847–53.

44. Wicher KB, Fries E. Haptoglobin, a hemoglobin-binding plasma protein, is present in bony fish and mammals but not in frog and chicken. Proc Natl Acad Sci U S A 2006;103(11):4168–73.

45. Iwasaki K, Morimatsu M, Inanami O, et al. Isolation, characterization, and cdna cloning of chicken turpentine-induced protein, a new member of the scavenger receptor cysteine-rich (SRCR) family of proteins. J Biol Chem 2001;276(12): 9400–5.

46. Wicher KB, Fries E. Evolutionary aspects of hemoglobin scavengers. Antioxid Redox Sign 2010;12(2):249–59.

47. Garcia K, Berchieri-Júnior A, Santana A, et al. Experimental infection of commercial layers using a Salmonella enterica serovar Gallinarum strain: Leukogram and serum acute-phase protein concentrations. Braz J Poult Sci 2009;11(4):263–70.

48. Goetting V, Lee KA, Woods L, et al. Inflammatory marker profiles in an avian experimental model of aspergillosis. Med Mycol 2013;51(7):696–703.

49. Adler KL, Peng PH, Peng RK, et al. The kinetics of hemopexin and a1-acid glycoprotein levels induced by injection of inflammatory agents in chickens. Avian Dis 2001;45(2):289.

50. Weiss G, Goodnough LT. Anemia of chronic disease. N Engl J Med 2005;352(10): 1011–23.

51. Lee KA, Goetting VS, Tell LA. Inflammatory markers associated with trauma and infection in red-tailed hawks (*Buteo jamaicensis*) in the USA. J Wildl Dis 2015; 51(4):860–7.

52. Briscoe JA, Rosenthal KL, Shofer FS. Selected complete blood cell count and plasma protein electrophoresis parameters in pet psittacine birds evaluated for illness. J Avian Med Surg 2010;24(2):131–7.
53. Heatley JJ, Mitchell MM, Roy A, et al. Disseminated mycobacteriosis in a bald eagle (*Haliaeetus leucocephalus*). J Avian Med Surg 2007;21(3):201–9.
54. Yamashita K, Fujinaga T, Miyamoto T, et al. Canine acute phase response : Relationship between serum cytokine activity and acute phase protein in dogs. J Vet Med Sci 1994;56(3):487–92.
55. Campbell TW. Peripheral blood of birds. In: Campbell TW, editor. Exotic animal hematology and cytology. Philadelphia: Wiley Blackwell; 2015. p. 37–66.
56. Malvat Z, Lynch SA, Bennison A, et al. Evidence of links between haematological condition and foraging behaviour in northern gannets (*Morus bassanus*). Roy Soc Open Sci 2020;7(5):192164.

Blood Lipid Diagnostics in Psittacine Birds

Hugues Beaufrère, DVM, PhD, Dipl. ACZM, Dipl. ABVP (Avian), Dipl. ECZM (Avian)

KEYWORDS

• Cholesterol • Triglycerides • Lipidomics • Lipoproteins • Parrots • Lipidology

KEY POINTS

- Lipid disorders such as atherosclerosis, hepatic lipidosis, obesity, and xanthomatosis are common in captive psittacine birds and are associated with a variety of dyslipidemias.
- Lipidologic diagnostic assays include routine tests such as total cholesterol, total triglycerides, lipoprotein testing using different methods, and clinical lipidomics.
- Lipoprotein abnormalities have been insufficiently described in psittacine birds and lipoprotein panels should be performed more commonly in sick birds.
- As low-density lipoprotein cholesterol measurements are generally not reliable, a lipid panel including cholesterol, triglycerides, high-density lipoprotein (HDL) cholesterol, and non-HDL cholesterol is recommended.
- The high numbers of lipid species present in parrot plasma can be measured comprehensively by lipidomics paving the way for discovering new biomarkers for lipid disorders in parrots.

INTRODUCTION

Lipids are central in metabolism and have many important functions such as structural in cell membranes and tissues, as energy source and storage, as mediators of inflammation and cell signaling, and thermal insulation. The diversity of biological lipid is staggering with more than 25,000 different lipids identified in biological systems (lipidmaps.org, accessed June 2022). In terms of diagnostic tests and monitoring tools for fatty disorders, blood lipid analysis is key. Most lipid-related disorders are either directly associated with dyslipidemic changes or secondarily through metabolic dysfunction and alterations of broad metabolic pathways. For these reasons, lipids are frequently used as diagnostic and prognostic biomarkers in medicine and to explore the pathogenesis of many diseases.

Lipid disorders reported in birds include common diseases such as atherosclerotic diseases, hepatic lipidosis, fatty tumors (lipoma, liposarcoma), xanthomatous

Department of Veterinary Epidemiology and Medicine, School of Veterinary Medicine, University of California-Davis, One Shields Avenue, Davis, CA 95616, USA
E-mail address: hbeaufrere@ucdavis.edu

Vet Clin Exot Anim 25 (2022) 697–712
https://doi.org/10.1016/j.cvex.2022.05.003
1094-9194/22/© 2022 Elsevier Inc. All rights reserved.

masses, and obesity and less common disorders such as corneal lipidosis, renal lipidosis, systemic xanthogranulomatosis, lysosomal storage disease, endogenous lipid pneumonia, adiponecrosis, and many others. Blood lipid abnormalities are associated with a wide range of diseases not directly involved with lipid accumulation or fatty tissues such as reproductive disorders in female birds (egg yolk peritonitis, yolk emboli, dysregulated vitellogenesis) and potentially other disorders such as acute pancreatic necrosis, hepatic diseases, nephrotic syndrome, and endocrine disorders.

To understand the pathophysiology and management of lipid-related disorders in birds, working knowledge of lipid biochemistry and lipoprotein metabolism is needed. For this reason, this review will review plasma lipid biochemistry and metabolism and then focus on current diagnostic tests in birds and their interpretation as well as potential new avenues for novel lipid biomarkers.

PLASMA LIPID DIVERSITY

Lipids represent approximately 40% of plasma biomolecules in psittacine plasma (on a molar basis) with, for comparison, carbohydrates and proteins representing another 30% each. Many different types of lipids occur and have many functions.

Some lipids of high concentration (measured in mmol/L or μmol/L) in the plasma are part of the macrolipidome and typically include constitutive (such as cholesterol, cholesteryl esters [CEs], glycerophospholipids, and sphingolipids) or storage lipids (such as triacylglycerols [TAGs]). Their plasma concentrations are affected by a variety of metabolic disorders and are also precursors of many bioactive and signaling lipid molecules. Notable lipid precursors include arachidonic acid and cholesterol. Many lipids have fatty acyl chains, which are typically abbreviated by their short-hand formula with first the number of carbon atoms followed by the number of carbon-carbon double bonds (eg, stearic acid is FA 18:0 and cholesteryl stearate is CE (18:0)).

Numerous other lipids are bioactive molecules that act as mediators in various functions and are in very low concentration (measured in nmol/L or pmol/L, so a thousandth or millionth less concentrated than other lipids). These bioactive lipids are part of the microlipidome or the mediator lipidome. Important lipid mediators include inflammatory mediators (prostaglandins, leukotrienes, eicosanoids), prothrombotic molecules (thromboxanes), vitamins (A, D, E), pain mediators (endocannabinoids: anandamide and 2-AG), and steroid hormones (corticosterone, estradiol). Most lipid species of the macrolipidome are transported within lipoproteins, but free fatty acids are bound to albumin and lipid mediators are typically free in the plasma, bound to albumin, or transported by specific proteins.

A comprehensive plasma lipidome of Quaker parrots (*Myiopsitta monachus*)[1] reported lipids found in the plasma from five groups of lipids: sterol lipids, fatty acyls, glycerolipids, glycerophospholipids (also called phospholipids), and sphingolipids. **Fig. 1** gives an overview of the relative abundance of respective lipid classes and species in the plasma of parrots. **Table 1** summarizes the basic classification of plasma lipids with their function and examples of common plasma lipid species. The metabolism of common plasma lipids is also discussed below:

-Sterol lipids include free cholesterol, CEs, bile acids, and steroid hormones and make up approximately two-third of all plasma lipids. Cholesterol and CEs are the predominant lipid species in parrot plasma (approximately 50%–60% on a molar basis). Approximately one-third of total cholesterol is nonesterified (free), whereas two-third is esterified to various acyl chains, the most abundant by far being linoleic acid (18:2). Linoleic acid constitutes more than 70% of all CEs. Cholesterol is synthesized in the liver through a process involving the key enzyme HMG-CoA reductase, the target of

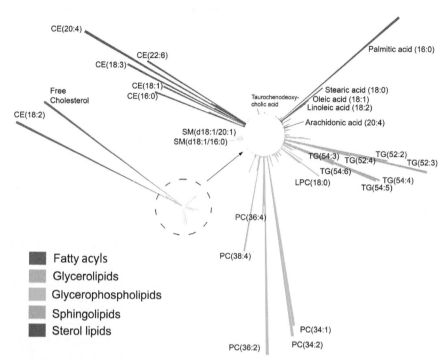

Fig. 1. Circular bar plot of mean concentrations of lipid species in five lipid categories measured by targeted lipidomics in Quaker parrots (*Myiopsitta monachus*). The dashed circle and arrow indicate a magnified portion of the left bar plot. Each lipid category is color coded and lipid species abbreviations follow the LIPIDMAPS nomenclature. Although lipid species were quantitively measured, comparisons of lipid categories should be made with caution. (*Reproduced from* Beaufrère H, Gardhouse SM, Wood RD, Stark KD. The plasma lipidome of the Quaker parrot (*Myiopsitta monachus*). PLoS ONE. 2020;15(12 December); with permission.)

statins. Exogenous sources of cholesterol are few in parrots as they are mainly frugivorous or granivorous animals and cholesterol does not occur in plants. Cholesterol is used for cellular membranes and as a precursor for other steroids. Bile acids are cholesterol derivatives produced by the liver that assist in the emulsion and digestion of fat in the digestive system. The most common bile acid in parrot plasma is taurochenodeoxycholic acid, which constitutes approximately 70% of all plasmatic bile acids. Bile acids are used as markers of liver health. Steroid hormones are synthesized from cholesterol and include hormones such as glucocorticoids (the main one being corticosterone in birds), mineralocorticoids (aldosterone), and sex hormones (produced by the gonads and adrenal glands) such as androgens (testosterone, androstenedione), estrogens (estradiol) and progestins (progesterone). They can affect the overall lipid metabolism and regulate vitellogenesis in hens. Estradiol is also linked to hepatic lipidosis in chickens.[2,3]

Fatty acyls include simple lipids such as free fatty acids and fatty acid derivatives and constitute approximately 5% of plasma lipids. They typically have an even carbon chain in vertebrates. Fatty acids can be saturated or unsaturated (presence of double bonds in the hydrocarbon chain). The location of the double bond is important in terms

Table 1
Important lipid groups of parrot plasma[1]

Lipid Class	Subclass	Common Lipid Species in Parrot Plasma	Function
Sterol lipids	Cholesterol	Cholesterol	Cellular membranes
	Cholesteryl ester	CE(18:2)	Cellular membranes
	Bile acids	Taurochenodeoxycholic acid	Lipid digestion
	Steroid hormones	Corticosterone	Stress, sexual hormones, and osmoregulation
Fatty acyls	Free fatty acids	Palmitic acid (16:0)	Energy source
		Stearic acid (18:0)	Eicosanoid precursors
		Oleic acid (18:1)	
		Linoleic acid (18:2)	
		Arachidonic acid (20:4)	
	Fatty acyl carnitine	Acetyl-carnitine	Fatty acid mitochondrial transport
	Eicosanoids	Prostaglandin F2a	Inflammation, coagulation, and egg laying
		Thromboxane B2	
	Fatty amides	Anandamide	Endocannabinoid
Glycerolipids	Monoacylglycerols		Metabolite
			Endocannabinoid (2-AG)
	Diacylglycerols	DG(36:3)	Metabolite
	Triacylglycerols	TG(16:0_18:1_18:2)	Energy storage
		TG(16:0_18:0_18:3)	
Glycerophospholipids	Glycerophosphates (PA)	PA(36:2)	Cellular membranes
			Signal transduction
	Phosphatidylcholines (PCs)	PC(36:2), PC(34:2), and PC(34:1)	Cellular membranes Signal transduction
	Phosphatidylethanolamides (PE), serines (PS), inositol (PI), and glycerol (PG)	PE(36:2), PG(36:2), PI(36:2), and PS(21:0)	Cellular membranes Signal transduction
	Lyso-PC, Lyso-PE, Lyso-PS, and Lyso-PI	Lyso-PC(20:2)	Metabolites
Sphingolipids	Free sphingoid bases	Sphingosine (d18:0)	Metabolites and backbone of sphingolipids
	Ceramides	Cer(d18:1/22:0)	Metabolites and signaling molecules
	Sphingomyelins	SM(d18:1/16:0)	Cellular membranes and myelin
	Glycosphingolipids (cerebrosides, globosides, and gangliosides)	Galactosyl(beta)ceramide (d18:1/24:0)	Cellular membranes and myelin

of diet and health (omega-3 such as alpha-linolenic acid, docosahexaenoid acid (DHA), eicosapentaenoic acid (EPA), and omega-6 fatty acids such as linoleic acid). Linoleic (18:2) and alpha-linolenic acid (18:3) are essential fatty acids and must be supplied to the diet. Fatty acids are used as energy through mitochondrial beta-oxidation. Very long-chain polyunsaturated fatty acids (PUFA) (DHA, EPA, arachidonic acid) are the precursors of the eicosanoid lipid mediators such as prostaglandins, leukotrienes, thromboxanes, and others. Nonesterified (free) fatty acids (NEFAs) in the plasma come from either intestinal absorption or lipolysis (from TAGs). To enter the beta-oxidation pathway occurring in the mitochondria, they are typically esterified to carnitine for transport through the mitochondrial membranes. Several acyl-carnitine species can be detected and quantified in parrot plasma. Beta-oxidation results in ketone bodies (with beta-hydroxybutyric acid being the most common in birds) that can get elevated in the plasma with some disease conditions. Plasma NEFA concentrations can also be used clinically to assess the degree of lipolysis and negative energy balance. Eicosanoids are not routinely measured but are useful to understand inflammatory pathways induced in various disease states. The most preponderant fatty acid in parrot plasma is palmitic acid (16:0). In much lower concentrations, oleic acid (18:1) is the most common monounsaturated fatty acid, and linoleic acid (18:2) is the most common polyunsaturated fatty acid. Fatty acids produced by the preen gland are particular in that they are branched-chain fatty acids.[4]

Glycerolipids include TAGs (commonly called triglycerides in medicine even though it is an outdated term), diacylglycerols (DAGs), and monoacylglycerols (MAGs) and their alkyl-glycerol (glyceryl ethers) counterparts. TAGs are the type of lipids stored by adipose cells and also the lipids found in hepatic cells in hepatic lipidosis. They are composed of a molecule of glycerol esterified to 1 to 3 fatty acids in a specific order. The first fatty acid tends to be a saturated fatty acid (typically palmitic acid), the second a monounsaturated fatty acid (typically oleic acid), and the third is more variable and where polyunsaturated fatty acids are typically located.[4] TAGs composition typically reflects the diet and the contribution of metabolism ("*de novo*" lipogenesis). *De novo* lipogenesis mainly occurs in the liver in birds with minimal contribution of the adipose tissues, unlike in mammals.[5] The main function of TAG is energy storage. Because of the large number of potential combinations of esterified fatty acids, glycerolipid species are very diverse in the plasma and hundreds of distinct lipid species occur in the plasma. Glycerolipids constitute approximately 10% of plasma lipids on a molar basis and TAG are by far the most abundant. TAGs with 52 or 54 carbons [commonly combinations of palmitic acid (16:0), stearic acid (18:0), oleic acid (18:1), linoleic acid (18:2), alpha-linolenic acid (18:3) and arachidonic acid (20:4)] predominate in parrot plasma. DAGs and MAG are in much lower concentrations and are metabolic intermediates. A MAG of particular significance is 2-arachidonoyl-glycerol or 2-AG, which is the main endocannabinoid present in parrot plasma (Beaufrère, unpublished).

Glycerophospholipids, commonly abbreviated as phospholipids, are a diverse group of amphiphilic molecules that serve as metabolic intermediates, signaling molecules and as part of cellular membrane. They are made of a glycerol backbone with usually 2 esterified fatty acids (like glycerolipids) and an esterified phosphoryl part. The phosphoryl part can simply be phosphoric acid (glycerophosphates) or additional head groups to form more complex glycerophospholipid such as choline [glycerophosphocholine, also known as phosphatidylcholine (PC) or lecithin], phosphatidylserines (PS), phosphatidylinositol (PI), phosphatidylglycerol (PG), phosphatidylethanolamines and others. Phospholipids are the second more abundant plasma lipid class in parrots after the sterols and constitute approximately 14% to 15% of lipids. Most phospholipids in plasma both in the number of lipid species and concentration are the PC. Lyso-PC (and other lysophospholipids) are metabolites generated by the loss of one of the 2 acyl chains. They occur in plasma in much lower concentrations and are considered metabolic intermediates.

Sphingolipids are incredibly diverse and complex structural lipids (membranes, myelin). They are in relatively low concentrations in the parrot plasma compared with other lipid class (around 0.6%). Sphingomyelins are the most abundant sphingolipids in parrot plasma. Although glycerolipids and phospholipids are based on glycerol, sphingolipids use long-chain sphingoid bases as backbones. Several sphingoid bases are possible, but sphingosine (abbreviated as d18:1) is the most common by far (as in mammals). When sphingosine is esterified to one fatty acyl chain, it is called a ceramide. Ceramides are intermediaries or byproducts of sphingolipid metabolism, but some may also serve as signaling molecules. On top of a fatty acyl chain (ceramides), other head groups may be found on the sphingosine backbone and determine the type of sphingolipid subclass such as the sphingomyelin (additional phosphocholine), sugars (cerebrosides, globosides, and gangliosides). Sphingomyelins are the most abundant sphingolipids in parrot plasma.

AVIAN LIPOPROTEIN METABOLISM

Almost all lipids in the plasma are transported in the form of macromolecular aggregates of mixed lipid species and proteins known as lipoproteins. The exception is NEFAs, which are transported bound to albumin. As avian lipoprotein metabolism has been comprehensively reviewed elsewhere,[5,6] only a brief recapitulative will be given here.

Lipoproteins are classified based on their density and size and are involved in different lipid transport pathways. They have a micellar lipid structure with a surface monolayer mainly composed of free cholesterol and phospholipids and a hydrophobic core composed of TAGs and CEs. Proteins called apolipoproteins also occur on the surface and have structural and signaling properties (**Fig. 2**). Apolipoproteins are used for lipoprotein trafficking. Lipoproteins are classified based on their density into portomicrons, very low density lipoproteins (VLDLs), intermediate-density lipoproteins (IDLs), low-density lipoproteins (LDLs), and high-density lipoproteins (HDLs). Portomicrons are the avian equivalent to mammalian chylomicrons. Portomicrons are not released into the minimal lymphatic system of birds, but into the portal vein. Portomicrons and VLDLs are very large lipoproteins that participate in the exogenous lipid pathway in birds, in which lipid absorbed through the intestinal walls are transported to the liver (**Fig. 3**). These molecules are high in triglycerides.

VLDLs and LDLs participate in the endogenous cholesterol/lipid pathway, in which cholesterol synthesized in the liver is transported into effector tissues. Lipoprotein lipase and hepatic lipase enzymes hydrolyze TAG within VLDL and IDL, reducing them to LDL at the effector sites. LDLs are particularly high in cholesterol and CEs. LDL particles are then picked up by the liver through LDL receptors for recycling. Apolipoprotein B100 is the main apolipoprotein of portomicrons, VLDL, and LDL. In humans, ApoB48 occurs in chylomicrons, but in birds ApoB100 is analogous in portomicrons.

HDLs participate in the reverse cholesterol transport pathway, in which cholesterol is returned to the liver from effector tissues. Cholesterol is then further recycled or excreted through the bile. High in phospholipids and proteins, HDLs have apolipoprotein A as their main apolipoproteins. The plasma enzyme cholesteryl ester transfer protein (CETP) can move cholesterol from HDL to LDL in exchange for triglycerides. In Quaker parrots, CETP increases with dyslipidemia (abnormal blood lipid

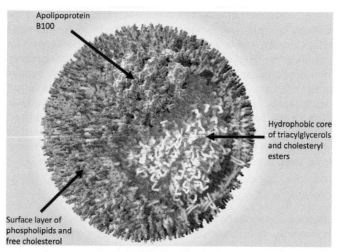

Fig. 2. Schematic representation of an LDL particle. Lipoproteins are made of a hydrophobic core containing cholesteryl esters and triacylglycerols (shown in *yellow*) surrounded by a hydrophilic surface monolayer made of phospholipids (shown in *orange with blue caps*) and free cholesterol (shown in *green*). Apolipoproteins such as apolipoprotein B100 in this LDL particle (shown in *blue*) occur in the surface layer and help with lipoprotein trafficking and structure. Modified from stock image (iStockphoto LP) and reprinted with permission.

concentrations).[7] In parrots, as in most birds and unlike humans, HDL is the main lipoprotein of the plasma. Most of parrot HDL particles are small to medium in size with a mean diameter of approximately 9.8 to 10.9 nm, much like in humans.[8] Female birds

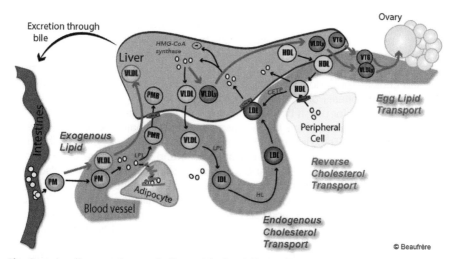

Fig. 3. Avian lipoprotein metabolism with the different lipid transport pathways. Differences from mammals are shown in red (portomicrons instead of chylomicrons, VLDL involved in exogenous pathway, movement of most portomicrons to the liver, and egg lipid transport pathway). CETP, cholesteryl ester transfer protein; HL, hepatic lipase; LPL, lipoprotein lipase.

have another lipid metabolic pathway, not present in mammals, the egg lipid transport pathway. In the egg-lipid pathway specialized VLDL, the phospholipid-rich vitellogenin and triglyceride-rich VLDLy (yolk VLDL), transport lipid to the developing oocyte under estrogenic influence. In chickens, vitellogenin and VLDLy have smaller diameters (around 30 nm) than regular VLDL (most being >31–36 nm) which allows transit of the granulosa basal lamina. These lipoproteins are not susceptible to lipoprotein lipase unlike other lipoproteins.[9] However, in other species than chickens, which have been heavily selected for egg production, a shift to smaller VLDLs during egg production is not necessarily seen and the trend may be reversed with a shift toward larger VLDLs as in passerine birds.[10] In Quaker parrots, the trend seems similar to that of passerine birds (Beaufrere, personal observation).

LIPIDOLOGIC DIAGNOSTIC METHODS

A variety of lipidologic diagnostic assays are available including those targeting a single lipid (cholesterol), low molecular specificity (triglycerides), a group of lipids (NEFAs), lipoproteins, or whole pathways (lipidomics). Some of these assays are not readily available in clinical reference laboratories and some are mostly used in research laboratories. Blood lipidologic tests characterize dyslipidemia and risk factors for some diseases, but do not directly diagnose lipid-accumulation disorders such as atherosclerosis and hepatic lipidosis. Although blood lipid changes may increase suspicion of these disorders, other diagnostic tests should be used to diagnose these conditions to include diagnostic imaging and tissue biopsies.

Total Cholesterol

Total cholesterol is the main lipid diagnostic test available in routine biochemistry panel and in many point-of-care veterinary analyzers. Most tests are based on enzymatic reactions that hydrolyze CEs into free cholesterol and fatty acids and then oxidize cholesterol to generate hydrogen peroxide that is measured using a colorimetric reaction.[11] Thus these tests are total cholesterol assays and do not differentiate between esterified and nonesterified cholesterol or between cholesterol contained within different lipoproteins. Enzymatic cholesterol assays can also react with other sterols. Other analytical techniques to measure cholesterol such as gas chromatography, liquid chromatography, and mass spectrometry can differentiate free from esterified cholesterol.[11] However, these are not available at most veterinary clinical diagnostic laboratories. Point-of-care analyzers such as the PTS-Diagnostics Cardio-Chek are unreliable for use in birds and lipemia and hemolysis increased bias.[12,13]

Some psittacine species have higher plasma cholesterol than others, which reflects their susceptibility to lipid disorders. For instance, Quaker parrots have much higher plasma cholesterol than most other parrot species and macaws (Ara spp.) tend to have lower cholesterol.[14] Quaker parrots are prone to lipid disorders and also have higher plasma triglycerides than other parrot species.[15] Although female parrots may have higher cholesterol levels than male parrots, conflicting reports,[14,16,17] suggest that blood cholesterol in non-reproductive female parrots may not differ from male parrots depending on species. Blood cholesterol concentration may also increase with age in parrots.[14]

Total cholesterol is the first line of diagnostics for dyslipidemia as most are characterized by hypercholesterolemia. The prevalence of hypercholesterolemia (total cholesterol >8 mmol/L (309 mg/dL)) is estimated to be 20% in psittacine birds (n = 5625, Beaufrère, unpublished). Severe hypercholesterolemia along with atherosclerosis can be induced via cholesterol diet in Quaker parrots.[7,18] Atherosclerosis was associated with an increase in plasma cholesterol in one study.[19] Psittacine species more susceptible to atherosclerosis also tend to have higher plasma cholesterol than less susceptible species on average.[14] In Quaker parrots, birds with higher body condition score and weight also have higher cholesterol levels.[17]

Elevation in cholesterol can also be seen with a variety of other conditions and physiologic status. For instance, it can also increase post-prandially and with cholestasis. Vitellogenesis and egg formation in hens is also strongly associated with hypercholesterolemia.[20,21] Endocrine disorders such as diabetes mellitus and hypothyroidism and hepatic lipidosis have also been associated with hypercholesterolemia in parrots.[22–25] In mammals, an increase in blood cholesterol is also seen with other conditions such as nephrotic syndrome, hyperadrenocorticism, infections, and genetic disorders.[26–28]

An increase in polyunsaturated fatty acid intake, in particular n3 fatty acids via dietary flaxseed oil or fish oil, lowered blood cholesterol in cockatiels (*Nymphicus hollandicus*).[29] However, in another study in Quaker parrots, supplementation of n3 polyunsaturated fatty acids with flaxseeds did not result in plasma cholesterol changes.[30] A seed-based diet has not been associated with hypercholesterolemia in two studies in parrots.[17,24] Seeds and other plant-based diet items do not contain cholesterol, which can only be obtained from animal products.

Total Triglycerides

Like total cholesterol, measurement of total triglycerides is available on a wide variety of laboratory analyzers. These assays target the glycerol backbone of the molecule, which is the same across species. Standard biochemistry assays are typically enzymatic colorimetric tests using a lipoprotein lipase to hydrolyze triglycerides into glycerol and fatty acids followed by oxidation reactions producing hydrogen peroxide. Hydrogen peroxide is then measured via colorimetric reaction.[31] Consequently, triglyceride assays do not distinguish between free glycerol, glyceryl ethers (DG-O), MAGs, DAGs, and TAGs, rendering it more of a total glycerides test than a TAG test. Although non-TAGs glycerolipids account for only approximately 3% to 4% of plasma glycerolipids in parrots, which could be considered negligible,[1] Backspace approximately 30% of that measured as triglycerides is actually free glycerol in normal parrots, on a molar basis.[8] This is about triple the expected values for humans where free glycerol constitutes only approximately 6% of total glycerides.[32,33] The relatively increased free glycerol of parrots can interfere with clinical interpretation of the triglycerides assay or use of the assay value to obtain calculated values such as VLDL or ratios. Pseudohypertriglyceridemia is caused by increased concentrations of blood-free glycerol in humans, but has not yet been described in parrots.

In birds, blood triglyceride concentrations mainly increase following a meal and in reproductive women with most plasma triglycerides composed of VLDL.[34–36] Hypertriglyceridemia has not been associated with atherosclerosis in psittacine birds in epidemiologic studies[14,19] or experimental studies.[7] In people, plasma triglyceride concentrations are a risk factor for atherosclerotic diseases. Increased plasma triglycerides occur in a variety of lipid-related diseases such as acute pancreatitis, endocrine disorders (mainly diabetes and metabolic syndrome), and fatty liver.[37] High amounts of dietary sugars, especially fructose, are also well known to be associated with hypertriglyceridemia in people,[37–40] but whether the same is true in parrots consuming a high quantity of simple sugars in fruits is unknown. Preliminary findings with fructose supplementation in macaws failed to find an effect.[41] Supplementation in n3 polyunsaturated fatty acids may decrease blood triglyceride concentrations in parrots.[29] Plasma triglycerides are also used in avian ecological studies as a marker of fat stores.

Lipoprotein Panel

Analytical techniques

As most lipids are transported within lipoproteins, lipoprotein testing and profiling are routine in human medicine and research. Avian lipoproteins have many differences from mammals and no lipoprotein diagnostic test has been validated for clinical use in birds. In addition, as lipoproteins tend to degrade with storage, the performance of lipoprotein analysis on fresh samples whenever possible is recommended.[42]

The gold standard for lipoprotein analysis is separation by density gradient ultracentrifugation, wherein lipoproteins are separated along a density gradient in a vertical tube. Lipoproteins will settle in different sections of the tube based on their differing density. Different lipoproteins fractions can then be pipetted out and analyzed. This technique is extremely time-consuming, requiring 6 to 30 h of very high-speed centrifugation and specialized equipment.[43] It is not offered commercially for animals, but has been used for research in pigeons, chickens, quails, geese, Quaker parrots, and cockatiels.[5,17,29,44–48] Although this method allows separation and isolation of lipoprotein classes and subclasses, it does not allow the determination of lipoprotein particle numbers and particle sizes. To analyze the lipid content of the lipoprotein classes, a relatively large volume of blood is necessary, and each fraction must be carefully collected from the centrifugal tubes before analysis. For this reason, ultracentrifugation of small volumes in parrots to obtain a lipoprotein panel is typically done by using analytical ultracentrifugation techniques. A lipid dye or fluorophore is typically added to the tube and then the optical density/fluorometry along the gradient is obtained using an optical system. This technique only allows the determination of relative distribution (% of total lipids). Absolute values are then determined from the total blood cholesterol levels and are not directly measured from each lipoprotein fraction.[17,29,45] Moreover, parrot-specific density gradient cutoff have not been established.[17] Other techniques to measure lipoproteins include electrophoresis and nuclear magnetic resonance (NMR) spectroscopy. Electrophoresis to obtain lipoprotein panels was used in Quaker parrots,[45] but NMR determination has not been applied to parrot lipoproteins yet.

Recently, a high-resolution technique using gel-permeation HPLC (Liposearch) has provided full lipoprotein profiling of parrots with a panel of 20 subclasses and particle sizes reported from just one drop of plasma.[8] Although particle numbers can be obtained through NMR, this method remains unavailable because the algorithm to analyze the NMR spectrum is proprietary and based on humans, or Liposearch panel. Most of these reference or high-resolution techniques allow the determination of subtypes of lipoproteins. However, the different lipid subtypes defined within the various techniques do not necessarily match or correspond. For instance, VLDL subtypes include large and small VLDLs, LDL includes a group of highly atherogenic lipoproteins called the "small, dense" LDL (or sdLDL), and HDL also includes several subtypes (eg, HDL 1–7 with Liposearch). In healthy Quaker parrots, most VLDLs are small, LDLs are large to medium in size with 37% being sdLDL, and HDL are mostly of the medium and small categories.[8]

Although these reference techniques are applicable to any animal species, they not use clinical reference laboratories that prefer rapid and more automated tests. Direct LDL and HDL wet-chemistry analytes were developed for human plasma and typically only measure cholesterol content. These tests focus on HDL and use selective precipitation or complexation methods. As direct LDL measurement is challenging, indirect formulas are used to include Friedewald formula:

LDL = Cholesterol − HDL − VLDL/x with x = 5 in US units and x = 2.18 in SI units, which assumes the ratio of triglycerides and VLDL is the same across species. Despite wide use, this formula is inaccurate in Quaker parrots[8] and suggests a similar lack of accuracy for lipids of psittacine species. The Friedewald formula is also inaccurate in the case of hypertriglyceridemia in mammals; avian vitellogenesis is similarly expected to prevent accurate calculations for LDL of female birds.

Preliminary research findings comparing the Liposearch technique to standard lipoprotein measurements show that direct LDL measurement is unreliable in parrots. Further, indirect estimation via the Friedewald formula and other equations are equally unreliable in the measurement of lipoproteins of Quaker parrots (Beaufrère, unpublished). However, HDL is measured reliably by standard analyzers and atherogenic lipoproteins can be estimated using non-HDL cholesterol that encompasses VLDL, IDL, and LDL. Hypertriglyceridemia increases bias in HDL (underestimation) and indirect LDL measurements (underestimation) (Beaufrère, unpublished). Total cholesterol/HDL ratio is also a useful biomarker that allows the assessment of the relative importance of atherogenic lipoproteins. Non-HDL cholesterol and total cholesterol/HDL ratios are effective biomarkers in people and better predict risks of cardiovascular disease than LDL alone.[49] As HDLs are the main plasma lipoproteins in parrots versus LDLs in humans, human guidelines are not likely as useful in psittacine species.

Apolipoproteins (apoB, apoB/apoA) are commonly measured in human medicine as they indicate lipoprotein particle numbers as there is a single apolipoprotein B molecule per non-HDL lipoprotein particle.[50] Birds lack Apo-E and ApoB-48. In addition, parrot ApoB-100, the predominant apolipoprotein in the portomicrons VLDL and LDL, has only approximately 50% sequence homology with human Apo-B100. Therefore, apolipoprotein diagnostic tests based on human plasma are unlikely useful in parrots, although this concept has yet to be directly investigated.

Interpretation

Dyslipidemias are common in Psittaciformes and are strongly associated with lipid-accumulation disorders in parrots such as atherosclerosis, hepatic lipidosis, fatty tumors, obesity and with chronic reproductive diseases in females.[17,51] Lipoprotein abnormalities in dyslipidemia have been poorly characterized in clinical patients and in published case studies, only reporting total hypercholesterolemia and/or hypertriglyceridemia.

Female birds undergoing vitellogenesis have increased cholesterol and triglyceride concentrations in the plasma. As vitellogenin and VLDLy are resistant to lipoprotein lipase degradation, the dyslipidemia of dysregulated vitellogenesis may last longer and be harder to control. Diet undoubtedly plays an important role in the emergence of dyslipidemia either through increased calorie or fat intake and through multiple deficiencies.

Studies on lipoproteins in parrots have proved inconsistent regarding sex differences for lipids: females had higher HDL than males in some studies,[16] higher LDL,[52] or most commonly no difference.[14] Lipoprotein values may also markedly differ between psittacine species. Quaker parrots have LDL concentrations almost double that of other parrot species. Macaws show the opposite trend, with one-third the concentrations of most other parrot species.[14] Concentrations of HDL seem to have less variability across psittacine species. Clinical experience suggests both non-HDL and HDL increase in dyslipidemia, but the ratio HDL/non-HDL tends to shift.

Strong dyslipidemia has been experimentally induced in Quaker parrots fed a 1% cholesterol pelletized diet.[7] In this study, a drastic increase in LDL along total cholesterol was observed, whereas HDL concentrations remained stable. In another study in the same species fed a 0.3% cholesterol pelletized diet, a sharp increase in plasma

VLDL and LDL concentration and particle numbers were seen concomitant to a mild increase in HDL.[18] Concentrations of LDL subtype distribution changes with a higher proportion of larger LDL (LDL1) than on the control diet, whereas HDL subtypes were not altered. In the same study, no effect of sunflower oil supplementation occurred for plasma lipoproteins in Quaker parrots. Overweight quaker parrots with spontaneous dyslipidemias also have a marked increase in VLDL, LDL (with a higher proportion of larger LDL) concentrations, and a shift in the LDL/HDL ratio.[17]

As lipoprotein panels, especially including non-HDL cholesterol, will become more commonplace in the future, as will our ability to better understand lipoprotein changes in bird, which differ greatly from those of human and other mammals. More information will undoubtedly become available on plasma lipoprotein changes in association with various diseases in parrots.

B-Hydroxybutyric Acid

As the main ketone of birds, B-hydroxybutyric acid (BHBA) is a marker of increased and overwhelmed fatty acid oxidation. Although not usually not part of standard biochemistry panels, most veterinary laboratories offer BHBA as a standalone test. Ketone blood meters are available, but their reliability is untested in psittacine birds. However, point-of-care ketone meters have shown good reliability in other birds.[53] BHBA can also be used as a marker of fasting.

Under certain circumstances such as diabetes or negative energy balance, TAGs of adipose tissue are hydrolyzed into fatty acids and glycerol. The NEFAs are transported in the blood bound to albumin and are then oxidized in the liver to generate energy through β-oxidation in mitochondria and peroxisomes generating acetyl-CoA. Acetyl-CoA is then used either in the tricarboxylic (TCA) cycle to generate energy or for ketogenesis in mitochondria. Ketones may be eliminated or further oxidized to produce energy via the TCA cycle. Ketoacidosis occurs in diabetes mellitus based on increased lipolysis along with stimulation of hepatic neoglucogenesis that increases ketogenesis. Concentrations of BHBA increase in diabetic parrots.[22]

In birds, starvation may also lead to changes in plasma BHBA as birds transition from stage II starvation (depletion of fat store) to stage III (depletion of muscles). During this transition, BHBA will decrease in plasma, whereas uric acid will increase.[54] In humans, ketogenesis is also altered with hepatic lipidosis and results in lower blood ketone bodies.[55] Therefore, further research on plasma BHBA concentrations in parrots in relation to hepatic lipidosis may show an associated decrease.

Nonesterified Fatty Acids

NEFAs are also a marker of lipolysis and negative energy balance. Hydrolysis of adipose TAG by hormone-sensitive lipase generates plasma NEFA. NEFAs can be used by the liver to generate energy, be re-esterified into TAG for hepatic storage or export in VLDL, and as substrates for ketogenesis. NEFAs are also used by other peripheral tissue for energy production. In wild birds, low plasma triglycerides and high NEFA indicate fat store utilization, and these markers are frequently used in ecological studies.[56,57]

Clinical Lipidomics

Most blood diagnostic tests in veterinary medicine and in avian medicine focus on plasma protein biomarkers, enzyme activities, electrolytes, or small metabolites instead of lipids. However, lipids are preponderant in the plasma and lipidomics studies reveal approximately 1000 to 1500 distinct lipid species detected in Quaker parrot plasma.[1] Some of these lipids could serve as novel biomarkers for several lipid-related and metabolic diseases.

Comprehensive lipid analysis by mass spectrometry, known as lipidomics, is revolutionizing the investigation of metabolic disorders. In the context of dyslipidemia, specific lipid species of complex lipids may be better targets or biomarkers than crude measurements of a single lipid class or subclass such as with cholesterol and glycerol (for triglycerides) analysis. Thousands of species of triglycerides, phospholipids, and CEs with a variety of saturated and unsaturated fatty acyl chains can be measured in plasma. Lipidomic analysis provides an important alternative approach that bypasses many limitations of conventional tests while providing considerably more information. The lipidome of male and female parrots also tend to be different.[1] Although it is not yet used on clinical patients, lipidomic research is underway in parrots and may lead to improved lipidologic diagnostic tests in the future. Specific biomarkers or lipidomic signatures for specific diseases may be discovered with these techniques.

Plasma concentrations of several lipid metabolites including many CEs, ceramides, PCs, and sphingomyelins increased in Quaker parrots following 0.3% dietary cholesterol supplementation.[18] Doubling the dietary fat to 20% using sunflower oil (high in n6 polyunsaturated fatty acids) also decreased glycerolipids and increased in acylcarnitines concentrations in these parrots.[18] Further studies investigating lipidomic profiling in association with various diseases are needed to explore and propose new biomarkers or combination of biomarkers as diagnostic for disease in avian species.

CLINICS CARE POINTS

- When ordering a lipid profile on a bird, include total cholesterol, triglycerides, and high-density lipoprotein (HDL) cholesterol. Non-HDL cholesterol can be calculated as a measure of atherogenic lipoproteins.

- Reproductively active female birds undergoing vitellogenesis and egg production will likely have high plasma cholesterol and triglycerides and non-HDL cholesterol concentrations.

- Although species-specific sex predispositions exist, female birds tend to have a higher prevalence of lipid accumulation disorders and dyslipidemia overall than male birds in many species.

DISCLOSURE

Some of the research results summarized in this handout were obtained from research projects funded by the Morris Animal Foundation (grant ID: D19ZO-301), the Association of Avian Veterinarians (SOAR fund), and the OVC Pet Trust. Part of this article was previously published as a masterclass handout for ExoticsCon 2020.

REFERENCES

1. Beaufrère H, Gardhouse SM, Wood RD, et al. The plasma lipidome of the Quaker parrot (*Myiopsitta monachus*). PLoS One 2020;15(12). https://doi.org/10.1371/journal.pone.0240449.
2. Haghighi-Rad F, Polin D. The Relationship of Plasma Estradiol and Progesterone Levels to the Fatty Liver Hemorrhagic Syndrome in Laying Hens. Poult Sci 1981; 60(10):2278–83.

3. Lee BK, Kim JS, Ahn HJ, et al. Changes in hepatic lipid parameters and hepatic messenger ribonucleic acid expression following estradiol administration in laying hens (Gallus domesticus). Poult Sci 2010;89(12):2660–7.

4. Gurr M, Harwood J, Frayn K. Fatty acid metabolism. In: Gurr MI, Harwood JL, Frayn KN, editors. Lipids: biochemistry, biotechnology and health. 6th edition. Chichester, West Sussex, UK: Wiley Blackwell; 2016. p. 44–123.

5. Alvarenga RR, Zangeronimo MG, Pereira LJ, et al. Lipoprotein metabolism in poultry. World Poult Sci J 2011;67:431–40.

6. Beaufrere H. Atherosclerosis: Comparative pathogenesis, lipoprotein metabolism and avian and exotic companion mammal models. J Exot Pet Med 2013;22(4):320–35.

7. Beaufrère H, Nevarez JGG, Wakamatsu N, et al. Experimental diet-induced atherosclerosis in Quaker parrots (*Myiopsitta monachus*). Vet Pathol 2013;50(6):1116–26.

8. Beaufrere H, Gardhouse S, Ammersbach M. Lipoprotein Characterization in Quaker Parrots (*Myiopsitta monachus*) Using Gel-Permeation High-Performance Liquid Chromatography. Vet Clin Pathol 2020;49:417–27.

9. Buyse J, Decuypere E. Adipose tissue and lipid metabolism. In: Scanes C, editor. Sturkie's avian physiology. 6th edition. San Diego, CA: Academic Press; 2015. p. 443–54.

10. Salvante KG, Lin G, Walzem RL, et al. Characterization of very-low density lipoprotein particle diameter dynamics in relation to egg production in a passerine bird. J Exp Biol 2007;210(6):1064–74.

11. Li LH, Dutkiewicz EP, Huang YC, et al. Analytical methods for cholesterol quantification. J Food Drug Anal 2019;27(2):375–86.

12. Barboza T, Beaufrère H. Comparison of a Point-of-care Cholesterol Meter with a Reference Laboratory Analyzer in Companion Psittaciformes. J Avian Med Surg 2019;33(1):7–14.

13. Morales A, Frei B, Leung C, et al. Point-of-care blood analyzers measure the nutritional state of eighteen free-living bird species. Comp Biochem Physiol A Mol Integr Physiol 2020;240:110594.

14. Beaufrère H, Vet DM, Cray C, et al. Association of plasma lipid levels with atherosclerosis prevalence in psittaciformes. J Avian Med Surg 2014;28(3):225–31.

15. Beaufrère H, Reavill D, Heatley J, et al. Lipid-Related Lesions in Quaker Parrots (*Myiopsitta monachus*). Vet Pathol 2019;56(2). https://doi.org/10.1177/0300985818800025.

16. Ravich M, Cray C, Hess L, et al. Lipid Panel Reference Intervals for Amazon Parrots (Amazona species). J Avian Med Surg 2014;28(3):209–15.

17. Belcher C, Heatley JJ, Petzinger C, et al. Evaluation of Plasma Cholesterol, Triglyceride, and Lipid Density Profiles in Captive Monk Parakeets (*Myiopsitta monachus*). J Exot Pet Med 2014;23(1):71–8.

18. Beaufrere H, Stark K, Wood R. Effects of a 0.3% Cholesterol Diet and a 20% Fat Diet on Plasma Lipids and Lipoproteins in Quaker Parrots (*Myiopsitta monachus*). Vet Clin Pathol 2022. https://doi.org/10.1111/vcp.13108.

19. Pilny AA, Quesenberry KE, Bartick-Sedrish TE, et al. Evaluation of Chlamydophila psittaci infection and other risk factors for atherosclerosis in pet psittacine birds. J Am Vet Med Assoc 2012;240(12):1474–80.

20. Beaufrere H. Dyslipidemia/hyperlipidemia. In: Graham J, editor. 5-Minute veterinary consult : avian. Ames, IA: Blackwell Publishing; 2016. p. 98–100.

21. Harr K. Diagnostic value of biochemistry. In: Harrison G, Lightfoot T, editors. Clinical avian medicine. Palm Beach, FL: Spix Publishing; 2006. p. 611–30.

22. Gancz AY, Wellehan JFX, Boutette J, et al. Diabetes mellitus concurrent with hepatic haemosiderosis in two macaws (Ara severa, Ara militaris). Avian Pathol 2007;36(4):331–6.

23. Oglesbee B. Hypothyroidism in a scarlet macaw. J Am Vet Med Assoc 1992; 201(10):1599–601.

24. Stanford M. Significance of cholesterol assays in the investigation of hepatic lipidosis and atherosclerosis in psittacine birds. ExoticDVM 2005;7(3):28–34.

25. Harms C, Hoskinson J, Bruyette D, et al. Development of an experimental model of hypothyroidism in cockatiels (Nymphicus hollandicus). Am J Vet Res 1994; 55(3):399–404.

26. Bruss ML. Lipids and ketones. In: Kaneko JJ, Harvey JW, Bruss ML, editors. Clinical biochemistry of domestic animals. 6th edition. Cambridge, MA: Academic Press; 2008. p. 81–115.

27. Klosterman ES, Moore GE, Galvao JF de B, et al. Comparison of Signalment, Clinicopathologic Findings, Histologic Diagnosis, and Prognosis in Dogs with Glomerular Disease with or without Nephrotic Syndrome. J Vet Intern Med 2011;25(2):206–14.

28. Sharma D, Hill AE, Christopher MM. Hypercholesterolemia and hypertriglyceridemia as biochemical markers of disease in companion rabbits. Vet Clin Pathol 2018;47(4):589–602.

29. Heinze CR, Hawkins MG, Gillies LA, et al. Effect of dietary omega-3 fatty acids on red blood cell lipid composition and plasma metabolites in the cockatiel, Nymphicus hollandicus. J Anim Sci 2012;90(9):3068–79.

30. Petzinger C, Heatley JJ, Bailey CA, et al. Lipid Metabolic Dose Response to Dietary Alpha-Linolenic Acid in Monk Parrot (*Myiopsitta monachus*). Lipids 2014; 49(3):235–45.

31. Klotzsch SG, McNamara JR. Triglyceride measurements: a review of methods and interferences. Clin Chem 1990;36(9):1605–13.

32. Stinshoff K, Weisshaar D, Staehler F, et al. Relation between concentrations of free glycerol and triglycerides in human sera. Clin Chem 1977;23(6):1029–32.

33. Li H, Dong J, Chen W, et al. Measurement of serum total glycerides and free glycerol by high-performance liquid chromatography. J Lipid Res 2006;47(9): 2089–96.

34. Cray C, Stremme DW, Arheart KL. Postprandial biochemistry changes in penguins (Spheniscus demersus) including hyperuricemia. J Zoo Wild Med 2010; 41(2):325–6.

35. Vergneau-Grosset C, Beaufrere H, Ammersbach M. Clinical biochemistry. In: Speer B, editor. Current therapy in avian medicine and surgery. St. Louis, MO: Elsevier; 2016. p. 486–500.

36. Nemetz L. Chronic hypertriglyceridemia as a marker for ovarian pathology. Proc Annu Conf Assoc Avian Vet 2010;49–52.

37. Packard CJ, Boren J, Taskinen MR. Causes and Consequences of Hypertriglyceridemia. Front Endocrinol 2020;252. https://doi.org/10.3389/FENDO.2020.00252.

38. Kolderup A, Svihus B. Fructose Metabolism and Relation to Atherosclerosis, Type 2 Diabetes, and Obesity. J Nutr Metab 2015;2015. https://doi.org/10.1155/2015/823081.

39. KL S, JM S, NL K, et al. Consuming fructose-sweetened, not glucose-sweetened, beverages increases visceral adiposity and lipids and decreases insulin sensitivity in overweight/obese humans. J Clin Invest 2009;119(5):1322–34.

40. Stanhope KL, Bremer AA, Medici V, et al. Consumption of fructose and high fructose corn syrup increase postprandial triglycerides, LDL-cholesterol, and apolipoprotein-B in young men and women. J Clin Endocrinol Metab 2011; 96(10). https://doi.org/10.1210/JC.2011-1251.

41. Béland k, Ferrell D, Beaufrère H, et al. Impact of Dietary Fructose on the Lipid Profile in Six Macaws. J Avian Med Surg 2021;35(2):196–203.

42. Zivkovic AM, Wiest MM, Nguyen UT, et al. Effects of sample handling and storage on quantitative lipid analysis in human serum. Metabolomics 2009;5(4):507–16.

43. Caslake M, Packard C. The use of ultracentrifugation for the separation of lipoproteins. In: Rifal N, Warnick G, Dominiczak M, editors. Handbook of lipoprotein testing. 2nd edition. Washington, DC: AACC Press, 2000. p. 025–40.

44. Langelier M, Connelly P, Subbiah MT. Plasma lipoprotein profile and composition in White Carneau and Show Racer breeds of pigeons. Can J Biochem 1976; 54(1):27–31.

45. Petzinger C, Larner C, Heatley JJ, et al. Conversion of α-linolenic acid to long-chain omega-3 fatty acid derivatives and alterations of HDL density subfractions and plasma lipids with dietary polyunsaturated fatty acids in Monk parrots (Myiopsitta monachus). J Anim Physiol Anim Nutr 2014;98(2):262–70.

46. Oku H, Ishikawa M, Nagata J, et al. Lipoprotein and apoprotein profile of Japanese quail. Biochemica Biophys Acta 1993;1167:22–8.

47. Barakat HA, St Clair RW. Characterization of plasma lipoproteins of grain- and cholesterol-fed White Carneau and Show Racer pigeons. J lipid Res 1985; 26(10):1252–68.

48. Hermier D, Saadoun A, Salichon MR, et al. Plasma lipoproteins and liver lipids in two breeds of geese with different susceptibility to hepatic steatosis: changes induced by development and force-feeding. Lipids 1991;26(5):331–9.

49. Pokharel Y, Negi S, Virani S. Cholesterol: concentration, ratio, and particle number. In: Ballantyne C, editor. Clinical Lipidology. 2nd edition. Philadelphia, PA: Elsevier; 2015. p. 91–8.

50. Okazaki M, Yamashita S. Recent Advances in Analytical Methods on Lipoprotein Subclasses: Calculation of Particle Numbers from Lipid Levels by Gel Permeation HPLC Using "Spherical Particle Model. J Oleo Sci 2016;65(4):265–82.

51. Beaufrere H. Avian atherosclerosis: parrots and beyond. J Exot Pet Med 2013; 22(4):336–47.

52. Gustavsen KA, Stanhope KL, Lin AS, et al. Effects of exercise on the plasma lipid profile in hispaniolan amazon parrots (amazona ventralis) with naturally occurring hypercholesterolemia. JZWM 2016;47(3):760–9.

53. Lindholm C, Altimiras J, Lees J. Measuring ketones in the field: rapid and reliable measures of β-hydroxybutyrate in birds. Ibis 2019;161(1):205–10.

54. Lumeij JT. Avian clinical biochemistry. In: Kaneko JJ, Harvey JW, Bruss ML, editors. Clinical biochemistry of domestic animals. 6th edition. Cambridge, MA: Academic Press; 2008. p. 839–72.

55. Fletcher JA, Deja S, Satapati S, et al. Impaired ketogenesis and increased acetyl-CoA oxidation promote hyperglycemia in human fatty liver. JCI insight 2019;5(11). https://doi.org/10.1172/JCI.INSIGHT.127737.

56. Graña Grilli M, Pari M, Ibañez A. Poor body conditions during the breeding period in a seabird population with low breeding success. Mar Biol 2018;165(9):1–9.

57. Price ER. Dietary lipid composition and avian migratory flight performance: Development of a theoretical framework for avian fat storage. Comp Biochem Physiol A Mol Integr Physiol 2010;157(4):297–309.

III. Clinical Pathology Diagnostic Overviews for Select Reptile Species

Diagnostic Clinical Pathology of the Bearded Dragon (*Pogona vitticeps*)

Clark Broughton, DVM[a],*, Kyle Lauren Webb, DVM, DACVP[b]

KEYWORDS

- Bearded dragon • Chemistry • Clinical pathology • Cytology • Diagnostics
- Hematology • Neoplasia

KEY POINTS

- Thorough physical examination and a clinicopathologic minimum database are invaluable for prompt diagnosis in bearded dragons, which are otherwise stoic or display nonspecific symptoms when ill, or lack clinical symptoms until late in the course of disease.
- Numerous factors including age, sex, environmental temperature, diet, and season influence hematologic and biochemical analytes in bearded dragons and should be considered when interpreting results.
- The most common diseases affecting bearded dragons are infectious, inflammatory, or chronic/degenerative conditions, typically involving the gastrointestinal or hepatobiliary systems.
- Neoplasia in bearded dragons is not uncommonly reported for integumentary, hepatic, and lymphoid and hematopoietic tissue.

INTRODUCTION

The bearded dragon (*Pogona vitticeps*), an omnivorous Agamid lizard native to the arid woodland and desert environments of inland Australia, is one of the most popular reptile pets due to their sociable behavior, tame demeanor, low-maintenance care, and relative ease of breeding.[1–3] Although the majority of health issues in bearded dragons are a result of poor husbandry, they are generally stoic creatures and illness may not be evident until the late stages of disease. For this reason, thorough physical examination in conjunction with routine clinicopathologic data can prove invaluable in identifying disease and implementing appropriate therapy in a timely manner. The goal of this article is to assist the practicing clinician, based on review of current

[a] Department of Veterinary Pathobiology, Texas A&M College of Veterinary Medicine & Biomedical Sciences, 660 Raymond Stotzer Parkway, College Station, TX 77843-4457, USA;
[b] Antech Diagnostics, 7415 Emerald Dunes Dr, Suite 1500, Orlando, FL 32822 USA
* Corresponding author.
E-mail address: cbroughton@cvm.tamu.edu

Vet Clin Exot Anim 25 (2022) 713–734
https://doi.org/10.1016/j.cvex.2022.06.002
1094-9194/22/© 2022 Elsevier Inc. All rights reserved.

vetexotic.theclinics.com

literature, on how to approach the diagnostic challenge encountered in everyday practice when working up various conditions in bearded dragons.

HEMATOLOGY

Hematologic assessment of bearded dragons in the form of a complete blood count (CBC) is often performed for both routine wellness evaluation and as part of the diagnostic workup in sick animals. Indications are similar to those in companion mammals but results may be difficult to interpret due to changes associated with ectotherm physiology, environment, and lack of baseline values and abundant reference material.[1] Therefore, annual or biannual wellness checks with the evaluation of hematologic and plasma biochemical analytes can be helpful in establishing baseline values that can be used for comparison in the event of illness later in life.[5] Hematology reference intervals for bearded dragons from a variety of sources are presented in **Table 1**.

Lithium-heparin is a commonly used anticoagulant for blood collection in lizards because it is amenable to both hematologic and plasma biochemical analysis. However, samples collected in ethylenediaminetetraacetic acid (EDTA) are less likely to cause leukocyte clumping and, therefore, are considered superior for evaluation of leukocyte count and morphology.[4] It is generally accepted that the collection of a volume of blood equivalent to approximately 0.5% to 0.8% of a lizard's weight in grams is sufficient for hematology testing but when only a small volume of blood is able to be collected, blood smear preparation for microscopic evaluation should be given priority.[5] For best results, blood smears should be made from blood unaltered by anticoagulant, air-dried quickly, fixed in methanol within 1 to 4 hours of preparation, and examined within 24 hours.[4,6] Exposure of smears to formalin must be avoided.

Table 1
Hematologic reference values for the bearded dragon (*P. vitticeps*) from various publications and the author's (KLW) institution

Measurements	Moichor	Ellman 1997	Howard 2021 ♂	Howard 2021 ♀	SPECIES360
N	43	21	83	47	30
PCV (%)	20–44	17–41	24–48	18–38	15–48
WBC (10^3/µL)	5.6–19.1	6.7–19.9	4.1–19.2	3.9–28.4	0–21.6
Hets (%)	5–60	17–43	—	—	—
Hets (10^3/µL)	0.8–7.4	1.6–7.3	0.8–11.3	1.3–15.5	0–6.1
Bands (%)	0–3	—	—	—	—
Bands (10^3/µL)	0–0.2	—	—	—	—
Lymphs (%)	14–90	47–69	—	—	—
Lymphs (10^3/µL)	1.5–12.4	4.0–12.0	1.0–9.0	0.9–8.4	0–16.2
Azurophils (%)	0–13	0–9	—	—	—
Azurophils (10^3/µL)	0–2.0	0–1.1.	—	—	—
Monocytes (%)	0–2	0–4	—	—	—
Monocytes (10^3/µL)	0–0.2	0–0.5	0.2–4.2	0.3–9.0	0–0.97
Basophils (%)	1–10	2–18	—	—	—
Basophils (10^3/µL)	0.2–1.3	0.2–3.2	0–1.7	0–2.3	0–1.8
Eosinophils (%)	0–1	—	—	—	—
Eosinophils (10^3/µL)	0–0.2	—	0–0.1	0–0.1	0–0.9

Parameters evaluated in a routine bearded dragon CBC are similar to other reptiles and generally include packed cell volume (PCV) and total solids (plasma protein), red blood cell (RBC) count, RBC indices, total white blood cell (WBC) count and differential, thrombocyte estimation, and morphologic evaluation of erythrocytes and leukocytes.[4,5]

Erythron

As with other reptiles, bearded dragon erythrocytes are nucleated ellipsoid discs with an average life span of 600 to 800 days.[5] Erythrocytes generally display minimal anisocytosis. Because they are nucleated and nonspherical, erythrocytes pose an analytical challenge for modern hematology analyzers. For this reason, indices such as mean corpuscular volume (MCV), mean corpuscular hemoglobin concentration (MCHC), mean cell hemoglobin (MCH), and hemoglobin concentration (Hb) may be difficult to determine without species-specific settings.[4] Furthermore, calculated hematocrit (HCT) should be interpreted with caution because the ellipsoid shape of erythrocytes may result in discrepant results when compared with a spun PCV, which is considered the gold standard in reptiles.[4] PCV of most healthy bearded dragons is between 20% and 40% and this lower range suggests a decreased oxygen-carrying capacity in reptiles as compared with mammals and birds.[5] Similarly, Hb is expected to be lower in reptiles.

Increases or decreases in PCV, termed erythrocytosis or anemia, respectively, have numerous causes that may be physiologic, artifactual, or associated with disease processes similar to those in mammals. In general, indices such as PCV, RBC, MCV, MCHC, MCH, and Hb tend to increase with age.[4] Although an increased PCV with a robust regenerative response may be observed posthibernation (brumation), erythrocytosis is more commonly a result of dehydration secondary to improper husbandry or gastrointestinal or renal pathologic conditions.[4] If an animal is anemic (**Fig. 1**), the presence or absence of a regenerative response can aid in prioritizing differentials. Pathologic causes associated with regenerative anemia in reptiles most often are a result of acute blood loss secondary to parasitism (endoparasites/hemoparasites, ectoparasites), hemolysis, gastrointestinal disease, or trauma, whereas animals suffering from chronic conditions such as systemic inflammation, infection, iron deficiency, malnutrition, bone marrow dysfunction, or neoplasia are more likely to exhibit a nonregenerative anemia.[4,7] Successful management of a bearded dragon with a PCV as low as 3% secondary to hemocoelom from an ovarian rupture has been described.[7] In

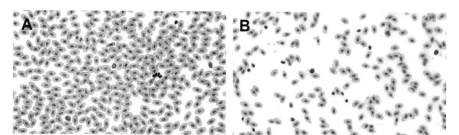

Fig. 1. (*A*) Monolayer of a blood smear from a nonanemic bearded dragon (*P. vitticeps*) with a PCV of 44%; RBCs abut each other with very little visible white space in the background. (*B*) Monolayer of a blood smear from an anemic bearded dragon (*P. vitticeps*) with a PCV of 15%; RBCs are dispersed far from one another with markedly increased white space in the background; 400× magnification, modified Wright's stain.

cases of iron deficiency anemia, erythrocytes often are hypochromic with a decreased MCV and MCHC. Although reptilian erythrocytes generally are sturdy and more resistant to fragmentation or morphologic changes when compared with mammalian erythrocytes, cells with a fusiform/spindle or teardrop shape (dacryocytes) can be seen in association with chronic disease, sepsis, or iron deficiency (**Fig. 2**).[5] Healthy bearded dragons normally have less than 5% polychromatophils (reticulocytes) in circulation, which are expected to increase with regeneration.[5] An important difference from mammals is that polychromatophils in reptiles are smaller than mature erythrocytes, thus the MCV may be decreased with regenerative anemia.[4] Polychromatophils in bearded dragons and other reptiles are more round, basophilic, and have a higher nuclear to cytoplasmic (N:C) ratio when compared with mature erythrocytes. Morphologic changes that can be observed in peripheral blood consistent with erythrocyte regeneration include basophilic stippling, polychromasia, anisocytosis and anisokaryosis, binucleation and mitotic figures, and/or increased erythroid precursors (left shift; **Fig. 3**).[4] Polychromasia can be increased in juvenile animals or during ecdysis, whereas basophilic stippling may also be observed with lead, zinc, or other heavy metal toxicity.[5] The amount of time necessary for a regenerative response to occur in reptiles is not well characterized but likely is longer than the 3 to 5 day time period for many mammals.

Another important component of the erythron is the evaluation for the presence of inclusions. Differential diagnoses for intraerythrocytic inclusions in bearded dragons are numerous and should include viral inclusions, erythrocytic parasites, bacteria, crystallized hemoglobin (**Fig. 4**), degenerate organelles (eg, clumped endoplasmic reticulum) associated with chronic disease, and drying artifact.[8] Hemoparasites rarely cause clinical illness unless the burden is severe, in which case hemolytic anemia may occur.

Leukon

The preferred method for total WBC determination in reptiles is a manual count, with the use of a hemocytometer chamber preferred over leukocyte estimation, although both methods are subject to error.[4] Romanowsky stains (Wright's, modified Wright's, Giemsa) can be used for the evaluation of bearded dragon blood smears. Methanolic-based Romanowsky stains are preferred because their aqueous counterparts (Diff-Quik) often fail to adequately stain basophil granules, which may cause confusion

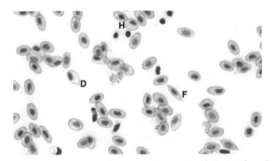

Fig. 2. Blood smear from same bearded dragon (*P. vitticeps*) as 1B showing microscopic evidence of iron deficiency. Note the hypochromic RBCs (H), dacryocytes (D), and fusiform RBCs (F). Dacryocytes are RBCs that take on a "teardrop" shape: one pole is rounded, whereas the other is tapered. Occasionally, the rounded end seems enlarged and bulbous. Fusiform RBCs are spindled cells that are tapered at both poles; 400× magnification, modified Wright's stain.

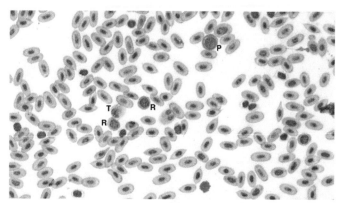

Fig. 3. Blood smear exhibiting an erythroid left shift. Prorubricytes follow rubriblasts in the RBC maturation sequence. They are large in size with a high N:C ratio, deep blue cytoplasm, and coarse chromatin. Nucleoli that were apparent in the rubriblast stage are no longer visible. Rubricytes represent the next stage in RBC maturation. They are smaller than prorubricytes with cytoplasm that is more medium blue and a slightly lower N:C ratio. The nucleus is characterized by lighter and darker areas of condensation. Note the toxic heterophil among the rubricytes. Toxic features seen here include cytoplasmic basophilia, partial degranulation, and a few atypical granules. P: prorubricyte, R: rubricyte, T: toxic heterophil; 400× magnification, modified Wright's stain.

when performing leukocyte differential counts.[6,9] Both staining methods result in good cytoplasmic detail but nuclear detail may be less clear.

Leukocytes in the bearded dragon generally are categorized as agranulocytic mononuclear cells such as lymphocytes, monocytes, and azurophils, or granulocytes including heterophils, eosinophils, and basophils (**Fig. 5**). Although recent reports describing morphology of leukocytes in the bearded dragon are not available to the best of the authors' knowledge, their characteristics have been described,[6] and cells are, for the most part, similar in cytologic appearance to those of other reptiles, which have been characterized elsewhere.[5] The predominant leukocyte present in the peripheral blood of healthy bearded dragons is the small lymphocyte, which can comprise up to 80% of the leukocyte differential. Lymphocytes in bearded dragons have similar morphology and function to those in birds and mammals. Cells are generally small but can range from 5 to 15 μm, display a high N:C ratio with a round to

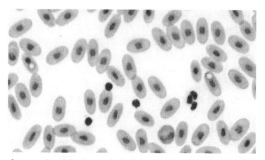

Fig. 4. Blood smear from a healthy bearded dragon (*P. vitticeps*) featuring 2 colorless, geometric erythrocyte inclusions consistent with hemoglobin crystallization. These inclusions are currently considered clinically insignificant; 400× magnification, modified Wright's stain.

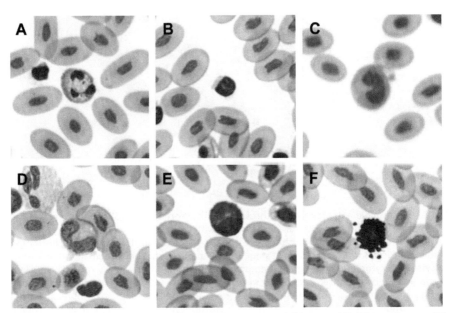

Fig. 5. Bearded dragon (*P. vitticeps*) leukocytes. Top row: (*A*) heterophil, (*B*) lymphocyte, (*C*) azurophil; Bottom row: (*D*) monocyte, (*E*) eosinophil, (*F*) basophil; 400× magnification, modified Wright's stain.

indented nucleus, and can be challenging to differentiate from nucleated thrombo-cytes on microscopic examination.[5,6] Lymphocytes may display irregular morphology in peripheral blood smears if they conform to or mold around adjacent cells. Lympho-cytosis can result from subacute or chronic antigenic stimulation, inflammation, infec-tion (bacterial, viral, parasitic), and wound healing, and increased proportions of large lymphocytes, reactive or plasmacytoid lymphocytes, granular lymphocytes, and rarely plasma cells may be observed.[4] Lymphoid leukemias have also been reported in bearded dragons. Lymphopenia may be associated with poor husbandry or malnutri-tion, acute bacterial infection, or exposure to excessive endogenous or exogenous hormones including corticosteroids or testosterone.[4]

Monocytes (see **Fig. 5D**) are generally large round to oval cells with moderate-to-high amounts of blue-gray cytoplasm and an irregular, pleomorphic nucleus, and typi-cally compose 0 to 10% of the leukocyte differential.[5] Cells may display cytoplasmic vacuoles when activated to perform phagocytic activity.[5] Azurophils are morphologi-cally similar to monocytes with the distinction of many fine dark blue to purple azuro-philic cytoplasmic granules and possibly a slightly smaller size. Azurophils are unique to reptiles and suspected to have functions similar to those of monocytes and hetero-phils, although their exact role remains to be determined.[4,5] Although typically only rarely observed in bearded dragons, increases of these cells may be associated with chronic antigenic stimulation or inflammation, infectious disease, dystocia, or leu-kemia.[4] A small proportion of monocytes in circulation may contain intracellular melanin pigment (melanomacrophages), erythrocytes, or hemosiderin pigment.[5] Pre-sumed chronic monocytic leukemia in a bearded dragon has been reported.

Heterophils are the predominant granulocyte in circulation in most bearded dragons and are considered functionally similar to mammalian neutrophils, although they gener-ally lack myeloperoxidase activity, which is responsible for the formation of liquid pus in many domestic mammals.[4,5] However, these activities have not been specifically confirmed for bearded dragons. Heterophils can exhibit variability in their size and staining characteristics but typically display moderate amounts of clear to light blue cytoplasm that contains a bilobed to multilobed nucleus and many rod-shaped granules that most often are pink to orange but may appear blue–green or fail to uptake stain altogether.[4,5] Heterophil granules may seem less eosinophilic or less distinct when stained with Diff-Quik compared with modified Wright's stain.[6] Heterophilia is most often a result of acute inflammation secondary to bacterial infection, tissue injury or necrosis secondary to trauma or neoplasia, excessive glucocorticoids, or rarely granulocytic leukemia.[4,5] With severe inflammation, toxic change may be observed in conjunction with a heteropenia and/or left shift. Toxic heterophils generally display increased cytoplasmic basophilia and degranulation and, with more severe disease, may exhibit cytoplasmic vacuolation and nuclear hypersegmentation (**Fig. 6**).[5] A small proportion of heterophils may display degranulation in normal reptiles, whereas a larger proportion exhibiting degranulation without cytoplasmic basophilia may occur based on inappropriate sample handling or prolonged storage.[5] Heteropenia has been associated with severe acute inflammation (eg, sepsis) and acute drug toxicity.[4]

Eosinophils are infrequently observed in healthy bearded dragons and are identified by visualization of abundant pink to dark gray, round, cytoplasmic granules and a central to eccentrically placed, round to oval to bilobed or band-shaped nucleus.[4–6] Among reptiles, lizards have the smallest eosinophils. Their exact function is not well characterized but similar to mammals, increases have been associated with parasitic diseases (helminths, protozoa) and antigenic stimulation.[5]

Basophils are characterized by their pale purple cytoplasm that contains abundant fine, round, metachromatic (dark purple) granules that often obscure the round nucleus. Similar to eosinophils, basophils tend to be smaller than heterophils in bearded dragons.[6] Cells can degranulate during sample collection, delayed processing, or as an artifact of preparation or their granules may fail to display metachromatic staining when aqueous-based stains (eg, Diff-Quik) are used.[4,5] The function of reptilian basophils is poorly understood but an increase in peripheral counts may be attributed to hemoparasites (eg, Hemogregarine, *Trypanosoma*; **Fig. 7**) or iridovirus infection.[4,5]

Thrombon

Thrombocytes in reptiles are similar to mammalian platelets with a few distinct differences. In mammals, platelets are derived from cytoplasmic fragments of

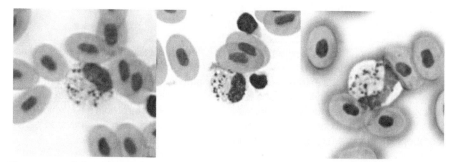

Fig. 6. Toxic, left-shifted (band) heterophils from a 3-year-old bearded dragon (*P. vitticeps*) presented with a forelimb abscess. The nucleus of each cell lacks segmentation and chromatin is more open. Features of toxic change include cytoplasmic basophilia, degranulation, and toxic granules; 400× magnification, modified Wright's stain.

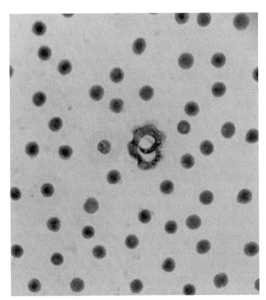

Fig. 7. Unspeciated Trypanosome in peripheral blood of a bearded dragon (*P. vitticeps*). To the left is an intact RBC. The background contains numerous free nuclei of lysed RBCs; 600× magnification, modified Wright's stain.

megakaryocytes in the bone marrow, whereas thrombocytes represent a unique cell line that arises from thromboblasts in hematopoietic tissue.[5] Thrombocytes are nucleated, ovoid cells with scant cytoplasm and a high N:C ratio that can be difficult to differentiate from small lymphocytes, although usually are smaller. These cells become rounded and may display a cytoplasmic pseudopod when activated and are also involved in wound healing and suspected to possess phagocytic capabilities.[4–6] Atypical thrombocytes with pleomorphic nuclei may occasionally be noted with severe inflammation. Because an adequate method for quantification of thrombocytes remains to be determined, numbers are typically estimated as adequate, increased, decreased, or clumped.[4] Platelet clumping can aid in morphologic evaluation and is commonly present in lithium-heparin anticoagulated samples. If thrombocytopenia is suspected, preanalytical errors including prolonged blood draw, delayed processing, and clotting of the sample should first be ruled out.[5]

Coagulation

Available studies characterizing hemostasis in reptiles are generally lacking and many aspects of coagulability testing remain to be well defined. Coagulation in reptiles is thought to involve predominantly the extrinsic and common pathways, whereas the intrinsic pathway is likely of little clinical significance due to low thromboplastin activity and a lack of other clotting factors from the intrinsic pathway.[10,11] As such, the prothrombin time, which evaluates the extrinsic and common pathways, will be of more use than the activated partial thromboplastin time, which evaluates the intrinsic and common pathways.

CLINICAL CHEMISTRY

The evaluation of plasma or serum biochemistry values can provide valuable information that is used to assess general wellness, metabolic abnormalities in sick animals, monitor response to therapy, or aid in the determination of prognosis.[12] A systematic approach based on clinician preference can aid in creating a prioritized problem list and differentials for any abnormalities present. For example, analytes in a biochemical panel may be grouped by organ or organ system (eg, hepatic, renal/urogenital, gastro-intestinal, and so forth) or by the class of analyte being measured (eg, enzymes, ions, proteins, lipids, and so forth). However, similar to hematologic changes, interpretation of chemistry values in bearded dragons can be complicated by individual variation or alteration based on the effect of age, sex, environmental temperature, or seasonal-ity.[3,11] Several studies have been performed to determine appropriate reference ranges for hematologic and biochemical values in wild bearded dragons in Australia,[13] as well as the effects of sex and season on biochemical values in captive bearded dragons.[3] Clinical chemistry reference intervals for bearded dragons from a variety of sources are presented in **Table 2**.

The sample of choice for a clinical chemistry panel in bearded dragons is lithium-heparin plasma because hemolysis is less common with this anticoagulant, and serum requires a larger volume of blood to be collected and an increased amount of time to analysis due to the necessity for complete clot formation.[12] Gel separator tubes are not recommended as incomplete separation or delayed processing can interfere with analysis. Plasma should be collected and ideally analyzed immediately after centrifugation but can be processed up to 24 hours after collection if refrigerated or frozen.[12] Before analysis, plasma characteristics should be noted for clarity, turbidity, and gross evidence of lipemia (opaque white), biliverdinemia (green), lymphatic

Table 2
Plasma biochemical reference values for the bearded dragon (*P. vitticeps*) from various publications and the author's (KLW) institution

Measurements	Moichor	Ellman 1997	Tamukai 2011 ♂	Tamukai 2011 ♀	Howard 2021 ♂	Howard 2021 ♀
N	43	21	35	65	83	46
Total Protein (g/dL)	3–6.9	4.5–9.5[a]	3.5–6.9	3.6–7.8	2.5–5.7	2.6–5.8
Albumin (g/dL)	1.8–5.7	—	1.6–3.1	1.5–3.0	1.4–3.5	1.0–30
Globulins (g/dL)	0.1–2.3	—	—	—	1.0–2.7	0.9–4.5
ALT (IU/L)	1–35	< 3–5	1–16	1–11	—	—
AST (IU/L)	7–51	4–40	3–28	2–26	5–52	5–62
Bile acids (μmol/L)	0–21	—	—	—	1–25	1–37
Bun (mg/dL)	0–3	<1–2	< 1	< 1	1–2	1–2
Uric Acid (mg/dL)	1–11.2	1.6–11.4	1.6–8.8	1.8–7.6	0–0.03	0–0.03
Phosphorus (mg/dL)	2.2–7.4	3.5–9.8	2.6–7.0	2.7–6.9	2.8–7.1	2.5–14.9
Calcium	10–21	8.6–19.4	10.3–14.9	8.6–23.2	8.0–17.4	8.5–86.6
Glucose	140–282	139–291	149–346	152–326	153–312	171–331
Sodium (mmol/L)	131 165	141–163	141–163	140–165	—	—
Potassium (mmol/L)	3.2–5.4	1.0–6.5	2.8–5.4	3.0–4.0	—	—
Chloride (mmol/L)	90–130	97–140	91–125	91–128	—	—
CK (U/L)	61–1500	—	43–3,580	26–4746	43–5637	13–5498
Cholesterol (mg/dL)	130–427	312–1129	125–294	142–476	77–305	112–440
Triglycerides (mg/dL)	12–404	—	44–325	19–373	9–310	18–1673

[a] Total solids.

contamination (clear to light yellow), and hemolysis (red, orange, pink), although the degree of interference induced by these changes is still not well understood. Fasting for a minimum of 24 hours up to several days is recommended to avoid lipemic samples but lipemia may still be present in bearded dragons with hepatic lipidosis or females undergoing vitellogenesis.[13]

Retrospective reviews[1,14] report that the systems most commonly affected by disease in the bearded dragon are the gastrointestinal, integumentary, hepatobiliary, and urinary systems, with a predominance of infectious or noninfectious inflammatory or degenerative etiologies over neoplastic conditions. In regards to neoplasia, other reports describe that the most commonly affected organs in lizards are the skin,[15] liver,[16] and hematopoietic tissue.[17] Therefore, a systems-based approach will be used to explain biochemical abnormalities in bearded dragons.

Gastrointestinal

Bearded dragons can suffer from several gastrointestinal conditions of infectious, inflammatory, or neoplastic cause. A review of 529 captive bearded dragons found that almost 43% of bearded dragons suffered from gastrointestinal conditions including endoparasitism, constipation, and sand ingestion.[14] In animals with constipation, 51.92% and 38.46% had evidence for endoparasitism (pinworms, coccidians [Fig. 9], flagellates) and metabolic bone disease (MBD), respectively, and MBD is a known contributing factor for constipation.[18] More than 80% of all fecal samples submitted were positive for parasites. Biochemical changes may be similar to those in mammals in the case of proximal gastrointestinal disease, in which case hypochloremic, hypokalemic metabolic alkalosis is a common finding.[19] If a necrotic lesion is present within the gastrointestinal tract, creatine kinase (CK) and aspartate aminotransferase (AST) may increase when released from damaged smooth muscle. However, AST can be released from other tissues and is not specific for muscle or hepatocellular injury. Nitrogenous waste products (urea, uric acid) can increase with dehydration or gastrointestinal hemorrhage but body condition should be considered because emaciated animals are likely in a state of increased tissue catabolism.[19]

Hepatobiliary

The usefulness of various enzymes as they relate to hepatic pathologic conditions is largely unknown, as to the authors' knowledge, no species-specific studies have investigated their utility in bearded dragons. Enzyme tissue distribution has yet to be specifically evaluated for the bearded dragon. Enzyme activities measured in lizards typically associated with hepatocellular injury in mammals include AST, alanine aminotransferase (ALT), sorbitol dehydrogenase (SDH), and lactate dehydrogenase (LDH), whereas those associated with cholestasis include alkaline phosphatase (ALP) and gamma glutamyltransferase (GGT). Measurement of these enzyme activities and their half-lives in lizards is of unknown accuracy or utility because the assays were developed for mammals and run at 37°C.[11] Furthermore, studies suggest these enzyme activities are present in a variety of other tissues, particularly muscle, or have isoenzymes (LDH) and thus are not specific for liver pathologic condition.[11] However, increases in plasma concentrations of AST, ALT, LDH, and SDH can be present in lizards with hepatitis or hepatic neoplasia.

Bile acids are synthesized in hepatocytes of all vertebrates and can be helpful in the assessment of liver function in bearded dragons. Bile acids are conjugated in hepatocytes and cholangiocytes before secretion into the biliary and intestinal systems to aid in lipid digestion. After deconjugation by gut flora, bile acids are reabsorbed in the ileum and transported back to the liver via portal circulation to be reconjugated. Bearded dragons should be fasted for a minimum of 48 hours before collection of a baseline preprandial sample (RI: 0.8–33.7 μmol/L).[10,11] A postprandial sample of plasma collected 4 to 24 hours later with increased bile acids (RI: 1.4–37.6 μmol/L) is consistent with decreased hepatic functional capacity, and causes including cirrhosis, lipidosis, and neoplasia should be investigated.[12]

Additional analytes that may decrease with chronic hepatic insufficiency include albumin, glucose, and urea and uric acid; however, these analytes can be affected by other variables such as nutrition, hydration, temperature, and gastrointestinal or renal disease. Therefore, the entire clinical picture should be considered before diagnosing liver disease.[12]

Fatty deposition within the liver (Fatty liver syndrome) is common in bearded dragons and can occur as normal physiologic change during vitellogenesis, before brumation, or based on several other reasons. Diagnosis of pathologic hepatic lipidosis should be reserved for when the entire clinical picture (age, sex, nutrition, reproductive status, season, clinicopathologic findings) can be considered.[1,10] The combination of factors that result in this clinical entity still remains poorly understood. Predisposing factors for hepatic lipidosis include animals with low activity level and a high fat diet (mice, wax worms, nongut-loaded insects), obese animals that develop acute anorexia, and aged females that have undergone seasonal cycles of lipogenesis for vitellogenesis before breeding season.[10,20] Clinicians should consider hepatic lipidosis when a lizard has a consistent clinical history and evidence for a persistent increase in plasma triglycerides, cholesterol, and lipoproteins. Hepatocellular enzymes may not be supportive of this diagnosis because hepatocellular injury is rarely significant with fatty change, and hyperbiliverdinemia would be unexpected because cholestasis is not a prominent feature of this syndrome.[14] However, hypoalbuminemia and increased bile acids suggest reduced hepatic functional capacity.[10,21] Stains that can be used to highlight lipid in cytologic preparations include Oil Red O or Sudan black B but cytology is an insensitive method for diagnosis and biopsy is considered the gold standard.

Renal and Urogenital

Bearded dragons lack a urinary bladder and can instead store urine in the colon, with most nitrogenous waste excreted in the form of urates. Therefore, urinalysis is of minimal diagnostic utility in this species. The majority of renal and urogenital diseases in bearded dragons include chronic renal disease/nephritis and dystocia.[14]

Uric acid may increase significantly only in the late stages of renal disease but can also be altered with nonrenal conditions including dehydration, a high-protein diet, or hypothermia.[12] Bearded dragons may experience a significant increase in plasma levels of uric acid between 4 and 24 hours after being fed 1% of their body weight in gut-loaded crickets.[22] This increase typically returns to baseline within 48 hours of the meal. Urea and creatinine are unreliable markers for renal disease in lizards due to their small amount of production, inconsistent elimination, and variability with hydration status.[11,23] Measurement of ammonia concentration is seldom practical due to its high volatility and the necessity for transport on ice preceding prompt analysis. Toxic nephropathy is not particularly common but can occur from treatment with aminoglycosides, exogenous dietary supplementation of vitamin D_3 (cholecalciferol), or heavy metal toxicity with lead.[23,24] Vitamin D_3 over supplementation, when severe, would be expected to cause hypercalcemia leading to metastatic mineralization of tissues, including the kidneys. Commercial assays for plasma vitamin D_3 concentration may be helpful in assessing for possibility of toxicosis, but to the authors' knowledge a consensus on the reference interval for this analyte is not available.[23]

Gout is among the most common systemic diseases in this species, and may be of the visceral form involving organs in the coelomic cavity including the spleen, liver, kidneys, or pericardial sac, or the articular form in the case that joints are affected.[1,20] Lizards with the articular form may be lethargic, anorexic, and have swelling of the limbs and pain causing reluctance to move.[25] Cytologically, variable numbers of inflammatory cells admixed with irregular, needle-like, refractile crystals that are highly birefringent under polarized light can be present within phagocytic cells and the background. Disease occurs due to decreased renal excretion of uric acid with subsequent hyperuricemia, ultimately resulting in deposition of monosodium urate crystals (tophi) in tissues and resulting granulomatous inflammation.[25] Risk factors include dehydration, cachexia, diets consisting predominantly of insects or other high protein food, chronic dehydration, and renal damage. Pseudogout has also been described[26] in a bearded dragon with a similar clinical presentation in which there was radiographic evidence of mineralization and decreased definition of the articular surfaces of the femorotibial joint, as well as lysis of the distal femur and proximal tibia. Cytologically, fine needle aspirates contained numerous rod-shaped to rhomboid crystals consistent in morphology with calcium pyrophosphate, a byproduct of numerous metabolic pathways that may be increased in a number of underlying conditions.

Musculoskeletal

CK activity can be high in the skeletal and cardiac muscle and suggestive of muscle damage if an elevated concentration is present in plasma. Similar to mammals, AST and LDH activity may also be increased with muscle injury but are found in other tissues and thus not specific.[11]

Lipid and Protein

The most clinically relevant lipids in bearded dragons include triglycerides and cholesterol, which similar to many other analytes in lizards, can increase or decrease for physiologic reasons (eg, seasonality) or as a result of pathologic conditions. Cholesterol and triglyceride concentrations are commonly increased in females during vitellogenesis or in lizards before brumation,[11,12] and in wild bearded dragons they were relatively increased in females compared with males irrespective of seasonality.[13] Pathologic increases in triglyceride concentrations are associated with obesity and hepatic lipidosis, whereas hypercholesterolemia may result from extrahepatic biliary obstruction and has been reported in one bearded dragon[27] with atherosclerosis and associated pericardial effusion. However, another bearded dragon[28] with severe atherosclerosis had a normal plasma cholesterol concentration. Increased plasma cholesterol concentration is a risk factor for vascular pathology in various animal species but was within the reference interval in a bearded dragon with a tail base aneurysm.[29] Decreased cholesterol concentration may occur based on stress, increased age, or egg laying in females.[3,12] Bearded dragons that are obese or fed a high fat diet (eg, predominantly insects) may be predisposed to cholelithiasis due to increased bile synthesis for lipid digestion, which may facilitate bile sludge formation. Choleliths in bearded dragons are likely underdiagnosed and often an incidental finding during surgery or at necropsy.[10,30] Bearded dragon choleliths are composed of predominantly proteinaceous material or calcium carbonate ($CaCO_3$) but choleliths composed of significant amounts of cholesterol have been identified in humans. The biliary coccidian parasite *Choleoeimeria pogonae* (formerly *Eimeria pogonae*) has been demonstrated to alter the bile composition in a central bearded dragon and caused a significant decrease in the amount of normally predominantly taurine-conjugated bile acids.[31] Although this decrease in taurine-conjugated bile acids may decrease bile acid solubility, decrease lipid emulsification, and promote calcium precipitation, an association with *C. pogonae* infection and development of cholelithiasis has not been characterized.

Blood proteins predominantly consist of albumin and globulins and are commonly quantified by refractometry or the colorimetric Biuret method, the latter of which is considered more accurate.[11] The bromocresol green method for measurement of albumin concentration is inaccurate in bearded dragons and has been demonstrated to overestimate albumin concentration, particularly at lower albumin concentrations as determined by protein electrophoresis (EPH). Therefore, EPH remains the gold standard for characterization of blood protein fractions in this species.[32] The preferred sample for EPH is plasma instead of serum, given that fibrinogen is a significant positive acute phase protein in reptiles. Unlike mammals, healthy reptiles tend to have an inverted albumin:globulin (A:G) ratio with higher globulins relative to albumin.[11,32] Alterations in plasma or serum protein concentrations are generally nonspecific. Increased protein most often results from dehydration or vitellogenesis, whereas hypoproteinemia is associated with protein-losing conditions including various enteropathies (eg, stricture), nephropathy, or dermatopathy (eg, thermal burns).[12] Globulins and albumin in reptiles likely act as positive and negative acute phase proteins (APP), respectively, and concentrations should be interpreted in conjunction with a CBC and in light of the patient's gastrointestinal, renal, and hepatic health.[11,12]

Electrolytes

Differentials for electrolyte abnormalities in bearded dragons are similar to those in mammals and generally include gastrointestinal disease, renal disease, dehydration, or iatrogenic causes (eg, fluid therapy). Derangements should be interpreted based on the patient's hydration status and husbandry conditions including diet and temperature.[11] Determination of plasma osmolality, the measure of solutes or particles in a solution regardless of their charge, is highly recommended for patients for which fluid therapy is indicated so as to prevent potential adverse effects related to fluid shifting.[33] The mean plasma osmolality among 11 healthy adult male bearded dragons was determined to be 295.4 ± 9.35 mOsm/kg and is similar to that of other domestic species.[33] Although other equations consider plasma glucose concentration and plasma uric acid concentration, based on this study, in the absence of an appropriate osmometer, the recommended equation for calculating osmolality in bearded dragons was $1.85 \times (Na^+ + K^+)$.

INFECTION, NEOPLASIA, AND SELECTED METABOLIC CONDITIONS

Although metabolic disease occurs with some regularity in bearded dragons, infectious and inflammatory disease are among the most common pathologic conditions affecting this species, with various bacterial, fungal, viral, and parasitic causes frequently implicated.[1] For this reason, it is recommended that new lizards undergo a quarantine period before introduction with other reptiles. Furthermore, normal flora from a particular anatomic site may cause pathologic condition at foreign sites or in other species. For example, one report[34] describes isolation of *Devriesea agamarum* bacteria from the oral cavity of wild agamid lizards (*Pogona, Uromastyx, Agama*) symptomatic for cheilitis. The organism was also isolated from clinically healthy bearded dragons but when inoculated at areas of compromised skin barrier, subsequently induced dermatitis.

Bacterial Infections

Bacterial infections in lizards are more often caused by Gram-negative bacteria than Gram-positive bacteria, with organisms implicated including *Salmonella*,

Pseudomonas, *Aeromonas*, *Proteus*, and *Klebsiella* spp, among others. Anaerobes including *Clostridium*, *Bacteroides*, and *Fusobacterium* spp may also be encountered. Affected lizards often have a heterophilia with a left shift and evidence of toxic change ± monocytosis/azurophilia. *Salmonella enterica* subsp. *enterica* serovar *Brandenburg* has been described to cause hepatobiliary inflammation, hepatic necrosis, and sepsis (**Fig. 8**) in bearded dragons.[1] A *Klebsiella* sp was demonstrated to cause infectious spondylitis in another, although the route of infection was unclear, and a CBC and biochemistry panel demonstrated no abnormalities.[35] A case of systemic mycobacteriosis[36] described a bearded dragon in which *Mycobacterium marinum* was detected in joint aspirates and lung tissue. On cytologic examination of joint aspirates, numerous negatively stained bacterial rods were observed within the extracellular environment and within vacuolated mononuclear cells, and later confirmed as acid-fast. Another bearded dragon was demonstrated to have an atypical presentation of mycobacteriosis causing bony lysis and proliferation and granulomatous osteomyelitis in the right stifle.[37] If mycobacterial infection is suspected, it is recommended to use a number of acid-fast stains and speciate the organism because different species may display variable staining characteristics and require different treatments.[1,37] In many cases, suboptimal environmental temperature may predispose to infection based on reduced immune function.

Viral Infections

Viral agents most commonly reported to infect bearded dragons include adenovirus, iridovirus, and ranavirus, and an overview of viruses infecting reptiles is available.[38] Adenovirus typically infects juveniles via the fecal-oral route or contact with oronasal secretions, and affected animals are often presented for failure to thrive but symptoms

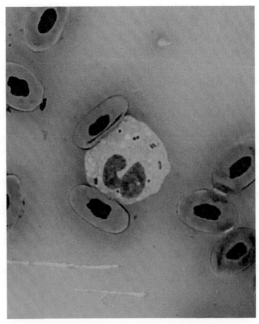

Fig. 8. Heterophil containing intracellular bacterial rods and cocci from a septic patient; 600× magnification, modified Wright's stain.

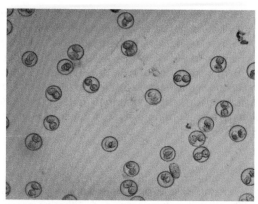

Fig. 9. Numerous *Isospora amphiboluri* oocysts in an unstained fecal wet mount; 400× magnification, modified Wright's stain.

such as head tilt, circling, and opisthotonus may also be present and suggest involvement of the central nervous system.[38] However, affected animals may not show clinical symptoms. Adenovirus infection can manifest in a variety of clinical presentations, and although specific clinicopathologic alterations have not been described in association with adenovirus, expected findings may include elevated enzyme activity of ALT and AST, suggesting hepatocellular injury due to hepatic necrosis. Hepatic insufficiency may also result in decreased plasma concentrations of albumin, blood glucose, or cholesterol, and an increase in total bilirubin.

Erythrocytic iridovirus infection in 11 captive central bearded dragons resulted in HCT decrease in all animals during a 2 month period but remained within the reference interval in all but one lizard. Approximately 40% to 50% of erythrocytes contained one to less often 2 intracytoplasmic viral inclusions approximately 1.4 to 2.8 μm, which demonstrated variable blue staining intensity.[8] Additional microscopic findings may include hypochromasia and polychromasia. Although the mechanism of RBC death for infected erythrocytes is not clear, proposed theories include increased osmotic fragility and immune-mediated phagocytosis.[8]

The pathogenesis of ranavirus infection in bearded dragons is poorly understood. One report[39] described ranavirus coinfection in a colony of inland bearded dragons with multifocal flat to nodular superficial skin lesions caused by the contagious and zoonotic bacteria *Dermatophilus chelonae* (*Austwickia chelonae*). Lesions contained branching filamentous bacteria and Gram-positive cocci present in 2 to 4 parallel rows, consistent with the "railroad tracks" classically associated with dermatophilosis but no clinicopathologic changes attributable to ranavirus were described. Differentials for ulcerative or necrotizing skin lesions in bearded dragons include dermatitis secondary to poor husbandry (thermal burns, unsanitary conditions, excessive humidity), trauma, bacterial or fungal dermatitis, parasitic infection (acariasis), and neoplasia (squamous cell carcinoma [SCC], melanoma).[15,39]

Fungal Infections

The most well-known fungal agents that infect bearded dragons are the Chrysosporium-related fungi *Chrysosporium* anamorph of *Nannizziopsis vriesii* and *N. guarroi*, causative agents of "yellow fungus disease." Microscopically, granulomatous inflammation is evident with abundant macrophages, fewer heterophils, and possibly occasional multinucleated giant cells (pyogranulomatous inflammation).[40] Organisms may be visualized as branching to undulating, septated hyphae 4 to 12 μm thick with variable length and a thin, clear cell wall, or as 5 to 8 μm long and 2 to 5 μm wide clavate to ovoid conidia with a central purple nucleus and thin clear capsule.[40,41] Animals may also have a heterophilia, lymphocytosis, and monocytosis in conjunction with anemia attributed to chronic disease. Although cytology of impression smears can be performed for a preliminary diagnosis, a combination of biopsy, fungal culture in appropriate conditions, and PCR are considered the gold standard.[41]

NEOPLASIA

Neoplasia of lizards is not uncommon and bearded dragons seem to be no exception, with more than 20 different tumor types reported. Although comprehensive reviews regarding neoplasia specific to the bearded dragon are not available, there are several reviews characterizing neoplasia with scope limited to lizards,[15,42] and others that encompass class *Reptilia* as a whole.[16,17,43] We will focus our discussion of neopasia of bearded dragons to those with reported clinicopathologic findings (eg, paraneoplastic syndromes) and description of those with supportive cytologic findings within the literature and our institutions' experience.

Hematologic changes in bearded dragons with neoplasia may be related to the chronic nature of disease or inflammation resulting from the neoplastic process or secondary infection, and plasma biochemical abnormalities may reflect dysfunction of the organ(s) affected. For example, one bearded dragon with liposarcoma of the fat body was described to have a severe leukocytosis characterized by a heterophilia with a left shift and monocytosis (attributed to secondary infection or tumor-associated inflammation/necrosis) as well as total and ionized hypercalcemia, hyperlactatemia, and azotemia.[44] Although humoral hypercalcemia of malignancy is common in mammals, it has not been reported in bearded dragons but was considered a differential for the hypercalcemia, among other causes. Cytologic examination of tissues and body fluids may be performed in-clinic or sent out to a diagnostic laboratory, and is often useful in differentiating inflammatory and neoplastic lesions. Publications describing the utility of cytology for reptiles can be consulted.[45,46]

Numerous case reports describing neoplasms in bearded dragons are available, and cases predominantly describe integumentary, hepatobiliary, or hematopoietic involvement. This species is overrepresented in the literature for developing SCC, which often arises in the periorbital/periocular area or in close proximity to a mucocutaneous junction.[15] A causative relationship between long-term exposure to high-intensity artificial ultraviolet light and the development of SCC or other skin tumors has been proposed but remains to be defined.[15] Other ocular or periocular neoplasms identified in bearded dragons include fibroma, papilloma, fibropapilloma, adenocarcinoma,[2] and myxosarcoma.[47] Additional neoplasms reported to arise within cutaneous and subcutaneous tissues include chromatophoromas, myxoma,[48] benign peripheral nerve sheath tumor,[49] anaplastic sarcoma of the gular region (presumed histiocytic sarcoma) in a bearded dragon with a Sertoli cell tumor,[50] and various soft tissue sarcomas.[1]

Of tumors arising within the hepatobiliary system, one report[51] describes a single bearded dragon with an intrahepatic cholangiocarcinoma, adenocarcinoma of the gallbladder, and 2 adenomas of the gallbladder. Although many IHC markers are of limited utility in exotic species, in this case, *claudin-7* was determined reliable to differentiate biliary cells (immunopositive) from cells of hepatocellular origin (immunonegative). However, well-differentiated hepatocellular proliferations in reptiles should be interpreted with caution because well-differentiated hepatocellular carcinomas may be challenging to discern from benign hepatomas.[43]

Hematopoietic neoplasms described include leukemias of the myeloid cell line and lymphoid neoplasms with and without leukemia (**Fig. 10**). A case series of lymphoid leukemia in 5 bearded dragons reported an initial leukocytosis ranging from 20.0 to 140.0 × 10^3 cells/μL and a lymphocyte count ranging from 3.2 to 135.8 × 10^3 cells/μL among the animals. Additional hematologic abnormalities included anemia in 3 lizards, heterophilia in 2 lizards, and monocytosis in 2 lizards.[52] The maximum lymphocyte count among the dragons ranged from 66.7 to 393.3 × 10^3 cells/μL and excluding the one dragon still alive 244 days after diagnosis, survival time ranged from 57 to 416 days. Biochemical abnormalities among these animals included hyperuricemia, hyperglycemia, hypoalbuminemia, and hyperkalemia, and in one patient for which EPH was performed, increased β-globulin and γ-globulin concentrations were evident. Neoplastic lymphocytes were described as being intermediate to large with increased amounts of clear to light blue cytoplasm, occasionally with few vacuoles, and round to indented nuclei with stippled to lightly clumped chromatin and variably distinct nucleoli. Plasmacytoid cells, cytoplasmic fragments, and mitotic figures were also occasionally observed in the blood smears.

Gastric neuroendocrine carcinomas in bearded dragons have been reported, and this species seems overrepresented among reptiles.[53–57] In one case series, all of the animals for which an age was reported (8/10) were ≤ 3 years old. Animals were presented for anorexia, weakness, weight loss, and vomiting, attributable to the neoplastic mass protruding into the gastric lumen. Clinicopathologic findings may include anemia, heterophilia, monocytosis, and hyperglycemia, which can be extreme (up to 1,682 mg/dL).[53,54] Expected cytologic findings include a highly cellular sample consisting of abundant bare nuclei and variably-sized aggregates of disorganized, high N:C ratio, round to cuboidal epithelial cells with scant light blue cytoplasm and only mild anisocytosis and anisokaryosis.[53] Interestingly, parallels can be drawn between these cases and humans with somatostatin syndrome, in which weight loss, anemia, and hyperglycemia are also common findings.

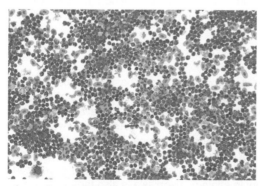

Fig. 10. Blood smear from a bearded dragon (*P. vitticeps*) with lymphoid leukemia. Lymphocytes range in size from 6 to 20 μm and are characterized by a round to lobulated nucleus, coarse chromatin, a high N:C ratio, and a small amount of dark blue cytoplasm that occasionally contains a few punctate vacuoles. Although confirmatory diagnostics such as immunochemistry were not performed the presence of larger lymphocytes suggests an acute lymphoblastic leukemia; 400× magnification, modified Wright's stain.

METABOLIC CONDITIONS

Derangements in normal metabolism are not uncommon in bearded dragons and often are multifactorial rather than resulting from a particular nidus. The most relevant conditions include MBD, hepatic lipidosis (see "Hepatobiliary" section), and gout (see "Renal and Urogenital" section).

Calcium and phosphorus concentrations are of particular importance in bearded dragons due to the prevalence of MBD, particularly secondary hyperparathyroidism that more often occurs due to poor husbandry rather than primary chronic renal disease. The pathogenesis of nutritional secondary hyperparathyroidism typically involves initial hypocalcemia due to deficiency of cholecalciferol (vitamin D_3) or an inadequate dietary Ca:P ratio. One retrospective study found that 57.71% of all bearded dragons for which bloodwork was available had an abnormal Ca:P ratio, with 63.98% having hypocalcemia and 26.71% having hyperphosphatemia.[14] Bearded dragons require vitamin D_3 through dietary supplementation and/or endogenous synthesis from exposure to artificial or natural ultraviolet B (UVB) radiation at a wavelength of 280 to 320 nm, although natural UVB is considered superior.[20,58] Furthermore, a study evaluating different UVB lamps found none of the lamps could induce plasma vitamin D_3 concentrations in captive growing bearded dragons comparable to those in free-living dragons.[58] Taking these factors into account, bearded dragons are at highest risk for the development of MBD when fed a diet with an excess of crickets or mealworms, which have an inverse Ca:P ratio and are calcium deficient when considering the needs of a growing dragon.[18] This is exacerbated by the absence of appropriate UVB lighting and dietary mineral supplementation. When ionized hypocalcemia is present, parathyroid hormone (PTH) is secreted from the parathyroid gland to stimulate resorption of calcium from bone and absorption from the gastrointestinal tract and kidneys. However, total and ionized calcium concentrations are often within reference intervals until stores are depleted.[20] Manifestations of disease can include decreased bone density, pathologic fractures, and replacement of bone with fibrous connective tissue (fibrous osteodystrophy).[20] Clinical symptoms that are suggestive of ionized hypocalcemia include muscle tremors, paresis, tetany, or seizures.[18,20] Hypercalcemia is a normal physiologic finding in reproductively active females but also is common in bearded dragons over supplemented with dietary vitamin D_3 and calcium.[11] Although an elevated PTH concentration is necessary for definitive diagnosis of hyperparathyroidism, a reliable assay for reptiles is not currently available.

SUMMARY

Despite bearded dragon popularity, many basic clinicopathologic diagnostics remain unstudied for this species. Coagulation studies, studies of APP, more accurate bench top protein determination, cardiac troponins, and evaluation of enzyme activity tissue distributions have yet to be performed but could prove invaluable for clinicopathologic determination of health in bearded dragons. These lizards are stoic creatures and may not display evidence of clinical illness until the late stages of disease, and symptoms are often nonspecific. Although most pathologic conditions in bearded dragons are infectious or inflammatory in etiology, neoplasia is also thought to occur with an incidence similar to that of domestic mammals. Improper husbandry can also predispose to several common metabolic conditions. Assessment of a thorough history and physical examination findings, in conjunction with clinicopathologic tests including bloodwork and cytology provide the best opportunity for the clinician to arrive at a diagnosis in a timely manner and implement potentially life-saving treatment.

CLINICS CARE POINTS

- The clinicopathologic minimum database is crucial for adequate evaluation of systemic health in bearded dragons. The majority of health problems in bearded dragons are a result of poor husbandry.

- Bearded dragons should have wellness check ups with a veterinarian biannually, or at minimum annually, to establish their baseline in health and potentially detect signs of illness early to allow prompt treatment.

- Many routine laboratory diagnostic tests commonly performed in domestic mammals have not been evaluated or are not well-characterized in bearded dragons, and further research is warranted.

- When cytologic examination cannot provide a definitive diagnosis, biopsy with histologic examination is recommended.

- Biopsy still may be unable to provide a definitive diagnosis due to lack of validation of immunohistochemistry (IHC) markers and special stains in bearded dragons.

DISCLOSURE

The authors have no conflicts to disclose.

REFERENCES

1. Crouch EEV, McAloose D, McEntire MS, et al. Pathology of the Bearded Dragon (Pogona vitticeps): a Retrospective Analysis of 36 Cases. J Comp Pathol 2021; 186:51–61.
2. Darrow BG, Johnstone McLean NS, Russman SE, et al. Periorbital adenocarcinoma in a bearded dragon (Pogona vitticeps). Vet Ophthalmol 2013;16(Suppl 1):177–82.
3. Tamukai K, Takami Y, Akabane Y, et al. Plasma biochemical reference values in clinically healthy captive bearded dragons (Pogona vitticeps) and the effects of sex and season. Vet Clin Pathol 2011;40(3):368–73.
4. Heatley JJ, Russell K. Hematology. In: Divers S, Stahl S, editors. Mader's reptile and amphibian medicine and surgery. 3rd. St. Louis, MO: Elsevier; 2019. p. 301–18.
5. Stacy NI, Alleman AR, Sayler KA. Diagnostic hematology of reptiles. Clin Lab Med 2011;31(1):87–108.
6. LeBlanc CJ, Heatley JJ, Mack EB. A review of the morphology of lizard leukocytes with a discussion of the clinical differentiation of bearded dragon, Pogona vitticeps, leukocytes. J Herpetological Med Surg 2000;10(2):27–30.
7. Aguilar LAB, Divers SJ, Comolli JR, et al. Successful management of hemocoelom and marked anemia in a central bearded dragon (Pogona vitticeps) following multiple blood transfusions and surgery. J Herpetological Med Surg 2021;31(2): 111–8.
8. Grosset C, Wellehan JF Jr, Owens SD, et al. Intraerythrocytic iridovirus in central bearded dragons (Pogona vitticeps). J Vet Diagn Invest 2014;26(3):354–64.
9. Allison RW, Velguth KE. Appearance of granulated cells in blood films stained by automated aqueous versus methanolic Romanowsky methods. Vet Clin Pathol 2010;39(1):99–104.
10. Divers SJ. Hepatology. In: Divers SJ, Stahl SJ, editors. Maders reptile and amphibian medicine and surgery, 3e. St. Louis, MO: Elsevier; 2019. p. 649–68.

11. Divers SJ, Camus MS. Lizards. In: Heatley JJ, Russell KE, editors. Exotic animal laboratory diagnosis. Hoboken, NJ: John Wiley & Sons, Inc; 2020. p. 319–46.

12. Heatley JJ, Russell K. Clinical chemistry. In: Divers S, Stahl S, editors. Maders reptile and amphibian medicine and surgery, 3e. St. Louis, MO: Elsevier; 2019. p. 319–32.

13. Howard JG, Jaensch S. Haematology and plasma biochemistry reference intervals in wild bearded dragons (Pogona vitticeps). Aust Vet J 2021;99(6):236–41.

14. Schmidt-Ukaj S, Hochleithner M, Richter B, et al. A survey of diseases in captive bearded dragons: a retrospective study of 529 patients. Veterinarni Medicina 2017;62(09):508–15.

15. Kubiak M, Denk D, Stidworthy MF. Retrospective review of neoplasms of captive lizards in the United Kingdom. Vet Rec 2020;186(1):28.

16. Sykes JM 4th, Trupkiewicz JG. Reptile neoplasia at the Philadelphia Zoological Garden, 1901-2002. J Zoo Wildl Med 2006;37(1):11–9.

17. Christman J, Devau M, Wilson-Robles H, et al. Oncology of reptiles: diseases, diagnosis, and treatment. Veterinary Clin North Am Exot Anim Pract 2017;20(1):87–110.

18. Wright K. Two common disorders of captive bearded dragons (Pogona vitticeps): Nutritional secondary hyperparathyroidism and constipation. J Exot Pet Med 2008;17(4):267–72.

19. DeVoe R. Gastroenterology – oral cavity, esophagus, and stomach. In: Divers S, Stahl S, editors. Maders reptile and amphibian medicine and surgery, 3rde. St. Louis, MO: Elsevier; 2019. p. 752–60.

20. Boyer TH, Scott PW. Nutritional diseases. In: Divers S, Stahl S, editors. Maders reptile and amphibian medicine and surgery, 3e. St. Louis, MO: Elsevier; 2019. p. 932–50.

21. Divers SJ. Hepatic lipidosis. In: Divers SJ, Stahl SJ, editors. Maders reptile and amphibian medicine and surgery. 3rd edition. St. Louis, MO: Elsevier; 2019. p. 1312–3.

22. Parkinson LA, Mans C. Investigation of the effects of cricket ingestion on plasma uric acid concentration in inland bearded dragons (*Pogona vitticeps*). J Am Vet Med Assoc 2020;257(9):933–6.

23. Divers SJ, Innis C. Urology. In: Divers S, Stahl S, editors. Mader's reptile and amphibian medicine and surgery, 3e. St. Louis, MO: Elsevier; 2019. p. 624–48.

24. Fitzgerald KT, Martínez-Silvestre A. Toxicology. In: Divers SJ, Stahl SJ, editors. Maders reptile and amphibian medicine and surgery. 3rd edition. St. Louis, MO: Elsevier; 2019. p. 977–91.

25. Pennick KE, Holicky RA, Wilkerson MJ. What is your diagnosis? Joint and associated tissue aspirates from a Bearded Dragon (Pogona vitticeps). Vet Clin Pathol 2017;46(2):363–4.

26. Perpiñán D. What's Your Diagnosis? Joint swelling in a bearded dragon (Pogona vitticeps). J Herpetological Med Surg 2009;19(3):72–5.

27. Schilliger L, Lemberger K, Chai N, et al. Atherosclerosis associated with pericardial effusion in a central bearded dragon (Pogona vitticeps). J Vet Diagn Invest 2010;22(5):789–92.

28. Schilliger L, Paillusseau C, Gandar F, et al. Hypertensive heart disease and encephalopathy in a central bearded dragon (Pogona vitticeps) with severe atherosclerosis and first-degree atrioventricular block. J Zoo Wildl Med 2019;50(2):482–6.

29. Furst N, Alexander A, Ossiboff RJ, et al. Tail base aneurysm in an inland bearded dragon (Pogona vitticeps). J Exot Pet Med 2020;33:34–7.

30. Gimmel A, Kempf H, Öfner S, et al. Cholelithiasis in adult bearded dragons: retrospective study of nine adult bearded dragons (Pogona vitticeps) with cholelithiasis between 2013 and 2015 in southern Germany. J Anim Physiol Anim Nutr (Berl) 2017;101(Suppl 1):122–6.

31. Johnston AN, Stöhr AC, Artiles C, et al. *Choleoeimeria pogonae* alters the bile acid composition of the central bearded dragon (Pogona vitticeps). J Herpetological Med Surg 2021;31(2):99–100.

32. Comolli J, Divers S, Lock B, et al. Comparison of protein electrophoresis and biochemical analysis for the quantification of plasma albumin in healthy bearded dragons (Pogona vitticeps). J Zoo Wildl Med 2021;52(1):253–8.

33. Dallwig RK, Mitchell MA, Acierno MJ. Determination of plasma osmolality and agreement between measured and calculated values in healthy adult bearded dragons (Pogona vitticeps). J Herpetological Med Surg 2010;20(2–3):69–73.

34. Hellebuyck T, Martel A, Chiers K, et al. Devriesea agamarum causes dermatitis in bearded dragons (Pogona vitticeps). Vet Microbiol 2009;134(3–4):267–71.

35. Vetere A, Bertocchi M, Pelizzone I, et al. Klebsiella sp.-related infectious spondylitis in a bearded dragon (Pogona vitticeps). BMC Vet Res 2021;17(1):230.

36. Girling SJ, Fraser MA. Systemic mycobacteriosis in an inland bearded dragon (Pogona vitticeps). Vet Rec 2007;160(15):526–8.

37. Kramer MH. Granulomatous osteomyelitis associated with atypical mycobacteriosis in a bearded dragon (Pogona vitticeps). Veterinary Clin North Am Exot Anim Pract 2006;9(3):563–8.

38. Marschang RE. Viruses infecting reptiles. Viruses 2011;3(11):2087–126.

39. Tamukai K, Tokiwa T, Kobayashi H, et al. Ranavirus in an outbreak of dermatophilosis in captive inland bearded dragons (Pogona vitticeps). Vet Dermatol 2016; 27(2):99–105e28.

40. Le Donne V, Crossland N, Brandão J, et al. Nannizziopsis guarroi infection in 2 Inland Bearded Dragons (Pogona vitticeps): clinical, cytologic, histologic, and ultrastructural aspects. Vet Clin Pathol 2016;45(2):368–75.

41. Minard HM, Burrell C, Delgado JD, et al. What's your diagnosis? Skin impression smear from a Bearded Dragon. Vet Clin Pathol 2016;45(3):505–6.

42. Hernandez-Divers SM, Garner MM. Neoplasia of reptiles with an emphasis on lizards. Veterinary Clin North Am Exot Anim Pract 2003;6(1):251–73.

43. Garner MM, Hernandez-Divers SM, Raymond JT. Reptile neoplasia: a retrospective study of case submissions to a specialty diagnostic service. Veterinary Clin North Am Exot Anim Pract 2004;7(3):653–vi.

44. Crews J, Gendron K, Sladakovic I, et al. Liposarcoma of the fat body in a bearded dragon (Pogona vitticeps). J Herpetological Med Surg 2021;30(4):232–6.

45. Harr KE, Romagnano A. Clinically pertinent cytological Diff-Quick and Gram stain evaluation for the reptilian practitioner. ExoticsCon 2015 Pre-conference Proceedings. August 29-September 2, 2015, San Antonio, TX; 173-180.

46. Alleman AR, Kupprion EK. Cytologic diagnosis of diseases in reptiles. Veterinary Clin North Am Exot Anim Pract 2007;10(1):155–86, vii.

47. Gardhouse S, Eshar D, Lee-Chow B, et al. Diagnosis and treatment of a periocular myxosarcoma in a bearded dragon (Pogona vitticeps). Can Vet J 2014;55(7): 663–6.

48. Shokrpoor S, Pedram M, Torjani N, et al. Occurrence of myxoma in a bearded dragon (*Pogona vitticeps*): Surgical and histopathological studies. Vet Res Forum 2021;12(1):129–31.

49. Lemberger KY, Manharth A, Pessier AP. Multicentric benign peripheral nerve sheath tumors in two related bearded dragons, Pogona vitticeps. Vet Pathol 2005;42(4):507–10.

50. Williams MJ, Wong HE, Priestnall SL, et al. Anaplastic Sarcoma and Sertoli Cell Tumor in a Central Bearded Dragon (*Pogona vitticeps*). J Herpetol Med Surg 2020;30(2):68–73.

51. Jakab C, Rusvai M, Szabó Z, et al. Claudin-7-positive synchronous spontaneous intrahepatic cholangiocarcinoma, adenocarcinoma and adenomas of the gallbladder in a Bearded dragon (Pogona vitticeps). Acta Vet Hung 2011;59(1):99–112.

52. Hepps Keeney CM, Intile JL, Sims CS, et al. Lymphoid leukemia in five bearded dragons (*Pogona vitticeps*). J Am Vet Med Assoc 2021;258(7):748–57.

53. Anderson KB, Meinkoth J, Hallman M, et al. Cytological diagnosis of gastric neuroendocrine carcinoma in a pet inland bearded dragon (Pogona vitticeps). J Exot Pet Med 2019;(29):188–93.

54. Levine BS. Gastric endoneurocrine carcinoma (somatostatinoma) in a bearded dragon (Pogona vitticeps). Proc Assoc Reptilian Amphibian Veterinarians 2011;149–51.

55. Lyons JA, Newman SJ, Greenacre CB, et al. A gastric neuroendocrine carcinoma expressing somatostatin in a bearded dragon (Pogona vitticeps). J Vet Diagn Invest 2010;22(2):316–20.

56. Perpiñán D, Addante K, Driskell E. What's Your Diagnosis? Gastrointestinal disturbances in a bearded dragon (Pogona vitticeps). J Herpetological Med Surg 2010;20(2–3):54–7.

57. Ritter JM, Garner MM, Chilton JA, et al. Gastric neuroendocrine carcinomas in bearded dragons (Pogona vitticeps). Vet Pathol 2009;46(6):1109–16.

58. Diehl JJE, Baines FM, Heijboer AC, et al. A comparison of Uvb compact lamps in enabling cutaneous vitamin D synthesis in growing bearded dragons. J Anim Physiol Anim Nutr (Berl) 2018;102(1):308–16.

Clinical Pathology of Box Turtles (*Terrapene* spp.)

Laura Adamovicz, DVM, PhD*, Matthew C. Allender, DVM, MS, PhD, Dipl. ACZM

KEYWORDS

- Hematology • Biochemistries • Protein electrophoresis • Acute phase proteins

KEY POINTS

- Blood samples may be collected from the subcarapacial sinus, jugular vein, or radiohumeral venous plexus in box turtles. Lithium heparin is the preferred anticoagulant.
- Seasonal changes in box turtle clinical pathology parameters include increased packed cell volume, total protein, albumin, albumin:globulin, uric acid, creatine kinase, partial pressure of CO_2 and lactate concentrations in the summer, decreased heterophils, monocytes, heterophil:lymphocyte ratio, pH, bicarbonate, total carbon dioxide, and base excess in the summer, and increases in eosinophils, bile acids, and total calcium as the active season progresses.
- Female eastern box turtles have relatively increased plasma concentrations of total solids, total protein, basophils, calcium, phosphorous, cholesterol, beta globulins, hemoglobin-binding protein, and erythrocyte sedimentation rate compared with males. Males have relatively increased packed cell volume and trend toward increased concentrations of uric acid.
- Adult box turtles have a relatively increased packed cell volume, total calcium, calcium:-phosphorous, beta globulins, and hemoglobin-binding protein concentrations compared with juveniles. Juveniles have relatively increased monocyte counts and concentrations of phosphorous and albumin.
- Despite a reasonable clinicopathologic database for eastern box turtles, additional work is needed to characterize clinical pathology parameters in other box turtle species.

INTRODUCTION

North American box turtles (*Terrapene* spp.) are a group of terrestrial to semi-aquatic omnivorous chelonians characterized by a hinged plastron. These species range from the eastern and central United States to Mexico (**Table 1**). Box turtle species are classified as near-threatened (*Terrapene ornata*), vulnerable (*Terrapene carolina*, *Terrapene mexicana*, *Terrapene triunguis*, *Terrapene yucatana*), critically endangered (*Terrapene coahuila*), or data deficient (*Terrapene nelsoni*) by the IUCN Tortoise and

Wildlife Epidemiology Laboratory, University of Illinois, College of Veterinary Medicine, 2001 South Lincoln Avenue, Urbana, IL 61802, USA
* Corresponding author.
E-mail address: adamovi2@illinios.edu

Vet Clin Exot Anim 25 (2022) 735–754
https://doi.org/10.1016/j.cvex.2022.05.004
1094-9194/22/© 2022 Elsevier Inc. All rights reserved.

Table 1
Currently recognized box turtle species[1]

Common Name	Scientific Name
Eastern box turtle	*Terrapene carolina carolina*
Gulf Coast box turtle	*Terrapene carolina major*
Florida box turtle	*Terrapene carolina bauri*
Ornate box turtle	*Terrapene ornata*
Three-toed box turtle	*Terrapene triunguis*
Coahuilan box turtle	*Terrapene coahuila*
Mexican box turtle	*Terrapene mexicana*
Southern spotted box turtle	*Terrapene nelsoni nelsoni*
Northern spotted box turtle	*Terrapene nelsoni klauberi*
Yucatan box turtle	*Terrapene yucatana*

Freshwater Turtle Specialist Group,[1] and many wild populations are declining. Recognized threats to box turtle conservation include habitat destruction, road mortality, nest predation, illegal trafficking, and diseases such as ranavirus. Box turtles are commonly presented for veterinary assessment as pets, members of zoologic collections, patients at wildlife rehabilitation centers, and as a result of confiscations. Veterinarians are also increasingly involved in health assessments of wild populations and conservation interventions including head-starting, translocations, and release of confiscated/rehabilitated individuals back into the wild. General health assessment tools are needed to support the management of these species at both the individual and population levels. This article will review current knowledge about box turtle clinical pathology testing and identify gaps for future research.

Sample Collection and Handling

Box turtles experience stress from handling which can alter clinical pathology parameters. Wild eastern box turtles have increases in plasma corticosterone, total leukocyte count (WBC), heterophil count, monocyte count, heterophil:lymphocyte (H:L), and decreases in lymphocyte count following capture, consistent with an acute stress response.[2] These changes are time-dependent, with WBC peaking at 83 minutes after initial contact, but corticosterone concentrations rising within 3 minutes of capture.[2] Blood samples should therefore be collected early in the examination process to minimize artifactual changes which could mask underlying pathology.

Blood collection in box turtles is similar to other chelonians. The most accessible venipuncture sites include the subcarapacial sinus, jugular vein, and radiohumeral venous plexus (aka brachial vein), although use of the post-occipital venous plexus, dorsal coccygeal vein, and femoral vein has also been reported in this genus.[3] The subcarapacial sinus is the easiest place to collect a large (>1 mL) blood sample in an adult box turtle and is the only practical venipuncture site in juveniles. It is also the only accessible venipuncture site for box turtles completely withdrawn into the shell ("boxed up", **Fig. 1**) and does not require an additional handler for restraint. Despite these advantages, the risk of sample contamination with lymphatic or cerebrospinal fluid is high due to sinus anatomy.[4] This venipuncture site also carries the risk of inadvertent puncture into the lung, subarachnoid space, or injury to spinal nerves resulting in temporary to prolonged limb and tail paresis.[5,6] Venipuncture from the radiohumeral venous plexus carries a lower risk of lymphatic contamination

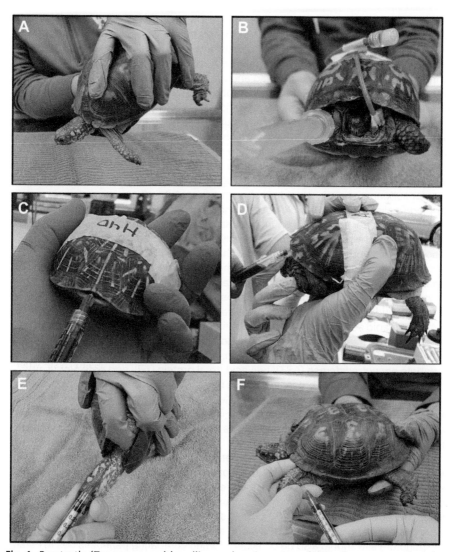

Fig. 1. Box turtle (*Terrapene* spp.) handling and venipuncture. (*A*) Turtles can sometimes be coaxed from their shells by holding them head-down over the exam table. (*B*) A 3 cc syringe case with cap can be inserted between the carapace and plastron to hold the turtle open. (*C*) Subcarapacial sinus venipuncture can be performed in completely closed box turtles. (*D*) The subcarapacial sinus is located on midline at the junction of the cervical vertebrae and the carapace. (*E*) The jugular vein is located along an imaginary line from the dorsal aspect of the tympanic membrane to the thoracic inlet. The turtle is placed in lateral recumbency and the head and neck are extended to access this venipuncture site. (*F*) The radiohumeral venous sinus, or brachial vein, is located on the ventral surface of the radiohumeral joint immediately above the biceps brachii tendon. The forelimb is extended and the needle is inserted above the tendon, then directed toward the joint.

compared with the subcarapacial sinus;[7] however, only small volumes of blood (0.1–0.25 mL) can be collected from this location.[3] Use of this venipuncture site also requires either a cooperative patient, skillful extraction of a forelimb from a boxed turtle, or chemical restraint. Moderate volumes of blood (0.5–1 mL) can be collected from the jugular vein in box turtles. The risk of lymphatic contamination is considered low;[8,9] however, use of this site requires an extension of the head and neck which can be challenging in a boxed-up turtle, sometimes necessitating sedation.

In the authors' experience, the head and forelimbs of uncooperative box turtles can be easily accessed by using a thin metal probe to gently open the anterior plastron and inserting a 3-cc syringe case (with cap) to hold the shell open (see **Fig. 1**). In addition, many turtles can be coaxed into sticking out a forelimb or their head by holding them perpendicular to the exam table with their head facing down (see **Fig. 1**). Positioning and landmarks for box turtle venipuncture sites are similar to other chelonians (see **Fig. 1**). Needle size and length depend on patient size, a 23–25 gauge 1″ needle is adequate for most venipuncture sites, though a 22 gauge 1.5″ needle may be necessary for subcarapacial sinus venipuncture in adults. A 1 to 3 cc syringe is appropriate for blood collection, and sample volume should be limited to less than 0.8% of body weight (0.8 mL per 100 g).[10] Lithium heparin is the anticoagulant of choice, as EDTA causes significant and unpredictable hemolysis in eastern box turtle blood samples.[11] Blood samples obviously contaminated with lymph or other fluids should be discarded and a new sample should be collected, although inapparent hemodilution is possible regardless of venipuncture site and visual appearance of the sample.

The effects of sample storage conditions have not been evaluated in box turtles, however, studies in other chelonians indicate that short-term blood sample storage at 4°C and rapid separation of plasma is optimal to avoid artifactual changes in several analytes (eg, decreases in heterophils, monocytes, sodium, glucose, gamma-glutamyl transferase [GGT], albumin, and albumin:globulin [A:G]; increases in potassium, aspartate aminotransferase [AST], uric acid, total protein [TP], and beta globulin).[12–17] Freezing plasma samples before analysis is frequently necessary in a research setting, and this likely creates changes in box turtle clinical pathology parameters similar to other chelonians (eg, increased variability in reported values, increased potassium, AST, uric acid, TP, and beta globulins; decreased albumin, A:G, and alpha globulins).[14,16]

Differences in clinical pathology parameters based on venipcunture site in chelonians are likely attributed to variable rates of hemodilution, which is generally considered least likely from the jugular vein, followed by the radiohumeral venous plexus and femoral veins, then the subcarapacial sinus and post-occipital venous plexus, and finally the coccygeal veins.[7–9,18–20] Thus serial samples should be collected from the same site to best facilitate direct comparison and evaluation of patient progress. Venipuncture site should also be considered when comparing patient values to established reference ranges.

Considerations for Interpretation of Results

Like other reptiles, box turtle clinical pathology values can vary significantly based on extrinsic (season, environmental quality, source population, captive vs wild) and intrinsic factors (sex, age class, reproductive status, health status). Research has characterized the effect of these factors on clinical pathology values in eastern and, to a lesser extent, ornate box turtles. However, comparatively sparse clinical pathology data are available for other box turtle species. Extrapolation from eastern box turtle data may provide a basis for interpreting bloodwork in other box turtle species, however, this should be done judiciously because of differences in biology and ecology within the genus *Terrapene*.

Reliable reference intervals are important for clinical interpretation of bloodwork in exotic species. The reference intervals we present in this article were generated following American Society for Veterinary Clinical Pathology guidelines[21] using data from at least 40 apparently healthy wild eastern and ornate box turtles. Additional clinical pathology values are reported in the box turtle literature;[22–24] however, many of these were collected with goals other than reference intervals in mind and their use for assessment of clinical data should be performed with caution. Sources which compile box turtle reference interval data from the literature are also available,[25,26] however, important factors such as sample size, venipuncture site, and methodology used to generate the data are not consistently reported. Clinicians are encouraged to investigate this information to judge the quality and clinical applicability of these tools before use.

Many veterinary reference intervals are produced using cross-sectional data from a large number of apparently healthy individuals. These population-based reference intervals are most useful for analytes in which intra-individual variation is large compared with inter-individual variation.[21,27] However, when inter-individual variation is large compared with intra-individual variation, that is, when a high degree of biological variation is present, population-based reference intervals can be insensitive for detecting pathologic change.[21,27] Box turtles and other reptiles have a high degree of biological variability in their clinical pathology parameters, potentially indicating that population-based reference intervals have limited clinical utility in these species. An alternative approach is the use of subject-based reference intervals, which are developed via serial sampling of apparently healthy individuals. Data from longitudinal sampling is used to calculate the index of individuality, which helps determine whether subject or population-based reference intervals are more appropriate, and the reference change value, which is the percent change in an analyte's value that is considered statistically different from normal.[21,27] Reference change values can identify clinically significant deviations in a patient's bloodwork that might not be detectable with population-based reference intervals.[27] Subject-based reference intervals have been investigated in a small number of reptiles,[28–30] and they seem to be useful for several analytes. Future research is needed to determine whether the use of subject-based reference intervals is warranted in box turtles.

Hematology

Complete blood counts are used to assess numbers of erythrocytes, leukocytes, and thrombocytes and to examine cellular morphology for evidence of general or specific disease processes. Box turtles possess nucleated erythrocytes and therefore require manual cell counting methods. Three of the most common approaches to leukocyte quantification include estimation from a blood film, Natt and Herrick's (NH) method, and Avian Leukopets (LO) which use phloxine stain. Discrepancies have been documented between all methods and there is no current gold standard leukocyte quantification method in reptiles.[17,31,32] In eastern box turtles the LO method produces greater leukocyte counts compared with blood film estimates.[2,11,33] Specifically, WBC, monocytes, and basophils are proportionally increased in the LO method, heterophils are constantly increased in the LO method, and lymphocytes are both constantly and proportionally increased in the LO method compared with blood film estimation.[33] These changes are potentially attributable to the use of a human-derived equation to calculate total leukocyte count; humans are a neutrophil-dominant species, whereas box turtles are lymphocyte predominant.[23] Thus the equation provided in the LO kit may not properly extrapolate leukocyte counts for box turtles. Indeed, agreement between LO and blood film WBC estimates is improved when heterophils and eosinophils make up greater than 15% of the differential (ie, when lymphocyte counts are lower).[2] The LO method has an intra-assay variability of 8.2% and an inter-assay variability of 12% in eastern box turtles, independent of biological variation, however, the variability of NH and blood film WBC estimates has not yet been determined in this species.[33] Owing to significant between-method variability and uncertainty about which is most accurate, we recommend selecting one leukocyte quantification method and using it to consistently evaluate serial samples. Methodology is also important to keep in mind when comparing patient values to reference intervals (**Tables 2** and **3**).

Regardless of leukocyte quantification method used, blood film review is recommended to evaluate cellular morphology and determine the presence of hemoparasites and intracellular inclusions. Blood smears should ideally be made immediately following venipuncture using fresh, non-anticoagulated blood. This avoids artifacts associated with sample storage and prolonged exposure to heparin such as cellular clumping and changes in thrombocyte morphology which can complicate differential counts (**Figs. 2** and **3**). Blood smears should be made without excessive downward pressure on the spreader slide as this can lead to cell lysis and impact the accuracy of the differential. A good quality blood smear has a thumbprint shape, a dense body that takes up about 2/3 of the smear, a thin monolayer where estimated counts and differentials can be performed, and a well-developed feathered edge (see **Fig. 2**).

Table 2
Hematology reference ranges for apparently healthy free-living eastern box turtles (*Terrapene carolina carolina*) in Illinois[21,37]

Parameter	Units	Partition	N	CT	Dispersion	Min	Max	Reference Interval
Packed	%	Female	162	23	6.3	7.5	45.5	9–33
cell	%	Male	146	26	6.2	10.5	45	13–36
volume	%	Juvenile	61	20	6.3	5	30	6–30
Total solids	g/dL	Female*	162	7	5.2–8.9	3.9	11.7	4.6–10.1
	g/dL	Male	146	6.7	1.38	3.8	9.7	4.2–9.1
Total white blood cells*	cells/µL		365	19,766	10,258–35,687	3259	168,080	7215–50,034
Heterophils	cells/µL	Spring*	226	2,594	921–5067	296	12,539	581–7039
	cells/µL	Summer*	58	1,896	872–3612	261	7691	450–4842
	cells/µL	Fall*	85	2,543	1,232–5190	585	9,433	743–8,405
Lymphocytes*	cells/µL		369	11,432	4,554–25,807	259	157,995	3,365–40,688
Monocytes	cells/µL	Adult*	313	364	0–1,124	0	2,728	0–1,763
	cells/µL	Juvenile*	61	417	0–1,647	0	2,953	0–2,860
Eosinophils	cells/µL	Spring*	220	2,041	836–3,904	0	11,812	641–5,361
	cells/µL	Summer*	61	2,429	1,180–5,126	619	7,109	622–6,735
	cells/µL	Fall*	84	2,653	1,459–6,769	380	12,635	1,153–12,201
Basophils	cells/µL	Female*	162	1,639	411–3,155	0	6,540	196–5,493
	cells/µL	Male*	146	1,339	301–2,980	0	5,670	140–4,955
Heterophil: lymphocyte*			367	0.2	0.07–0.58	0.01	12	0.036–0.99

Blood samples were collected from the subcarapacial sinus and stored in lithium heparin. Leukocyte quantification was performed with Avian Leukopets. Data distribution is normal unless indicated by an *. CT = measure of central tendency, mean for normally distributed data, median for nonnormally distributed data. Dispersion = standard deviation for normally distributed data or 10th–90th percentiles for nonnormally distributed data.

Table 3
Hematology reference ranges for apparently healthy free-living ornate box turtles (*Terrapene ornata*) in Illinois sampled in May[21,37]

Parameter	Units	Partition	N	CT	Dispersion	Min	Max	Reference Interval
Packed cell volume	%	Male	34	25	4.4	14.5	36	17–32
	%	Female	18	23	4.5	15	34	–
Total solids	g/dL		66	6.55	1.05	4	9.6	4.87–8.12
Total white blood cells	cells/μL	*	72	18,053	10,904–26,675	7323	41,507	8048–41,310
Heterophils	cells/μL		72	4,767	1,691	1,491	8,615	1,548–8,464
Lymphocytes	cells/μL	*	72	9,605	4,867–18,717	2,709	24,349	3,316–24,122
Monocytes	cells/μL	Adult*	52	621	207–1,420	0	2,490	171–1,956
	cells/μL	Juvenile	16	1,225	815	0	2,889	–
Eosinophils	cells/μL	*	70	1,320	468–4,237	73	7,471	169–5,505
Basophils	cells/μL	*	72	483	84–1,286	0	2,781	0–2,189

Blood samples were collected from the subcarapacial sinus and stored in lithium heparin. Nonnormal data distribution is indicated *. CT = measure of central tendency, mean for normally distributed data, median for nonnormally distributed data. Dispersion = standard deviation for normally distributed data or 10th–90th percentiles for nonnormally distributed data. Reference intervals were not calculated for fewer than 20 turtles.

The ability to make high-quality blood smears is an essential skill for exotics clinicians and technical staff and is worth perfecting through abundant practice.

Blood films should be air-dried completely, then stained before review. Modified Wright-Giemsa stains are recommended, as rapid stains (eg, Diff-Quik) can fail to stain basophil granules.[10] Box turtle leukocyte morphology is similar to other chelonians, and cells are classified as heterophils, eosinophils, basophils, lymphocytes, and monocytes (see **Fig. 2**). As part of the blood film review, cells should be evaluated for evidence of immaturity, toxicity, parasitism, and inclusions such as those occurring with ranavirus infection[34] (**Fig. 4**). Whip-like heterophil projections can also be visualized (see **Fig. 4**). These likely represent heterophil extracelluar traps, the nonmammalian equivalent of neutrophil extracellular traps, which function to combat microbial infection and can be identified in both infectious and noninfectious inflammatory conditions.[35,36] Heterophil extracellular traps seem to be markers of systemic inflammation in reptiles.[35,36]

As previously stated, box turtle hematology values can vary based on extrinsic and intrinsic factors including year, season, sex, and age class. Although many associations have been detected, this article will focus on those identified by studies with a large sample size and/or those that are repeatable between studies. Many hematology parameters differ by year, which is probably attributable to inter-annual differences in temperature, rainfall, and resource availability which influence box turtle stress, movement patterns, and overall wellness.[37] This is not an uncommon finding in multi-year chelonian health studies,[38,39] and highlights why alternative tools such as subject-based reference intervals may be more useful in a clinical setting than population-based reference intervals, especially in species with a high degree of biological variation in clinical pathology parameters such as box turtles.[21,27] Generally, box turtle PCV is highest in summer, heterophils, monocytes, and H:L are lowest in summer, and

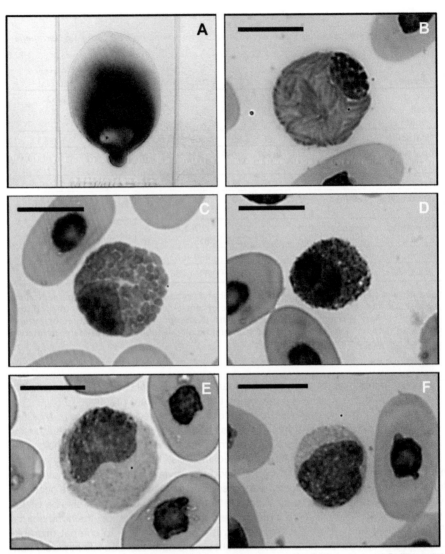

Fig. 2. Box turtle (*Terrapene* spp.) blood smears and normal leukocyte morphology. (*A*) Appearance of a high-quality blood smear showing a thumbprint shape, a dense body that takes up about 2/3 of the smear, a thin monolayer where estimated counts and differentials can be performed, and a well-developed feathered edge (*B*) Heterophil (*C*) Eosinophil (*D*) Basophil (*E*) Monocyte (*F*) Lymphocyte. Cells from eastern box turtles (*Terrapene carolina carolina*), 1000x magnification, oil immersion, Hema-3 stain (Fisher Scientific, Waltham, MA 02451, USA). Scale bars = 10 μm.

eosinophils rise throughout the active season.[22,37,40] Increased PCV in summer months occurs in other chelonians[38,39,41,42] and is presumably due to changes in hydration status and/or metabolic activity. Seasonal leukocyte variation may reflect shifts in health status due to changes in temperature, resource availability, pathogen exposure, or reproductive cycle. Although seasonal leukocyte changes have been

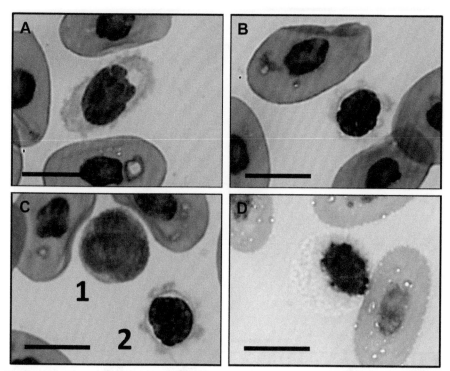

Fig. 3. Common artifacts in box turtle (*Terrapene* spp.) blood smears. (*A*) Thrombocyte appearance in non-anticoagulated blood. (*B*) Thrombocyte appearance in blood samples exposed to lithium heparin. (*C*) Lymphocyte (1) and thrombocyte (2) in a heparinized blood sample. (*D*) Degranulated basophil. Cells from eastern box turtles (*Terrapene carolina carolina*), 1000x magnification, oil immersion, Hema-3 stain. Scale bars = 10 μm.

identified in other chelonians the patterns of change are rarely consistent, potentially indicating that these are species-specific differences.[38,39,41,42]

Sex-based changes in box turtle hematology are similar to those of other chelonian species.[38,41,42] Specifically, female eastern box turtles have relatively increased plasma TS concentrations and basophil counts and males have a relatively increased PCV.[2,23,24,37,40,43] Male ornate box turtles also have higher PCV than females.[37,40] Interestingly, an increasing red iris color positively correlates to PCV in male eastern box turtles, providing a subjective means of assessing patient status without repeated venipuncture.[44] Adult eastern box turtles have relatively increased PCV and relatively decreased monocyte counts than juveniles.[23,37] Monocyte counts are also relatively decreased in adult ornate box turtles compared with juveniles.[37] Although the provided reference intervals for wild eastern and ornate box turtles are an important tool for box turtle clinicians, these values may not be reflective of bloodwork from captive individuals, especially those maintained indoors (see **Tables 2** and **3**).[41,45–47]

Plasma Biochemistries

Biochemistry panels are used to evaluate glucose, electrolytes, proteins, and organ function via the measurement of enzyme activities, metabolites, and cellular products. Although interpretation of glucose, electrolyte, and, to a lesser extent, protein

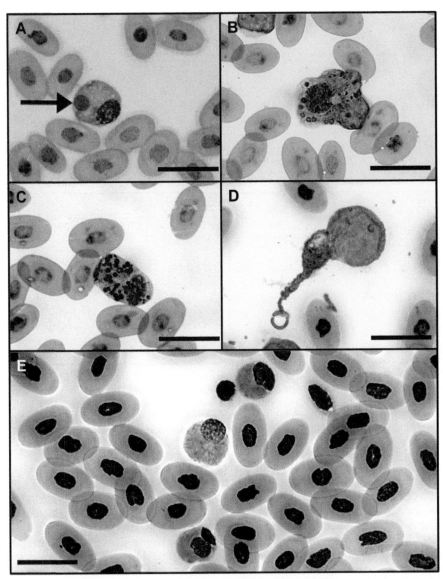

Fig. 4. Abnormalities in box turtle (*Terrapene* spp.) leukocytes. (*A*) Intracytoplasmic inclusion (*arrow*) associated with ranavirus infection in an eastern box turtle (*Terrapene carolina carolina*) monocyte. (*B, C*) Immature heterophils with mild toxic change, note cytoplasmic basophilia, mild degranulation, and the presence of immature (large, dark purple) granules. (*D*) Heterophil with a whip-like projection, presumptively consistent with an extracellular trap.[35,36] (*E*) Variation in heterophil morphology; from top to bottom: immature heterophil, mature heterophil, and a heterophil with a segmented nucleus—often associated with chronic inflammation. Image is 1000x magnification, oil immersion, Hema-3 and Wright stain. Scale bars = 20 μm. Image A adapted with permission.[34] Images D & E courtesy Nicole Stacy.

concentrations is straightforward in reptiles, most biochemistry panel enzymes were originally developed for use in humans and their clinical utility seems variable in chelonians.

Tissues of origin have been determined for six biochemistry panel enzymes in eastern box turtles.[48] Creatine kinase (CK) activity is highest in skeletal muscle, cardiac muscle, and gastrointestinal tract; glutamate dehydrogenase (GLDH) and alanine aminotransferase (ALT) activities are highest in liver, kidney, and gallbladder; alkaline phosphatase (ALP) and GGT activities are relatively increased in kidney and gastrointestinal tract tissues; and AST is relatively nonspecific, with significantly higher activity in the cardiac muscle, liver, kidney, skeletal muscle, and gallbladder compared with other tissues.[48] These findings indicate that no enzymes are fully specific to a single tissue type, but do provide a framework for the interpretation of enzyme changes. Leakage enzymes can be associated with the cytosol (CK, ALT, AST) or mitochondria (GLDH, AST), with cytosolic enzyme activities typically increasing based on less severe tissue insults (eg, inflammation) compared with mitochondrial enzymes (eg, necrosis).[49,50] Enzymes with high activities in the kidney (GGT, ALT, ALP, AST, and GLDH) or gastrointestinal tract (ALP & CK) tend to be expelled as waste products instead of circulating in the blood following insult.[49,50] The activities of induction enzymes such as GGT and ALP can be massively up-regulated during disease states, and their tissues of origin in health may not reflect the source of these enzymes in disease.[49,50] Given this, in box turtles ALT and GLDH activities may primarily indicate liver disease/damage, with ALT activity being more sensitive for mild hepatocyte insult. AST may be a good (but nonspecific) marker for muscle and liver insult, and increases in plasma CK activity most likely indicate skeletal and smooth muscle damage. Additional research is needed to clarify the clinical utility of GGT and ALP in box turtles. Further investigation is also needed to assess analytes such as bile acids and cardiac troponins in box turtles.

Season, sex, and age class are powerful drivers of select biochemistry panel analytes in box turtles. Thus reference ranges created for these species may be wide and difficult to interpret without adjustment for season, sex, and age class (**Tables 4** and **5**). In eastern box turtles, uric acid concentrations and CK activities peak in the summer, whereas bile acid and calcium concentrations increase as the active season progresses.[37] Increased uric acid concentrations could result from dietary changes during the summer months, or be associated with decreased rainfall and resulting water availability.[38] Increased plasma CK activities are likely consistent with increased movement and mate competition during the active season.[41,42] Progressive increases of bile acid and calcium concentrations are likely related to reproductive physiology, specifically in females producing greater than one clutch per year. Female box turtles have significantly increased plasma concentrations of calcium, phosphorous, and cholesterol compared with males, whereas uric acid concentrations tend to be increased in males; importantly, there is no difference in calcium:phosphorous between the sexes.[23,24,37,43] Increased concentrations of calcium, phosphorous, and cholesterol are consistent with egg formation, and these sex differences are highly conserved among chelonians.[38,41,42,51] Increased plasma concentrations of uric acid are also common in male chelonians, though the reason why is not entirely clear.[41,42,51] Adult eastern box turtles have greater total calcium concentrations and calcium:phosphorous than juveniles, whereas juveniles have higher plasma phosphorous concentrations,[23,37] likely based on differences in physiology between growing and reproductively active turtles. Reference intervals for eastern and ornate box turtle plasma biochemistry panels are provided in **Tables 4** and **5**.

Table 4
Plasma biochemistry reference ranges for apparently healthy free-living eastern box turtles (*Terrapene carolina carolina*) in Illinois[21,37]

Parameter	Units	Partition	N	CT	Dispersion	Min	Max	Reference Interval
Calcium	mg/dL	Female*	165	13.55	9.9–21.53	7.1	37.3	8.25–28.79
	mg/dL	Male*	124	10.45	7.49–12.43	4.8	24.1	7.1–14.11
	mg/dL	Juvenile	37	10.4	2.26	5.1	15.2	5.1–15.2
Phosphorous	mg/dL	Female*	165	4.2	2.9–5.61	2	8.8	2.3–7.75
	mg/dL	Male*	124	3.1	2.3–4.51	1.5	6.6	1.8–5.29
	mg/dL	Juvenile	37	3.95	0.84	2.8	8.3	2.02–0.2
Calcium:phosphorous		Adult*	314	3.39	2.34–4.39	1.65	6.4	2–4.87
		Juvenile	61	2.93	0.78	1.2	4.38	1.2–4.38
Bile acids	µmol/L	Spring*	229	4.9	2.6–12	1.1	42.3	2.1–18.3
	µmol/L	Summer*	61	7	2.7–15.6	2	28.9	2–27
	µmol/L	Fall*	85	8.2	4.2–15.3	2.6	27.8	2.7–26
Uric acid	mg/dL	Spring*	228	1.4	0.9–1.5	0.8	3	0.8–1.8
	mg/dL	Summer*	61	1.4	0.8–2.6	0.8	3.1	0.8–3.04
	mg/dL	Fall*	84	1.5	0.9–2.3	0.8	4.4	0.8–2.7
Creatine kinase	U/L	Spring*	230	307	125–777	31	2521	85–1424
	U/L	Summer*	56	373	156–699	42	4,268	118–1,058
	U/L	Fall*	83	304	121–661	17	5,163	61–1,165
Aspartate aminotransferase*	U/L		371	65	38–123	19	1230	32–199

Blood samples were collected from the subcarapacial sinus and stored in lithium heparin. Plasma samples were frozen before analysis. Data distribution is normal unless indicated by an *. CT = measure of central tendency, mean for normally distributed data, median for nonnormally distributed data. Dispersion = standard deviation for normally distributed data or 10th–90th percentiles for nonnormally distributed data.

Table 5
Plasma biochemistry reference ranges for apparently healthy free-living ornate box turtles (*Terrapene ornata*) in Illinois sampled in May.[21,37]

Parameter	Units	Partition	N	CT	Dispersion	Min	Max	Reference Interval
Calcium	mg/dL	Male	36	8.74	1.17	6.8	12.1	6.8–12.1
	mg/dL	Female*	20	13.9	9.07–22.52	9	28.4	9–28.4
Phosphorous	mg/dL	Male*	36	2.35	1.95–3.1	1.9	4.2	1.9–4.2
	mg/dL	Female	18	4.06	1.3	2.2	7.6	–
Calcium:phosphorous			48	3.6	0.64	2.52	4.84	2.53–4.82
Bile acids*	µmol/L		48	4.5	2.7–8.6	2	12.7	2–12.6
Uric acid*	mg/dL		38	1.4	0.9–2	0.8	5.6	1–2.2
Creatine kinase*	U/L		48	188	46–697	10	3002	11–2698
Aspartate aminotransferase*	U/L		48	77	48–159	33	222	33-222

Blood samples were collected from the subcarapacial sinus and stored in lithium heparin. Plasma samples were frozen before analysis. Data distribution is normal unless indicated by an *. CT = measure of central tendency, mean for normally distributed data, median for nonnormally distributed data. Dispersion = standard deviation for normally distributed data or 10th–90th percentiles for nonnormally distributed data. Reference intervals were not calculated for fewer than 20 turtles.

Protein Electrophoresis and Inflammatory Markers

The acute phase response is a highly coordinated but nonspecific physiologic reaction to combat infection, inflammation, stress, and neoplasia. Multiple testing modalities are available to assess single or multiple acute phase reactants; those that have been evaluated in box turtles include plasma protein electrophoresis, hemoglobin-binding protein (HBP), erythrocyte sedimentation rate (ESR), and fibrinogen. Protein electrophoresis has been investigated in eastern[37,52] and ornate[37] box turtles with reference intervals generated (**Tables 6** and **7**). Generally, TP, albumin, and A:G values are highest in the summer, likely consistent with changes in resource availability and the reproductive cycle.[37,52] Female box turtles have relatively increased TP and beta globulin concentrations compared with males, with inconsistent increases in other protein fractions.[37,52] This is likely attributable to vitellogenesis, as proteins are mobilized for egg formation. Increased beta globulins have also been documented in other female turtles and tortoises.[30,41] Adult box turtles have relatively increased concentrations of beta globulins, whereas juveniles have increased albumin concentrations.[37,52] Differences in antigenic stimulation and the acute phase response between the age classes may contribute to a difference in protein fractions based on age.

Hemoglobin-binding protein scavenges free hemoglobin, prevents oxidative damage, and interferes with bacterial growth. This acute phase reactant is higher in adult eastern and ornate box turtles compared with juveniles, and higher in female eastern box turtles compared with males.[40,52] Concentrations of HBP are also relatively increased in sick and injured turtles.[40] Interestingly, HBP values do not seem to

---

Table 6
Plasma protein electrophoresis and erythrocyte sedimentation rate reference ranges for apparently healthy free-living eastern box turtles (*Terrapene carolina carolina*) in Illinois[21,37,40]

Analyte	Units	Partition	N	CT	Dispersion	Min	Max	Reference Interval
Total protein	g/dL	Female	32	3.74	1.44	1.4	6.8	1.4–6.5
	g/dL	Male*	35	3.2	2–6	1.4	7.2	1.4–7.0
Prealbumin*	g/dL		75	0	0–0.07	0	0.11	0–0.09
Albumin	g/dL	Adult	63	1	0.43	0.3	1.94	0.31–1.85
	g/dL	Juvenile	12	1.2	0.4	0.66	1.74	–
Alpha 1 globulins*	g/dL		75	0.48	0.25–0.65	0.18	0.82	0.2–0.72
Alpha 2 globulins*	g/dL		75	1.25	0.66–1.75	0.46	2.09	0.56–2.05
Beta globulins	g/dL	Female	32	1.76	0.53	1.04	2.99	1.04–2.99
	g/dL	Male	35	1.5	0.5	0.63	2.63	0.63–2.63
	g/dL	Juvenile	12	1.3	0.32	0.77	1.85	–
Gamma globulins	g/dL		75	0.43	0.15	0.14	0.9	0.16–0.72
Albumin:globulin		Spring	75	0.43	0.15	0.14	0.9	0.16–0.72
Erythrocyte sedimentation rate*	mm		85	4.7	3.1–7.3	1.1	14	2.6–8.4

Blood samples collected from the subcarapacial sinus, stored in lithium heparin. ESR values determined using hematocrit tubes. Plasma samples frozen before analysis. Data distribution is normal unless indicated by an *. CT = measure of central tendency, mean for normally distributed data, median for nonnormally distributed data. Dispersion = standard deviation for normally distributed data or 10th–90th percentiles for nonnormally distributed data. Reference intervals not calculated for less than 20 turtles.

Table 7
Plasma protein electrophoresis, hemoglobin-binding protein, and erythrocyte sedimentation rate (ESR) reference ranges for apparently healthy free-living ornate box turtles (*Terrapene ornata*) in Illinois sampled in May[21,37,40]

Parameter	Units	Partition	N	CT	Dispersion	Min	Max	Reference Interval
Total protein	g/dL		102	4.55	3–7.19	2.2	9.8	2.32–8.94
Prealbumin	g/dL		101	0.07	0.02–0.15	0	0.27	0–0.23
Albumin	g/dL		102	1.19	0.77–1.94	0.57	2.92	0.62–2.34
Alpha 1 globulins	g/dL		102	0.39	0.27–0.67	0.07	0.93	0.23–0.82
Alpha 2 globulins	g/dL		102	1.22	0.73–2.12	0.51	3.1	0.56–2.78
Beta globulins	g/dL		102	1.32	0.84–2.28	0.54	2.8	0.61–2.53
Gamma globulins	g/dL		102	0.38	0.23–0.63	0.16	0.75	0.17–0.74
Albumin:globulin*			102	0.39	0.069	0.23	0.6	0.27–0.54
Hemoglobin-binding protein	mg/dL	Adult	102	0.359	0.272–0.49	0.092	1.25	0.228–0.532
	mg/dL	Juvenile*	9	0.26	0.097	0.169	0.472	–
Erythrocyte sedimentation rate	mm		105	4.4	1.1	2	7.3	2.6–6.8

Blood samples were collected from the subcarapacial sinus and stored in lithium heparin, ESR was determined using hematocrit tubes. Plasma samples were frozen before analysis. Data distribution is normal unless indicated by an *. CT = measure of central tendency, mean for normally distributed data, median for nonnormally distributed data. Dispersion = standard deviation for normally distributed data or 10th–90th percentiles for nonnormally distributed data.

vary by year, potentially indicating a more stable baseline (and more reliable reference intervals) than other box turtle clinical pathology analytes.[40]

ESR measures the distance that erythrocytes settle out of an undisturbed blood sample after 60 minutes. These values are positively associated with fibrinogen concentrations, with increased values corresponding to higher levels of inflammation. ESR is negatively correlated with PCV and is higher in female eastern box turtles compared with males.[40] Similar values for ESR throughout seasons and populations of wild turtles suggest a lower biological variability than many other box turtle diagnostics. In addition, ESR values are higher in sick/injured turtles vs. healthy conspecifics, and the test is economical and easy to perform in-house using hematocrit tubes.[40] Thus, ESR may be diagnostically useful in this genus, similar to gopher tortoises (*Gopherus polyphemus*).[53]

Fibrinogen is an acute-phase protein and the final protein in the mammalian clotting cascade. Fibrinogen concentrations have been investigated in ornate box turtles using a modified Clauss method.[54] Turtles without evidence of inflammation had significantly decreased fibrinogen concentrations than those with suspected or confirmed inflammatory conditions. Fibrinogen concentrations did not vary by sex, season, animal source (wild vs. captive), or venipuncture site, though this study was relatively small (N = 48) and the method is unlikely to be available to most practitioners.[54]

Additional Clinical Pathology Tests

Venous blood gas and lactate concentrations have been explored in eastern box turtles using point-of-care analyzers (**Table 8**).[55,56] Most blood gas analytes of box turtles vary seasonally, with decreased pH, bicarbonate, total carbon dioxide (TCO_2) and

Table 8
Venous blood gas reference ranges for apparently healthy free-living eastern box turtles (*Terrapene carolina carolina*) in Illinois[21,56]

Analytes	Units	Season	N	Mean	SD	Min	Max	Reference Range
pH		Spring	38	7.49	0.18	7.18	7.84	7.18–7.84
		Summer	41	7.36	0.2	7	7.78	7.00–7.78
		Fall	17	7.59	0.14	7.29	7.8	–
pO$_2$	mm Hg	Spring	38	57	19	18	87	18–87
		Summer	41	58	21	8	98	8–97
		Fall	17	58	11	34	77	–
pCO$_2$	mm Hg	Spring	38	32.8	12.1	15.1	64.9	15.1–64.9
		Summer	41	43.9	16.8	16.5	75.1	16.5–74.7
		Fall	17	25.3	7	16.4	40.2	–
HCO$_3$	mmol/L	Spring	38	29.4	4.8	22.6	41.8	22.6–41.8
		Summer	40	28.2	5.1	17.7	40.6	20.4–40.6
		Fall	17	32	4.6	23	41.5	–
TCO$_2$	mmol/L	Spring	38	31	4.7	24	43	24–43
		Summer	41	30	5	20	43	20–43
		Fall	17	33	4.5	25	43	–
Lactate	mmol/L	Spring	38	4.97	2.84	1.23	11.78	1.23–11.78
		Summer	40	7.4	2.72	2.43	14.17	2.45–12.16
		Fall	16	4.61	3.21	1.04	11.36	–
Base excess	mmol/L	Spring	37	1.9	4.9	−7	11	−18
		Summer	40	−0.5	5.6	−13	14	−27
		Fall	17	3.5	4.2	−5	10	–

Blood samples were collected from the subcarapacial sinus and blood gas analysis was performed immediately using a CG4+ blood gas cartridge and an iSTAT 2 portable analyzer (iSTAT, Abbott, North Chicago, Illinois). Reference intervals were not calculated for fewer than 20 turtles.

base excess, and an increased partial pressure of CO$_2$ (Pco$_2$) and lactate concentrations in the summer. These changes are likely mediated by temperature and/or increases in activity level and metabolic rate.[56] Turtles that remain withdrawn into their shells have lower pH and Po$_2$ and higher Pco$_2$ than active individuals. This is consistent with a relative respiratory acidemia, potentially associated with impaired ventilation because of limited movement of the limbs within the shell.[56] Lactate concentrations have been assessed in eastern box turtles using a hand-held lactate meter.[55] Blood lactate concentrations increase following capture in wild eastern box turtles, with peak concentrations reached at 129 minutes.[55] Turtles that remain in their shells have increased lactate concentrations, again consistent with increased anaerobic respiration secondary to breath-holding. Taken together, these studies indicate that box turtles should not be taped into their shells for prolonged periods of time as a means of restraint.

Future Directions

Diagnostic clinical pathology testing is relatively well-described in the eastern box turtle compared with other species of turtle, however, many important research questions remain unanswered for this and other box turtle species. For example, the analytical variability of many clinical pathology analytes has yet to be characterized. Determining this information for total leukocyte estimates from blood films and for leukocyte counts using NH's method would help support clinical decisions about which leukocyte quantification method to use. Understanding the effects of venipuncture site and sample storage on box turtle clinical pathology parameters would also inform diagnostic test interpretation. Investigating the proteome of sick and injured box turtles could help clarify the utility of routine biochemistry enzymes and identify novel enzymes for future assessment. Indeed, many box turtle clinical pathology tests need to be explored in turtles with known duration illness and injury to uncover their use for differentiating sick and health animals. Some tests, such as urinalysis and coagulation factor testing, have been largely ignored and deserve to be examined to improve medical management of box turtles and other reptiles. Biological variation in box turtle clinical pathology parameters should also be investigated to determine whether subject-based or population-based reference intervals are most appropriate. Finally, clinical pathology research should be expanded to other species in the genus *Terrapene*.

SUMMARY

Box turtles are a unique group of charismatic chelonians commonly presented for veterinary care. Although our understanding of reptile clinical pathology remains rudimentary compared with birds and mammals, knowledge about box turtle diagnostics has increased dramatically over the last 15 years. Here we summarized the current literature about clinical pathology testing in box turtles and identified directions for future research. Continued advancement in this field has the potential to improve box turtle health assessments and veterinary care, ultimately benefitting species conservation and captive management.

CLINICS CARE POINTS

- Lithium heparin is the preferred anticoagulant in box turtles, as EDTA causes hemolysis.
- Many clinical pathology analytes vary based on year, season, sex, and age class in addition to health status.
- Venipuncture site, sample handling, and analytical methodology can also significantly influence clinical pathology values.
- Biological and analytical factors must be considered during interpretation of clinical pathology values. We recommend that clinicians utilize the same venipuncture site and analytical methods for serial patient assessments.

DISCLOSURE

The authors work in a laboratory that provides infectious disease testing for reptile clinicians. This role has not influenced the structure or content of this article.

REFERENCES

1. Rhodin A, Iverson J, Bour R, et al, Turtle Taxonomy Working Group. 9th edition. Turtles of the world annotated checklist and atlas of taxonomy, synonymy, distribution, and conservation status, vol. 8. Rochester, NY, USA: Mercury Print Productions; 2021. p. 1–472.
2. Boers KL, Allender MC, Novak LJ, et al. Assessment of hematologic and corticosterone response in free-living eastern box turtles (*Terrapene carolina carolina*) at capture and after handling. Zoo Biol 2020;39(1):13–22.

3. Heatley JJ, Russell KE. Box turtle (*Terrapene* spp.) hematology. J Exot Pet Med 2010;19(2):160–4.

4. Hernandez-Divers S, Hernandez-Divers S, Wyneken J. Angiographic anatomic and clinical technique descriptions of a subcarapacial sinus in chelonians. J Herpetol Med Surg 2002;12:32–7.

5. Innis C, DeVoe R, Mylniczenko N, et al. A call for additional study of the safety of subcarapacial venipuncture in chelonians. In: Proceedings of the association of reptile and Amphibian veterinarians. South Padre Island, TX; 2010:8-10.

6. Rockwell K, Rademacher N, Osborn M, et al. The subcarapacial vessel in chelonians: safe for intravenous injections? In: Proceedings of ExoticsCon. September 29 – October 3, St Louis, MO; 2019:559.

7. Neiffer DL, Hayek LAC, Conyers D, et al. Comparison of subcarapacial sinus and brachial vein phlebotomy sites for blood collection in free-ranging gopher tortoises (*Gopherus polyphemus*). J Zoo Wildl Med 2021;52(3):966–74.

8. Gottdenker N, Jacobson ER. Effect of venipuncture sites on hematological and clinical chemistry values in the desert tortoise, *Gopherus agassizii*. Am J Vet Res 1995;56(1):19–21.

9. Bonnet X, El Hassani MS, Lecq S, et al. Blood mixtures: impact of puncture site on blood parameters. J Comp Physiol B 2016;186(6):787–800.

10. Sykes JM, Klaphake E. Reptile hematology. Vet Clin North Am Exot Anim Pract 2015;18(1):63–82.

11. Klein K, Gartlan B, Doden G, et al. Comparing the effects of lithium heparin and dipotassium ethylenediaminetetraacetic acid on hematologic values in eastern box turtles (*Terrapene carolina carolina*). J Zoo Wildl Med 2021;51(4):999–1006.

12. Abou-Madi N, Jacobson ER. Effects of blood processing techniques on sodium and potassium values: a comparison between Aldabra tortoises (*Geochelone gigantea*) and Burmese Mountain tortoises (*Manouria emys*). Vet Clin Pathol 2003; 32(2):61–6.

13. Kunze PE, Perrault JR, Chang YM, et al. Pre-/analytical factors affecting whole blood and plasma glucose concentrations in loggerhead sea turtles (*Caretta caretta*). PLoS One 2020;15(3). https://doi.org/10.1371/JOURNAL.PONE. 0229800.

14. Eshar D, Kaufman E. Effects of time and storage temperature on selected biochemical analytes in plasma of red-eared sliders (*Trachemys scripta elegans*). Am J Vet Res 2018;79(8):852–7.

15. Eisenhawer E, Courtney CH, Raskin RE, et al. Relationship between separation time of plasma from heparinized whole blood on plasma biochemical analytes of loggerhead sea turtles (*Caretta caretta*). J Zoo Wildl Med 2008;39(2):208–15.

16. Alberghina D, Marafioti S, Spadola F, et al. Influence of short-term storage conditions on the stability of total protein concentrations and electrophoretic fractions in plasma samples from loggerhead sea turtles, *Caretta caretta*. Comp Clin Path 2015;24(5):1091–5.

17. Sheldon JD, Stacy NI, Blake S, et al. Comparison of total leukocyte quantification methods in free-living Galapagos tortoises (*Chelonoidis* spp.). J Zoo Wildl Med 2016;47(1):196–205.

18. López-Olvera JR, Montané J, Marco I, et al. Effect of venipuncture site on hematologic and serum biochemical parameters in marginated tortoise (*Testudo marginata*). J Wildl Dis 2003;39(4):830–6.

19. Werner RE, Lindley LC. Comparison between femoral and dorsal coccygeal venipuncture techniques on packed cell volumes and hemoglobin concentration in

the diamondback terrapin, *Malaclemys terrapin*. J Herpetol Med Surg 2005; 15(4):19–20.

20. Stewart K, Mitchell MA, Norton T, et al. Measuring the level of agreement in hematologic and biochemical values between blood sampling sites in leatherback sea turtles (*Dermochelys coriacea*). J Zoo Wildl Med 2012;43(4):719–25.

21. Friedrichs KR, Harr KE, Freeman KP, et al. ASVCP reference interval guidelines: determination of de novo reference intervals in veterinary species and other related topics. Vet Clin Pathol 2012;41(4):441–53.

22. Kimble SJA, Williams RN. Temporal variance in hematologic and plasma biochemical reference intervals for free-ranging eastern box turtles (*Terrapene carolina carolina*). J Wildl Dis 2012;48(3):799–802.

23. Rose BMW, Allender MC. Health assessment of the free-ranging eastern box turtle (*Terrapene carolina carolina*) in east Tennessee. J Herpetol Med Surg 2011; 21(4):107–12.

24. Lloyd TC, Allender MC, Archer G, et al. Modeling hematologic and biochemical parameters with spatiotemporal analysis for the free-ranging eastern box turtle (*Terrapene carolina carolina*) in Illinois and Tennessee, a potential biosentinel. EcoHealth 2016;13(3):467–79.

25. Klaphake E, Gibbons PM, Sladky KK, et al. Chapter 4 reptiles. In: Carpenter J, Marion C, editors. Exotic animal formulary. Elsevier; 2018. p. 81–166.

26. Gibbons PM, Whitaker BR, Carpenter JW, et al. Hematology and biochemistry tables. In: Divers S, Stahl S, editors. Mader's reptile and amphibian medicine and surgery. Elsevier; 2019. p. 333–50.

27. Walton RM. Subject-based reference values: Biological variation, individuality, and reference change values. Vet Clin Pathol 2012;41(2):175–81.

28. Bertelsen MF, Kjelgaard-Hansen M, Howell JR, et al. Short-term biological variation of clinical chemical values in Dumeril's monitors (*Varanus dumerili*). J Zoo Wildl Med 2007;38(2):217–21.

29. Mumm LE, Winter JM, Andersson KE, et al. Hematology and plasma biochemistries in the Blanding's turtle (*Emydoidea blandingii*) in Lake County, Illinois. PLoS One 2019;14(11). https://doi.org/10.1371/JOURNAL.PONE.0225130.

30. Andersson KE, Adamovicz L, Mumm LE, et al. Plasma electrophoresis profiles of Blanding's turtles (*Emydoidea blandingii*) and influences of month, age, sex, health status, and location. PLoS One 2021;16(10). https://doi.org/10.1371/JOURNAL.PONE.0258397.

31. Deem SL, Norton TM, Mitchell M, et al. Comparison of blood values in foraging, nesting, and stranded loggerhead turtles (*Caretta caretta*) along the coast of Georgia, USA. J Wildl Dis 2009;45(1):41–56.

32. Deem SL, Dierenfeld ES, Sounguet GP, et al. Blood values in free-ranging nesting leatherback sea turtles (*Dermochelys coriacea*) on the coast of the Republic of Gabon. J Zoo Wildl Med 2006;37(4):464–71.

33. Winter JM, Stacy NI, Adamovicz LA, et al. Investigating the analytical variability and agreement of manual leukocyte quantification methods in eastern box turtles (*Terrapene carolina carolina*). Front Vet Sci 2019;6. https://doi.org/10.3389/fvets.2019.00398.

34. Allender MC, Fry MM, Irizarry AR, et al. Intracytoplasmic inclusions in circulating leukocytes from an eastern box turtle (*Terrapene carolina carolina*) with iridoviral infection. J Wildl Dis 2006;42(3):677–84.

35. Flanders AJ, Ossiboff RJ, Wellehan JFX, et al. Presumptive heterophil extracellular traps recognized cytologically in nine reptile patients with inflammatory conditions. Vet Q 2021;41(1):89–96.

36. Stacy NI, Fredholm DV, Rodriguez C, et al. Whip-like heterophil projections in consecutive blood films from an injured gopher tortoise (*Gopherus polyphemus*) with systemic inflammation. Vet Q 2017;37(1):162–5.

37. Adamovicz L. Modeling the health of free-living Illinois herptiles: an integrated approach incorporating environmental, physiologic, spatiotemporal, and pathogen factors. [PhD Thesis]. Urbana, Illinois: University of Illinois; 2019.

38. Christopher MM, Berry KH, Wallis IR, et al. Reference intervals and physiologic alterations in hematologic and biochemical values of free-ranging desert tortoises in the Mojave Desert. J Wildl Dis 1999;35(2):212–38.

39. Dickinson VM, Jarchow JL, Trueblood MH. Hematology and plasma biochemistry reference range values for free-ranging desert tortoises in Arizona. J Wildl Dis 2002;38(1):143–53.

40. Adamovicz L, Baker SJ, Kessler E, et al. Erythrocyte sedimentation rate and hemoglobin-binding protein in free-living box turtles (*Terrapene* spp.). PloS One 2020;15(6). https://doi.org/10.1371/JOURNAL.PONE.0234805.

41. Zaias J, Norton T, Fickel A, et al. Biochemical and hematologic values for 18 clinically healthy radiated tortoises (*Geochelone radiata*) on St Catherine's Island, Georgia. Vet Clin Pathol 2006;35(3):321–5.

42. Yang PY, Yu PH, Wu SH, et al. Seasonal hematology and plasma biochemistry reference range values of the yellow-marginated box turtle (*Cuora flavomarginata*). J Zoo Wildl Med 2014;45(2):278–86.

43. Adamovicz L, Bronson E, Barrett K, et al. Health assessment of free-living eastern box turtles (*Terrapene carolina carolina*) in and around the Maryland Zoo in Baltimore 1996-2011. J Zoo Wildl Med 2015;46(1):39–51.

44. Cerreta AJ, Mehalick ML, Stoskopf MK, et al. Assessment of a visual scoring system for identifying and quantifying anemia in male eastern box turtles (*Terrapene carolina carolina*). J Zoo Wildl Med 2018;49(4):977–82.

45. Brenner D, Lewbart G, Stebbins M, et al. Health survey of wild and captive bog turtles (*Clemmys muhlenbergii*) in North Carolina and Virginia. J Zoo Wildl Med 2002;33(4):311–6.

46. Keller KA, Guzman DSM, Paul-Murphy J, et al. Hematologic and plasma biochemical values of free-ranging western pond turtles (*Emys marmorata*) with comparison to a captive population. J Herpetol Med Surg 2012;22(3):99–106.

47. Rangel-Mendoza J, Weber M, Zenteno-Ruiz CE, et al. Hematology and serum biochemistry comparison in wild and captive Central American river turtles (*Dermatemys mawii*) in Tabasco, Mexico. Res Vet Sci 2009;87(2):313–8.

48. Adamovicz L, Griffioen J, Cerreta A, et al. Tissue enzyme activities in free-living eastern box turtles (*Terrapene carolina carolina*). J Zoo Wildl Med 2019;50(1):45–54.

49. Boyd JW. Serum enzymes in the diagnosis of disease in man and animals. J Comp Pathol 1988;98(4):381–404.

50. Boyd JW. The mechanisms relating to increases in plasma enzymes and isoenzymes in diseases of animals. Vet Clin Pathol 1983;12(2):9–24.

51. Chung CS, Cheng CH, Chin SC, et al. Morphologic and cytochemical characteristics of Chinese striped-necked [corrected] turtle (*Ocadia sinensis*) blood cells and their hematologic and plasma biochemical reference values. J Zoo Wildl Med 2009;40(1):76–85.

52. Flower JE, Byrd J, Cray C, et al. Plasma electrophoretic profiles and hemoglobin binding protein reference intervals in the eastern box turtle (*Terrapene carolina carolina*) and influences of age, sex, season, and location. J Zoo Wildl Med 2014;45(4):836–42.

53. Rosenberg JF, Hernandez JA, Wellehan JFX, et al. Diagnostic performance of inflammatory markers in gopher tortoises (*Gopherus Polyphemus*). J Zoo Wildl Med 2018;49(3):765–9.

54. Parkinson L, Olea-Popelka F, Klaphake E, et al. Establishment of a fibrinogen reference interval in ornate box turtles (*Terrapene ornata ornata*). J Zoo Wildl Med 2016;47(3):754–9.

55. Klein K, Adamovicz L, Phillips CA, et al. Blood lactate concentrations in eastern box turtles (*Terrapene carolina carolina*) following capture by a canine search team. J Zoo Wildl Med 2021;52(1):259–67.

56. Adamovicz L, Leister K, Byrd J, et al. Venous blood gas in free-living eastern box turtles (*Terrapene carolina carolina*) and effects of physiologic, demographic and environmental factors. Conserv Physiol 2018;6(1). https://doi.org/10.1093/CONPHYS/COY041.

Diagnostic Clinical Pathology of Tortoises

Cheryl Moller, BSc, BVMS, MS, DACVP(Clinical)[a],*,
J. Jill Heatley, DVM, MS, DABVP (Avian, Reptilian, Amphibian), DACZM[b]

KEYWORDS

- Tortoise • Clinical pathology • Reptile • Hematology • Biochemistry • Urinalysis

KEY POINTS

- Clinical pathology of terrestrial tortoises is useful for health assessment and monitoring.
- Multiple preanalytical factors influence clinical pathology, especially the hematology, of tortoises, including season/time of year, age, sex, diet, and captive versus wild.
- Hematology reference intervals are often wide owing to preanalytical influences and also reliance on manual methods because all blood cells are nucleated.

INTRODUCTION

Reptiles of the family Testudinae, order Testudines, commonly known as tortoises, are distinguished from other turtles based on multiple characteristics to include being very long lived, mainly to exclusively herbivorous, land-dwelling, having domed thick shells, and clublike forelegs and elephantine hindlegs. Most are reclusive and diurnal or crepuscular. Thus, in many cultures, the tortoise is symbolic of longevity, endurance, and being grounded. Common species of tortoises maintained in captivity, their origins, and dietary habits are provided in **Table 1**. Clinicopathologic evaluation of blood and urine provides typically a low invasive means of evaluating health status in tortoises just like other species. In this article, the authors refer specifically to terrestrial tortoises because box turtles and aquatic turtles are discussed by other authors in this issue.

Data from clinical pathology tests: complete blood count (CBC), biochemistry, urinalysis, are compared with reference data from what is considered normal for a healthy individual. There is a wealth of information available on the American Society for Veterinary Clinical Pathology Web site published by the Quality Assurance and Laboratory Standards committee on how to construct clinical pathology reference

[a] ANTECH Diagnostics, 17260 Mt Herrmann Street, Fountain Valley, CA 92708, USA;
[b] Department of Small Animal Clinical Sciences, College of Veterinary Medicine & Biomedical Sciences, Texas A&M University, College Station, TX 77843, USA
* Corresponding author.
E-mail address: cheryl.moller@gmail.com

Vet Clin Exot Anim 25 (2022) 755–783
https://doi.org/10.1016/j.cvex.2022.05.007
1094-9194/22/© 2022 Elsevier Inc. All rights reserved.

Table 1
Common pet tortoise species natural range, preferred temperature and humidity, and dietary habits

Species	Origin	Preferred Temperature, Relative Humidity (RH)	Natural Dietary Habits
African spurred tortoise *Centrochelys (Geochelone) sulcate*	Southern Sahara, from Senegal and Mauritania east through Mali, Niger, Chad, Sudan, Ethiopia, along the Red Sea in Eritrea	Day, 29°C–40°C (85°F–105°F). Night, 21°C–26°C Day, RH, 40%–60%. Night, RH, 70%–80%	Herbivore: grass 90%
Leopard tortoise *Stigmochelys pardalis*	Savannas of Southern and Eastern Africa, from Ethiopia to Sudan, from Natal to southern Angola, South Africa, part of southwestern Africa. Semi-arid to grasslands	Day, between 75°F and 95°F. Night, not <70°F. Day, RH, 40%–60%. Night, RH, 70%–80%	Savanna grass graze. Strict herbivores; will eat grass, but prefer to graze on succulents, flowers, fungi, berries, and other fruits. Sometimes ash or carrion
Russian tortoise *Testudo (Agrionemys) horsfieldii*	Caspian Sea south through Iran, Pakistan, and Afghanistan, and east across Kazakhstan to Xinjiang, China. Arid, barren places, rocky hillsides, deserts, sandy steppes, grassy regions close to springs. Winter temperatures below freezing	Winter lows, 20°F, summer highs, 120°F. Most active at 60°F–90°F maintained indoors, 68°F–80°F basking spot 90°F–100°F. Night low, 50°F. RH, 30%–50%.	Herbaceous and succulent vegetation, green and dried, flowers, fruits, twigs eaves, and stems of both native and cultivated plants
Hermann's tortoise *Testudo hermanni*	Spain, France, Italy, Greece, Turkey, and the countries of the Balkans. Mediterranean evergreen and oak forests, arid, rocky hill slopes, scrubby vegetation, herbaceous scrub, grassy hillsides	Day, 15°C–30°C (60°F–85°F) basking spot 32°C–35°C (90°F–95°F). Night, 5°C–25°C (40°F–75°F). RH, 40%–75%. Natural climate tends to be moist during spring and fall, dry summers	~90% herbivorous diet of succulent and herbaceous plants. Favors legumes, clovers to grass. Opportunistic omnivores: invertebrates, worms, snails, carrion
Mediterranean tortoise *Testudo (graeca) ibera T g graeca*	Arid regions in Mediterranean Europe, Africa, parts of the Middle East	Day, 26°C–30°C (78.8°F–86°F) basking spot of 30°C–33°C (85°F–90°F). Night temperature should exceed 18°C (64.4°F)	Mainly herbaceous and succulent vegetation: grasses, flowers, twigs, occasionally fallen fruit

Red-footed tortoise *Geochelone carbonaria*	Dry and wet forests and grasslands of Central and South America	Day, 85°F–90°F, basking spot of 95°F. RH, 50%–70%	Wide variety in natural diet. 60% dark leafy greens and grasses, 15% vegetables, 15% fruit, 10% tortoise pellets or animal protein
Gopher tortoise *Gopherus polyphemus*	Southeastern United States	70°F –95°F. RH, ~80%	Herbivore scavengers, opportunistic grazers of a wide range of plants. Mainly broad-leaved grass, regular grass, wiregrass, legumes, but also mushrooms, gopher apple, pawpaw, blackberries, saw palmetto berries, nettle flowers, and Spanish and ball mosses
Desert tortoise *Gopherus agassizii* *G morafkai* *G evgoodei*	Deserts of SW United States and NW Mexico, Arizona, southeastern California, southern Nevada, southwestern Utah	Brumation: 40°F –55°F (4.5°C–13°C). RH, 30%–40% Nonbrumation: 80°F–85°F (27°C–30°C)	Herbivore: Grasses are the main diet, but also herbs, wildflowers, new growth of cacti, and their fruit and flowers. Rocks and soil are also ingested

intervals.[1] A group of at least 40, but ideally more than 120 healthy individuals, are sampled, and reference intervals are generated. The more specific the selection criteria for the group, the more robust the data. Reaching those numbers and sampling such a homogenous group becomes problematic when dealing with veterinary species, especially nonmammalian animals.

Limited published studies provide reference data for tortoises. Study methods should be reviewed to determine how the population was defined and how the data were obtained. Tortoises, like all reptiles, are ectotherms, so their metabolic processes are dependent on the environment. This will then influence many clinicopathologic results, especially in the CBC. Methods should specify reference population selection criteria, including sex, age, time of year/season, reproductive status, diet, captive versus wild, and geographic location. Collection methods, storage methods, and analyzer types should also be provided. Although a useful reference where published data are not available, especially for rare species, sources including the Species360 Zoological Information Management System may not provide information about selection criteria or methodology. Where methodology is not outlined or not applicable to the individual, then as a general rule of thumb, do not overinterpret small changes on either side of the reference data. To help address this, a baseline healthy clinical pathology data set can be obtained for an individual to which to compare future samples, and where applicable, follow over time. Concurrent sampling of a healthy conspecific can also be helpful.

Herein, the authors describe sample collection and methodology, CBC, biochemistry, and urinalysis considerations for terrestrial tortoises.

SAMPLE COLLECTION

Indications for sample collection from tortoise species include obvious illness, injury, or clinical signs of infectious disease. However, because of the widely varying and poorly explored physiology of many of these species and their natural seasonal and reproductive cycles and expected longevity, the authors advocate clinicopathologic assessment of most tortoise species a minimum of once yearly, with a recommended CBC and biochemistry panel before the season of hibernation (more correctly termed brumation). Animals that lose excessive weight or have other signs of illness upon emergence from brumation should be reassessed postemergence, or upon wakening should brumation be prematurely halted based on health concerns. In those species that do not brumate based on temperature drop, sampling before the season of lack of food intake (dry season) or before breeding season on a yearly schedule could also be elected. Independent of the season choice, yearly health check samples must be obtained at similar times during the year (same season) to allow better assessment of seasonal yearly and individual health.

Challenges to sample collection are many in tortoise species and include lymphatic contamination, temperature, animal temperament, defenses, and strength. The jugular vein of some tortoises can sometimes be visualized based on gravity and constrictive-assisted fill under the skin based on a vessel filling. However, most vessels are covered by skin and muscle, are relatively deep, and cannot be observed or palpated. Therefore, most approach these vessels based on local landmarks and careful blind sticks. However, the practitioner should always be aware of local nerves, vessels, and tendons and reflect upon the possibility of damage caused by multiple needle sticks. One boon to sample collection in tortoises is that practitioners need not be in a hurry or worried about clotting. Clotting appears to be a slow process in these species (~20 minutes or more), although this timeline has not been well determined in these species. Therefore, hurried sample collection or handling, or the preheparinizing of syringes, is usually not a necessity for tortoises.

Equipment needed for clinicopathologic sample collection will vary depending on the species, sample to be collected (blood, urine, feces, cerebrospinal fluid [CSF]), and collection conditions, but the technician should ensure the following needs are attended:

- Sample collection site cleaning and disinfection
- Needle size and length should be appropriate for patient size, vessel size, and depth, yet large enough to avoid cell lysis. Always have multiple needles and syringes put together and ready. Multiple syringes "set up" are extremely useful in the case of obtaining lymph, in case of the need for resampling, or for choosing another site.
- Tube size is dictated by patient and blood volume. Microtainers are appropriate for small species, but standard pediatric tubes, commonly used for small animal medicine or even human/large tubes, can be used for adult African spurred (sulcata) and larger tortoises. For larger species, lack of sample volume collection should not be a hindrance in the diagnosis.

To the authors' knowledge and based on recent literature search, the blood volume of any tortoise species remains unpublished. Blood volume determination of chelonian species, determined by various methods, appears limited to the aquatic turtles *Pseudemys* spp, *Chrysemys* spp, and *Chelydra* spp, which ranged from 3.3 to 9.08/100 g of body weight, or 3% to 10%.[2] As many tortoises presented for sampling may be overtly or covertly ill, the authors suggest erring on the conservative side for safe sample collection and using the following calculation for determination of a single safe blood draw volume. Tortoise body weight (TBW*) should be used before rehydration to err on conservative side of blood volume estimation.

(0.05) (TBW* g) = Estimated tortoise blood volume, mL (0.05) = single safe maximum blood draw of 5% of total estimated tortoise blood volume, mL.

OR

(0.0025) (TBW* (g)) = single safe maximum blood draw of 5% of total estimated tortoise blood volume, mL

Thus, the estimated blood volume of a 2-kg tortoise would be

(0.05) (2000) = 100 mL

and the single safe maximum blood draw from this 2-kg tortoise would be

(0.05) (100) = 5 mL

SAMPLE COLLECTION SITES

Sample collection sites reported for tortoise blood include the jugular veins, which are preferred based on likelihood of obtaining adequate sample volume uncontaminated by lymph.[3,4] Lymph contamination can cause alterations in many clinicopathologic values.[5–7] Other clinically acceptable sites of venipuncture include the tail or ventral coccygeal vein, the dorsal coccygeal sinus, the brachial vein, and the femoral veins. The occipital sinus and subcarapacial venous plexus may be acceptable in immobilized animals but have the concerns of central nervous system damage and sample contamination with central nervous system fluid.[8] Similarly, cardiac sampling is generally reserved for perimortem or research use.[9] Toenail clipping to obtain samples is inhumane and provides a contaminated sample, which is likely poorly representative of circulating blood.

CSF collection, both purposeful and accidental, has been described for the Galapagos tortoise (*Geochelone nigra*) and the gopher tortoise (*Gopherus polyphemus*).[10] Reptiles lack a true arachnoid space, necessitating that CSF be collected from the subdural space. However, the venous sinus positioned dorsal to the spinal cord is likely to cause blood contamination of collected samples. In all cases, animals should be anesthetized, and strict asepsis followed.[11] Contact your reference laboratories (REF) for particular requirements for CSF submission *before* sample collection. An approach for CSF collection from the gopher tortoise was described with the tortoise positioned in lateral recumbency, the neck extended, and the head ventroflexed. A 25-G, 19-mm needle is advanced paramedial to the sagittal plane, at a point 50% of the supraoccipital protuberance length and at a 45° angle toward the midline for entry to the subdural space.[10] Gradual advancement of the needle is continued in this direction until fluid flows into the needle hub. Literature review failed to reveal published CSF data for any tortoise species.

Tortoise bone marrow is found in medullary bone throughout the body to include the carapace and plastron on the shell.[12] In a postmortem study, bone marrow was obtained from the pelvis, proximal portion of the humerus, femur, and thickened portions of the cranial to craniolateral and caudal to caudolateral margins of the carapace and plastron from desert tortoises (*Gopherus agassizii*).[13] Although a standardized method of bone marrow collection from tortoises has not been described, collection of samples from the proximal humerus and or femur would likely be challenging based on local anatomy and shell obstruction. Collection of bone marrow from the caudolateral margins of the carapace and plastron appears preferable in the live patient based on accessibility and lesser likelihood of causing harm. Sample collection techniques and equipment for the live patient would be similar to those used for companion mammal bone marrow collection in most cases, with consideration of patient size.

SAMPLE HANDLING AND PRESERVATION

For biochemical samples, plasma is the diagnostic sample of choice, and the increased plasma harvest is facilitated by use of lithium heparin-coated tubes. The use of clot tubes and serum remnants, or gel separator tubes and their effect on plasma or serum analytes, has not been investigated in tortoises. Thus, the use of these tubes is not recommended. Lithium heparin is the preferred anticoagulant for tortoises based on the hemolysis noted for EDTA and citrate upon tortoise blood (Heatley, personal communication, 2022). However, the use of alternate anticoagulants for tortoise blood has received minimal investigation. Early separation of plasma is recommended particularly when measuring electrolytes, because potassium concentration may increase and sodium may decrease over time in some tortoises, especially if the sample is not refrigerated.[14]

For hematology, lithium heparin is also used, but "fresh" blood smears, created from blood that has not contacted anticoagulant and then rapidly air dried, are preferred to best facilitate cell differential count and for assessment of blood cell morphology, especially cellular changes associated with inflammation. Avoid allowing slides to share space with formalin-fixed tissues, as the slide fogging created will irreparably damage slide cellular morphology and color, rendering that blood smear to less than useless.

ANALYZER CHOICE

Although studies confirm that point of care (POC), in-house analyzers (INH), and REF may each be useful for clinicopathologic diagnostic purposes in tortoises, many values from these analyzers do not agree. Values from POC, INH, and REF should not be viewed as equivalent or interchangeable for tortoises.[15] Analyzer choice should include knowledge of reference intervals available for the species for that particular platform, cost of analysis, and necessary sample volume and type for the preferred or desired analytes for diagnosis of the suspected malady. Contact your REF for information related to the species of interest before collecting samples. Be wary should the laboratory suggest all tortoise species are the same.

COMPLETE BLOOD COUNT

A CBC is a useful diagnostic and monitoring tool for tortoises, although there are differences compared with domestic mammals, which must be considered. The reptilian ectothermic metabolism means that the environment (eg, season, rainfall, geography) affects hormonal regulation and therefore erythropoiesis and leukocyte levels. Tortoises may also brumate in winter, whereby metabolic processes downregulate, and this affects erythrocyte and leukocyte levels (ie, seasonal effects). Red blood cell (RBC) counts and white blood cell (WBC) counts use manual methods because all blood cells are nucleated and cannot be reliably differentiated by automated analyzers. There is more inherent variability of manual methods with coefficients of variation (CV) reported between 13% and 40%, compared with automated methods, which should have a CV of less than 5% to 10%.[16–18] CBC reference data for common tortoise species have been summarized in **Table 2**.

Erythrocytes

Erythrocytes are most commonly evaluated by measurement of packed cell volume (PCV) and blood smear evaluation. RBC counts are rarely requested or performed based on the technical foibles and time investment required. Tortoise erythrocytes are large ($\sim$17–21 $\times$ 10–12 µm), are elliptical, and have a central oval to mildly irregular nucleus with condensed chromatin, and the cytoplasm stains red/orange on Romanowsky-type stains, like commercial rapid stains and Wright-Giemsa–based stains. Tortoise erythrocytes are presumed to have a long lifespan; however, RBC lifespan has not been reported for tortoises. On a blood smear from a healthy adult tortoise, there are usually only rare polychromatophils (elliptical erythrocytes with a blue hue to the cytoplasm) and immature erythrocytes (round cells with higher nuclear to cytoplasm ratio and blue hue to the cytoplasm) (**Figs. 1** and **2**, also see **Fig. 5**). A normal PCV is usually 20% to 40%, although many reference values include minimums of less than 10% and as low as 6% in healthy individuals. Less than a 10% PCV in an otherwise healthy tortoise could suggest lymph dilution and must be correlated with the collection characteristics (was lymph seen flowing into the needle?) and the WBC differential (higher than expected small mature lymphocytes?).

PCV and RBC count are often higher in males, thought to be due to testosterone.[19] PCV and RBC count may also be higher in summer and lower in winter (especially if brumating).[20] The PCV and RBC count is typically lowest at the end of brumation, right before the metabolism starts to increase again, although there could be concurrent dehydration, especially in species in arid climates.

The same broad causes of anemia and erythrocytosis/polycythemia apply in tortoises as other species. Anemia may be nonregenerative or regenerative. This can be determined by evaluation of a blood smear for polychromasia and more immature erythrocytes. Mitotic figures may be seen in immature erythrocytes in regenerative anemias (**Fig. 3**). Because of the slower production of erythrocytes in tortoises,

Table 2
Hematology data for select tortoise species

Species	Data Format, n, Reference	PCV (%)	RBC Count (×10⁶/µL)	WBC Count (×10³/µL)	Heterophils (×10³/µL)	Lymphocytes (×10³/µL)	Monocytes (×10³/µL)	Azurophils (×10³/µL)	Eosinophils (×10³/µL)	Basophils (×10³/µL)
African spurred tortoise Centrochelys (Geochelone) sulcate	MD[70,a]	28 (9–43)	0.61 (0.08–1.15)	4.41 (0.87–13.23)	1.92 (0.23–7.43)	1.41 (0.17–6.06)	0.01 (0.01–0.37)	0.04 (0–0.84)	0.10 (0.01–0.43)	0.12 (0.01–0.36)
Russian tortoise Testudo (Agrionemys) horsfieldii	MD PCV[71,b] MN WBCs[72,c]	23 (22–34)	—	—	3.72 (1.30–4.56)	4.67 (3.61–7.56)	0.12 (0.01–0.21)	0.51 (0.33–1.20)	0.48 (0.2–0.59)	0.5 (0.20–0.76)
Greek tortoise (Testudo graeca)	MN[73,d]	28 (20–35)	0.67 (0.46–0.84)	7.1 (5.5–12.5)	4.30 (1.87–4.80)	2.86 (1.20–3.91)	0.1 (0–0.20)		0.06 (0–0.33)	Not reported
Hermann tortoise (Testudo hermanni)	MD[48,e]	24 (11–32)	0.8 (0.42–1.02)	9.4 (4.1–14.0)	2.31 (0.79–4.74)	4.44 (1.44–8.49)	0.48 (0.18–1.34)		0.97 (0.36–2.4)	0.0085 (0–0.19)
Red-footed tortoise (Chelonoidis carbonarius)	MN PCV RI WBCs[74,f]	F 20.3 (13–27) M 17 (9–32)	—	4.3–29.7	0–4.4	1.8–20.5	0.1–9.9		0–8.9	0–4.4

| Leopard tortoise (*Stigmochelys pardalis*) | MD[70,a] | 23 (8–37) | 0.52 (0.15–1.06) | 4.24 (0.6–10.0) | 1.92 (0.11–4.87) | 1.61 (0.05–4.74) | 0.08 (0.02–0.62) | 0.02 (0–0.51) | 0.15 (0.02–0.37) | 0.11 (0.01–0.34) |

Data presented as reference intervals (RI), medians (MD), or means (MN), and minimum to maximum (MM) values or confidence intervals (CI) in parentheses.

[a] No data available for selection criteria or methodology.

[b] Eight captive adults, 6 females and 2 males, 3 locations in Germany, spring to late summer, dorsal coccygeal vein, no anticoagulant.[71]

[c] Twenty captive adults, 7 females and 13 males, Brno Czech Republic, time of the year not specified, dorsal coccygeal vein, fresh blood smears without anticoagulant.[72]

[d] Six to 12 captive adults, sex unspecified, England, June presented, samples from January, March, October, November, December revealed seasonal variation, dorsal coccygeal vein, blood smears–anticoagulant not specified, Natt & Herrick's solution for manual RBC and WBC cell counts.[73]

[e] Eastern, 23 captive adults, both sexes but not further specified, northern Italy, September, jugular vein, fresh blood smears without anticoagulant, lithium heparin for other analytes, Natt & Herrick's solution for manual RBC and WBC cell counts.[48]

[f] Forty captive juveniles, 22 females and 18 males, one location, Georgia USA, November, variable venipuncture site, lithium heparin. Sexes stratified for PCV not WBCs.[74]

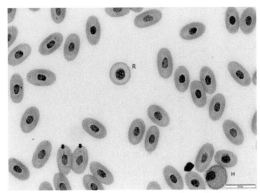

Fig. 1. Blood smear from an African spurred (sulcata) tortoise showing a rubricyte (R). Note also the erythrocyte inclusions (*arrows*), representing degenerate organelles. Also pictured is a heterophil (H) (Wright-Giemsa, original magnification ×600).

an apparently nonregenerative anemia may actually be preregenerative, that is, the bone marrow has not yet responded. To the authors' knowledge, no studies on the duration of the erythrocyte regenerative response in tortoises have been published, but is presumed to be many weeks, and likely affected by the season. Therefore, monitoring PCV and the blood smear over several weeks may be indicated in some cases.

Polychromatophils are rare in healthy adult tortoises, usually less than 1% of the erythrocytes. Polychromasia and increased immature erythrocytes in the absence of anemia may be seen in young tortoises, or may reflect a compensated or emerging

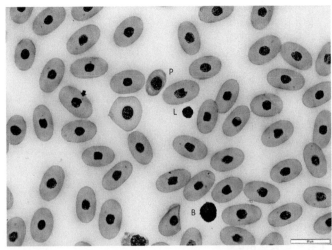

Fig. 2. Blood smear from a radiated tortoise showing a polychromatophil (P). Note also the erythrocyte inclusions (*arrow*), representing degenerate organelles. Also pictured is a small lymphocyte (L) and basophil (B) (Wright-Giemsa, original magnification ×600).

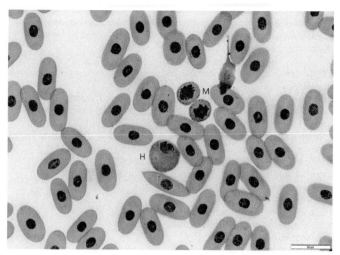

Fig. 3. Blood smear from a desert tortoise showing a mitotic rubricyte (M). Also pictured is a heterophil (H) (Wright-Giemsa, original magnification ×600).

anemia, bone marrow stimulation, including as a normal physiologic change, for example, emerging from brumation, or hypoxia, including from respiratory tract disease.

In general, poikilocytes (abnormally shaped erythrocytes) are most often artifacts of smear preparation. Erythroplastids, which are erythrocytes without nuclei, may be occasionally seen on normal smears and are generally insignificant.

Various types of inclusions may be seen within the cytoplasm erythrocytes. One- to 2-μm pale or light blue inclusions in the erythrocyte cytoplasm are degenerate organelles and considered insignificant (see **Figs. 1** and **2**). Sources may refer to Pirhemocyton, which was supposed to be a type of infection but seems in most cases to represent these degenerate organelles, or possibly iridovirus inclusions. Iridovirus is more commonly reported in the erythrocytes of lizards and snakes.[21] Bacterial and protozoal inclusions may be found in erythrocytes of terrestrial tortoises, including *Anaplasma* morulae, *Hemolivia*, or other hemogregarine protozoa gametocytes, *Haemoproteus* stages especially the gametocytes that contain brown hemozoin pigment, *Plasmodium* spp.[22–27] All these organisms may not be clinically significant, or may cause anemia, especially if there are concurrent stressors.

Extracellular trypanosomes or microfilaria may also occasionally be seen, again, usually thought to be nonpathogenic.[21]

Severe anemia was reported in 2 radiated tortoises with intranuclear coccidiosis, although organisms were not reported within erythrocytes. The mechanism of anemia was not clear.[28]

Causes of anemia

Regenerative
  Blood loss/hemorrhage
  • Trauma
  • Internal or external disease including inflammation, neoplasia

- Gastrointestinal disease, including parasites, ulcers, inflammation, neoplasia
- Potential coagulopathy from thrombocytopenia, disseminated intravascular coagulation (not well documented)

Hemolysis
- Artifact: EDTA anticoagulant in some species, sampling, sample aging, sample exposure to heat or freezing
- Infectious: *Anaplasma*, haemogregarines, *Haemoproteus*, *Plasmodium*
- Oxidative hemolysis, for example, ramson (*Allium ursinum*) toxicosis; no Heinz bodies or eccentrocytes reported[29]
  (Immune-mediated hemolysis has not been documented to the authors' knowledge)

Nonregenerative
- Artifact: lymph dilution, CSF dilution, anticoagulant dilution
- Preregenerative anemia (bone marrow not yet responded)

Anemia of inflammation/chronic disease
- Inflammation
- Chronic disease of any cause including hepatic, renal

Decreased bone marrow production/suppression
- Brumation, that is, normal physiologic
- Decreased nutrient intake, for example, due to prolonged entrapment[30]
- Bone marrow necrosis, for example, viral, such as adenovirus[31,32]
- Potentially drugs or toxins (although not well described in tortoises)
- Neoplasia

Chronic renal insufficiency[33]

Causes of erythrocytosis/polycythemia

- Artifact: Plasma evaporation
- Dehydration

Leukocytes

Leukocytes are most commonly evaluated by blood smear evaluation and manual cell counts. As for all species requiring manual cell counting methods, tortoise WBC count reference intervals may be very wide, so it is difficult to interpret mild changes on the basis of the CBC alone. Blood smear WBC count estimates are less reliable than manual counts in a hemocytometer, with Natt and Herrick's solution the favored hemocytometer stain/diluent.[34,35] Evaluation may also be challenging because thrombocytes (the nonmammalian equivalent of platelets) are nucleated, and both thrombocytes and immature erythrocytes can look similar to small lymphocytes. It is helpful to familiarize oneself with the species and expected differential, and to scan the blood smear to identify all the cell types before counting. Increases or decreases in leukocyte numbers should always be interpreted based on the absolute counts, that is, cells per microliter, not the percentage differential. Most animals have either heterophils/neutrophils or lymphocytes as the predominant leukocyte. However, some tortoises may have a large proportion of basophils.

Hematopoietic neoplasia is rarely reported in tortoises, with lymphoma with peripheralization (leukemia) reported in a Hermann tortoise and Burmese star tortoise.[36,37]

Intracytoplasmic iridovirus (ranavirus) inclusions have been reported in the WBCs of multiple reptile species.

Heterophils

Heterophils are considered the functional equivalent of neutrophils and behave in a similar way. They have an ovoid nucleus in tortoises (rarely bilobed), with dense chromatin, pale cytoplasm filled with usually large numbers of rice or short rod-shaped bright pink/orange granules (**Fig. 4**). Immature heterophils (left shift) will also have small dark pink/purple granules (**Fig. 5**). Toxic changes are seen because of increased marrow production as in mammals, with the same features (cytoplasmic basophilia, cytoplasmic vacuolation, Döhle bodies; see **Fig. 5**). Abnormal granulation may also be seen.[38,39] Heterophil degranulation can be difficult to interpret because it can be an in vitro change but can be a toxic change. Whiplike cytoplasmic projections in heterophils, the same color as the granules, have been reported in a gopher tortoise with inflammation.[40]

Heterophil numbers are usually highest during summer and lowest during brumation and may increase during gravidity/pregnancy.[41] During stress (including captivity), heterophil numbers may be relatively higher and lymphocyte numbers relatively lower, although they may not shift outside the reference intervals. It can be useful to evaluate heterophil to lymphocyte ratios in conjunction with cortisol and other data to investigate stress. Inflammation may alter heterophil numbers or cause left shifting or toxic changes, so other leukocyte changes or other data, such as protein electrophoresis, and possibly lactate or erythrocyte sedimentation rate, must be considered in interpretation.[42]

Causes of heterophilia

- Physiologic: seasonal, gravidity
- Inflammation
- Stress

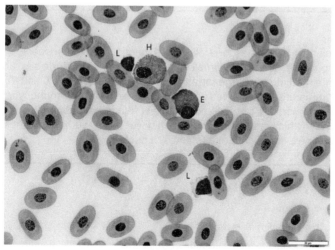

Fig. 4. Blood smear from an Indian star tortoise showing a mature heterophil (H) adjacent to an eosinophil (E), and 2 small lymphocytes also pictured (L) (Wright-Giemsa, original magnification ×600).

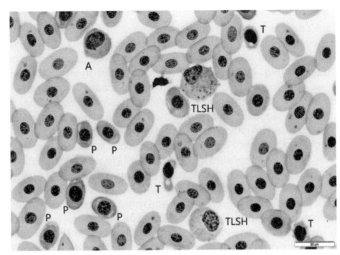

Fig. 5. Blood smear from a desert tortoise showing immature heterophils with primary granules and toxic changes: cytoplasmic basophilia (TLSH), an azurophil (A), polychromatophils (P), and thrombocytes (T) (Wright-Giemsa, original magnification ×600).

Causes of heteropenia

- Normal, actually is a low heterophil species
- Brumation (may be relative and not actually below reference interval)
- Overwhelming inflammation or infection
- Bone marrow suppression, for example, drugs, such as fenbendazole[43]
- Bone marrow necrosis, for example, sepsis, viral, such as adenovirus[32]

Lymphocytes

Lymphocytes have the same morphology and function as in other species, with B and T cells. Lymphocytes are usually small mature forms in healthy tortoises, although occasionally intermediate and large forms could also be seen (**Figs. 6** and **7**). Increased numbers of immature lymphocytes could be reactive or reflect lymphocytic neoplasia. Lymphocyte numbers are physiologically lowest during brumation owing to involution of splenic and thymic lymphoid tissue, and highest during summer.[44] There may also be sex differences, although it differs across species.

Causes of lymphocytosis

- Artifact: lymph dilution
- Antigenic stimulation/inflammation
- Lymphocytic neoplasia (peripheralization of lymphoma or leukemia): significant number of immature lymphocytes, or lymphocyte count greater than 30,000/μL mainly small mature lymphocytes; rule out lymph dilution

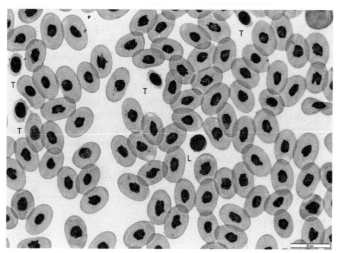

Fig. 6. Blood smear from a Greek tortoise. Compare the small lymphocyte (L) to the thrombocytes (T), which have paler and here more ruffled cytoplasm and are slightly elongated (Wright-Giemsa, original magnification ×600).

Causes of lymphopenia

- Stress
- Viral infection, for example, ranavirus[45]

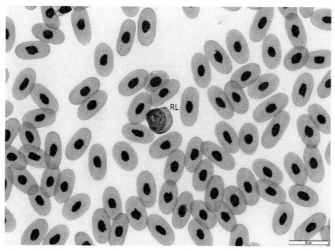

Fig. 7. Blood smear from a Russian tortoise with a reactive intermediate to large-sized lymphocyte (RL) (Wright-Giemsa, original magnification ×600).

Monocytes/azurophils

Monocytes appear similar to those of mammals, with an ovoid to indented or bilobed nucleus, dense chromatin, and pale blue gray cytoplasm. Azurophils appear similar to monocytes, with a purple ("azurophilic") dusting in the cytoplasm (**Figs. 8** and **9**). Despite debate regarding azurophils as a subtype of monocyte, the need to split azurophils and monocytes within a WBC differential is not necessary because the interpretation of azurophilia and monocytosis is the same. As a general rule, a monocytosis/azurophilia of greater than 2000/μL indicates inflammation. Azuropenia and monocytopenia lack clinical significance. Minimal seasonal variability in monocyte/azurophil numbers occurs, although numbers increase in the desert tortoise during brumation.[46] Monocytes or azurophils may phagocytose cells, melanin (melanomacrophages), or debris (**Fig. 10**), during blood sample storage, or with inflammation.[47]

Causes of monocytosis/azurophilia

Inflammation or infection

Eosinophils

Eosinophils have an ovoid nucleus with dense chromatin, slightly blue cytoplasm with usually large numbers of plump pink round granules. When present, degranulation is thought to be an in vitro change. In tortoises, eosinophil granules are generally round, and heterophil granules are elongated and more fluorescent-appearing and smudged (see **Fig. 4**; **Fig. 11**). The function of eosinophils has not been well studied in reptiles. Some species of tortoises may normally have a higher proportion of eosinophils, for example, the upper end of a reference interval for eastern Hermann tortoise was 25.1%, but the absolute numbers are typically low (<3000/μL).[48] Eosinopenia is typically difficult to identify, as the reference interval often starts at zero, but could reflect stress in high eosinophil species. Eosinophils are generally lowest in summer and highest during brumation.[49]

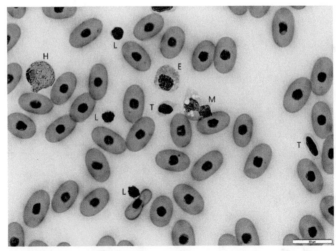

Fig. 8. Blood smear from a radiated tortoise showing a monocyte (M), with an eosinophil (E), heterophil (H), small lymphocytes (L), and thrombocytes (T) (Wright-Giemsa, original magnification ×600).

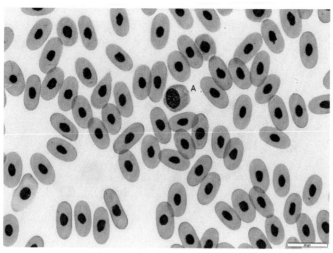

Fig. 9. Blood smear from a Russian tortoise showing an azurophil (A) (Wright-Giemsa, original magnification ×600).

Causes of eosinophilia

- Normal for the species
- Brumation (may only be a relative increase in eosinophils)
- Parasites
- Infections

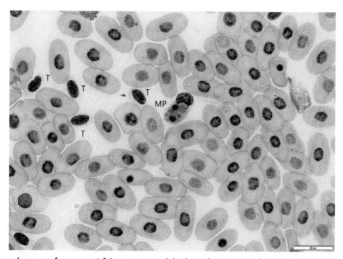

Fig. 10. Blood smear from an African spurred (sulcata) tortoise showing a macrophage (MP) containing material with the appearance of hemosiderin. Also pictured are thrombocytes (T) (Wright-Giemsa, original magnification ×600).

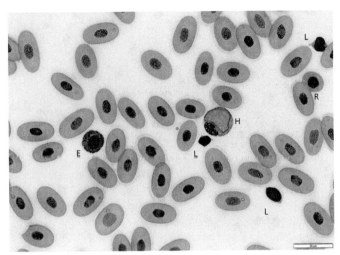

Fig. 11. Blood smear from an African spurred (sulcata) tortoise comparing an eosinophil (E) to a heterophil (H). Also pictured are small lymphocytes (L) and a rubricyte (R) (Wright-Giemsa, original magnification ×600).

Basophils

Basophils contain an ovoid nucleus with dense chromatin, pale cytoplasm, and variable but usually moderate to large numbers of dark purple, small round granules (**Fig. 12**). Degranulation is considered an in vitro change. In some species, such as the desert tortoise, basophils may be 30% of the WBC differential.[50] The function of basophils in tortoises is not well understood. Seasonal variation is usually mild. Basopenia is typically difficult to identify, as the reference interval often starts at zero, and in any case, given the lack of knowledge, the significance would be difficult to interpret, even in high basophil species.

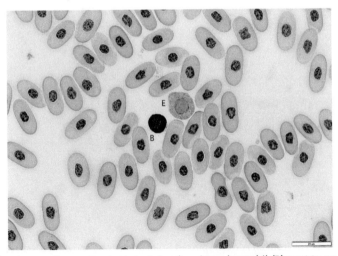

Fig. 12. Blood smear from a Forsten's tortoise showing a basophil (B) next to an eosinophil (E) (Wright-Giemsa, original magnification ×600). Slide provided by Fort Worth Zoo.

Thrombocytes

Thrombocytes are analogous to the mammalian platelet, involved in hemostasis. They are nucleated in nonmammalian animals. Thrombocytes in tortoises are elliptical or ovoid, with an elliptical or ovoid nucleus with very dense chromatin, and clear to pale blue cytoplasm (**Fig. 13**). The ovoid forms can resemble small lymphocytes, but lymphocyte chromatin is slightly less dense, and the cytoplasm is bluer (see **Fig. 5**). It is uncommon to count thrombocytes because they readily clump when heparin is used as the anticoagulant. Hence, counts are usually inaccurate, and it is difficult to identify a thrombocytopenia. Evidence of disseminated intravascular coagulation has been reported at necropsy, including of a desert tortoise.[52] However, as thrombocytes likely play a role in not only clotting but also the immune defenses for these species, the authors advocate research discovery and refinement of a method for thrombocyte enumeration for this species as needed to better evaluate health.

BIOCHEMISTRY

At this time, no foundational studies of tissue enzyme distribution for a tortoise species are published. Furthermore, proteins (total protein, albumin, globulins) of tortoises are seldom validated for assessment for most reference or INHs. Refractometry for determination of total solids or protein electrophoresis is recommended in these species for more accurate separation and determination of protein concentrations and relative percentages. Nonetheless, clinicians generally use similar analytes as those recommended for other shell-bearing reptiles for assessment of general health for these

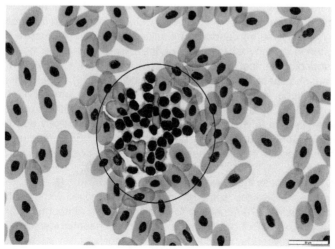

Fig. 13. Blood smear from a Russian tortoise showing a thrombocyte clump (*circle*) (Wright-Giemsa, original magnification ×600).

species: aspartate aminotransferase (AST), alanine aminotransferase (ALT), alkaline phosphatase (ALP), glucose, sodium, potassium, chloride, calcium, ionized calcium, phosphorus, albumin, globulins, total protein, fibrinogen, bile acids, blood urea nitrogen (BUN), uric acid.

Proteins

In tortoises, total proteins appear adequately measured via refractometer barring lipemia and rare hyperglycemia (Heatley, personal communication, 2022). Measurement of proteins is most accurate via electrophoresis. Expected values for healthy tortoises have only been described for a few species, and values are species-specific.[53] Protein electrophoresis values appear affected by sample site, sex, season, and possible other variables. In Hermann's tortoises, albumin concentration measured by bromocresol green (BCG) was only moderately correlated with protein electrophoresis measurements for healthy tortoises, whereas for diseased tortoises, the methods failed to correlate.[54] Even more concerning, for diseased tortoises, albumin concentrations measured by BCG were falsely elevated compared with values from electrophoresis. Plasma proteins are reasonably expected to increase based on acute inflammation (fibrinogen), chronic inflammation (globulins), and vitellogenesis (albumin), and may decrease, with albumin lost first, based on kidney/gut (loss), or liver (lack of production) disease. However, documentation of these expected pathologic changes in tortoises appears relatively rare, likely based on the poor measurements provided by many standard assays.

Liver Biomarkers

Absent known tissue distributions of enzymes or specific investigation of bile acids present in tortoise species, diagnosis of liver disease via clinical pathology remains challenging. The enzymes AST, ALT, ALP, gamma-glutamyl transferase (GGT), and lactate dehydrogenase may be used but are not of known sensitivity or specificity for the liver in these species. Values for bilirubin, uric acid, and BUN are unlikely helpful for the diagnosis.[55] Proteins (determined via electrophoresis and/or refractometry), hepatic enzymes, bile acids, and the presence of biliverdin in the urate/feces are more likely candidates for hepatic disease or dysfunction diagnosis but have been minimally studied for these species. Comparison to an apparently healthy conspecific is highly recommended: of similar age, sex, reproductive status, and season. Systemic adenoviral infection of the Sulawesi tortoise was associated with the plasma biochemical abnormalities of elevated AST activity (28%), elevated creatinine phosphokinase activity (5%), hypoglycemia (21%), hyperglycemia (58%), elevated BUN concentration (92%), hyperkalemia (22%), and elevated uric acid concentration (21%).[31] Although some of these abnormalities may have been related to liver disease (glycemic abnormalities), most were likely due to systemic inflammation, muscle/tissue disease, and dehydration.[55] Bile acids may be useful diagnostically in some tortoises, based on measurable presence in some species (**Table 3**).[56]

Very low values (all less than zero) and few greater than zero (4 and 7, respectively) from greater than 40 tortoises, some of which were diagnosed with hepatic lipidosis, suggest that GGT and ALP are unlikely to be diagnostic.[57] Although no correlation of serum AST, GGT, or ALT of red-footed tortoises with hepatic steatosis was found, increased serum triglycerides indicated hepatic lipidosis or severe hepatic disease: mean (SE) SD of those not suffering hepatic lipidosis of 0.572 (0.089) 0.356 and those affected by hepatic lipidosis with triglycerides of 2.474 (0.348) 1.56 mmol/L.[57]

Table 3
Plasma bile acids of apparently healthy tortoises[56]

Species	μmol/L	N
Hermann's tortoise, *Testudo hermanii*	17.64 ± 27.26	32
Greek tortoise, *Testudo graeca*	17.86 ± 15.37	30
Hingeback tortoise, *Kinixis belliana*	6 ± 0.1	8
Russian tortoise, *Testudo (Agrionemys) horsfieldii*	20 ± 24.65	8

Samples obtained within 2 d of fasting from jugular vein or subcarapacial vein and frozen at −20°C up to 12 d. (Multistat F.L.S- III centrifugal analyzer, with an enzymatic kit for spectrometric endpoint determination (Sterognost 3-alpha; Flu, Nyergard & Co, Norway). Test sensitivity of 0.1 umol/L. no significant difference between the sexes of each species.)

Muscle Biomarkers

As for other reptiles, creatine kinase is hoped to be muscle specific, whereas AST is likely widespread in tissues and in the liver for tortoises. Cardiac troponins have yet to be investigated/reported for these species, despite multiple cases of cardiac disease reported for multiple species.[58–60]

Renal Biomarkers

For tortoises, nitrogenous end products include minimal ammonia (3%–18%), intermediate BUN (9%–50%), and mainly uric acid (20%–56%).[55] Thus, both plasma BUN and uric acid are recommended diagnostic renal analytes for tortoises. In the free-living state, desert tortoises maintain a relatively increased BUN in the dry season.[61,62] For tortoises, uric acid is a main end product of the nitrogenous cycle; however, it remains neither a sensitive nor a specific indicator of renal function for these species. In captive tortoises, a persistently increased BUN and/or uric acid, despite adequate hydration, should create concern for renal function, urinary tract dysfunction, or gout. Calcium, phosphorus, and potassium may also be increased in these cases and should be reassessed after adequate hydration. To the authors' knowledge, symmetric dimethylarginine has not yet been investigated in these species.

Calcium, Phosphorus, Magnesium

The expected plasma calcium:phosphorus (Ca:P) ratio and ionized calcium were recently investigated in multiple species of captive tortoises **(Table 4)**.[63] Females had statistically higher levels of phosphorus and higher calcium and total calcium levels compared with males. Although solubility ratios of Ca:P have been advocated to determine renal disease in reptiles, this study showed differing ratios (and therefore solubility index) for males and females despite apparent health in both groups. However, persistently increased concentrations of Ca and/or P, despite adequate hydration and lack of active egg creation, does suggest renal dysfunction and/or gout as rule-outs in these species. Magnesium has received little if any investigation in these species. Plasma 25-hydroxyvitamin D3 can be measured, which may be useful for evaluation for metabolic bone disease.[64]

Electrolytes

Electrolyte disturbances can be difficult to evaluate for these species in which few reference intervals are available. However, a recent case of gastrointestinal obstruction in a red-footed tortoise with acute onset of frequent vomiting demonstrates similar clinicopathologic abnormalities as those expected for companion mammals.[65]

Table 4
Calcium and phosphorus values for *Testudo* spp[63]

Analyte	All = 25	Male (n = 11)	Female (n = 14)
Ionized calcium (mmol/L)	1.32 ± 0·14 1·32 (1·26–1·38)	1·31 ± 0·17 1·28 (1·19–1·42)	1·33 ± 0·12 1·37 (1·26–1·40)
Total calcium (mmol/L)	3·13 ± 0·45 3·10 (2·95–3·32)	3·24 ± 0·54 3·12 (2·93–3·55)	3·00 ± 0·27 3·07 (2·81–3·18)
Phosphorus (mmol/L)	1·01 ± 0·21 1·02 (0·93–1·10)	0·86 ± 0·17 0·86 (0·70–0·97)	1·13 ± 0·14 1·12 (1·05–1·22)

Data presented as mean ± SD; median (95% CI).[63]

Plasma biochemistry and blood gas abnormalities included hyperproteinemia, hyperglycemia, hypochloremia, and metabolic alkalosis.

URINALYSIS

The anatomy of the urinary tract for terrestrial tortoises comprises paired kidneys, which terminate into paired ureters. The urine moves through the ureters and empties into the bladder. There are often accessory bladders present. The bladder empties into the urodeum region of the cloaca via the urethra, and the urine is excreted through the cloaca. Note that the urethra does not traverse the penis in males. Urine may be collected as a voided sample on a clear surface, where it is likely to be contaminated with feces, via catheterization, or cystocentesis preferably with ultrasound guidance via femoral inlet or fossa.[66]

Urine-Specific Gravity

Tortoise kidneys cannot concentrate urine, but some water resorption can occur in the bladder and cloaca.[66,67] Urine-specific gravity (USG) is typically low, 1.003 to 1.012, and has been reported up to 1.017 in desert tortoises emerging from brumation with dehydration.[21,61]

Urine Dipsticks

Urine dipsticks can be used for the chemical evaluation of urine in tortoises; however, pads for USG, nitrate, urobilinogen, and leukocytes are not applicable/reliable. Urine ketones do not appear clinically relevant in tortoises. Bilirubin is not usually relevant because such low amounts are produced (the main product of heme breakdown in tortoises is biliverdin).

pH

In general, herbivorous terrestrial tortoises produce alkaline urine, and omnivorous tortoises consuming animal proteins may produce acidic urine. Acidic urine can also be present in herbivorous tortoises during brumation, with high protein diets, or in illness.[66]

Proteinuria

A positive result on the protein pad of the dipstick can be a false positive owing to alkaline pH (as in other species). Proteinuria could be due to the presence of spermatic fluid, mucus, or hematuria. Hematuria could be iatrogenic or pathologic. Pathologic proteinuria could be a result of glomerular or tubular disease, inflammation, or infection.

"Hematuria"

The occult "blood" or heme pad is nonspecific as in all species and is best interpreted in light of urine sediment findings. A positive result could be due to hematuria (erythrocytes in the urine), hemoglobinuria (pathologic, or from in vitro lysis of erythrocytes), or myoglobinuria from muscle damage.

Glucosuria

Normal tortoise urine does not contain glucose. Glucosuria has not been well reported in tortoises but may be a result of hyperglycemia (iatrogenic or pathologic) or renal tubular disease.

Urine Sediment

Normal urine sediment of terrestrial tortoises should be virtually acellular, or with few epithelial lining cells, as well as uric acid crystals. Typically, a wet mount preparation is evaluated, but slides can also be air dried and stained with Romanowsky stains for further evaluation, especially for cells and organisms.

Hematuria

Hematuria may be iatrogenic if the urine was collected via catheterization or cystocentesis. It can be pathologic secondary to inflammation, infection, neoplasia, trauma, and uroliths.

Pyuria

Pyuria (leukocytes in the urine) indicates inflammation and can be further evaluated on an air-dried and stained smear as to the type or types of leukocyte, usually heterophils. The inflammation could be within the urinary tract, or if the urine was voided, it could also be from the intestinal or reproductive tracts, or within the cloaca.

Organisms

The urine often contains bacteria and is usually a mixed population. Occasionally, yeast forms may be seen as contaminants from the colon. The presence of a monotypic population of organisms in large numbers (in a fresh sample, especially if obtained by cystocentesis) and pyuria supports infection. Parasites may be occasionally seen, with the most significant *Hexamita* (may also be called *Spironucleus*). *Hexamita* are protozoa approximately 8 μm in diameter with long flagella, normally found in the intestine but via ascending infection from the cloaca, can infect the renal tubules and cause inflammation.[68]

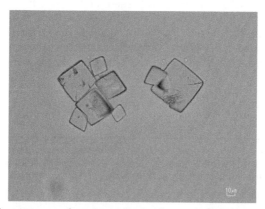

Fig. 14. Unstained wet mount of a urine sediment from a bobtail lizard with uric acid crystals. The crystals appear the same in tortoises (original magnification ×400).

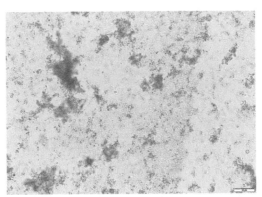

Fig. 15. Unstained wet mount of a voided urine sediment from an African spurred (sulcata) tortoise with a large number of pale brown amorphous crystals (probably uric acid) admixed with cloacal bacteria and debris (original magnification ×400).

Crystalluria
Uric acid crystals are considered normal in the urine of tortoises. They are typically flat, clear, elliptical, or rhomboid (**Fig. 14**). They can also be seen as amorphous crystals (**Fig. 15**). Calcium oxalate crystals may be seen, typically dietary in origin. A variety of other crystals have been reported in the urine of tortoises.[66]

Uroliths
Uroliths may be found in the urinary tract, and most are radiopaque. Uroliths in tortoises are predominantly composed of uric acid/urate, but calcium complexes and mixed uroliths may also be present. The type of urine crystals present in urine sediment does not necessarily indicate the composition of the urolith, with urolith analysis required to determine the composition. Dehydration, high protein diets/acidic urine, and high ambient temperatures have been reported as predisposing factors.[52] Ectopic eggs may also be found in the bladder and can act as a nidus for urolith formation.[66,69]

Casts
Hyaline and cellular casts have been reported with renal tubular disease in tortoises, including from *Hexamita* infection.[68]

Epithelial cells
Low numbers of epithelial cells may be present in the urine from the cloaca or the bladder (depending on the method of urine collection). The urinary bladder is lined by ciliated epithelium.[66] Increased numbers of epithelial cells could be from iatrogenic exfoliation during sampling, or from hyperplasia secondary to any cause of chronic irritation or inflammation, including uroliths. Urinary tract neoplasms have not been reported in tortoises.

CLINICS CARE POINTS

- Clinicopathologic evaluation is part of the general health assessment of tortoises, and must be interpreted in light of preanalytical factors, as well as any previous data available for the individual, a healthy conspecific, or published data.
- Be cautious when interpreting small changes outside reference data.

DISCLOSURE

Drs C. Moller and J.J. Heatley lack commercial or financial conflicts of interest, and no funding sources were necessary.

REFERENCES

1. ASVCP (American Society of Veterinary Clinical Pathologists). ASVCP Quality Assurance and Laboratory Standards Guidelines. 2021. Available at: https://www.asvcp.org/page/QALS_Guidelines. Accessed November 14, 2021.
2. Thorson TB. Body fluid partitioning in Reptilia. Copeia 1968;1968:592–601.
3. Naguib M. How to take blood from a tortoise. Companion Anim 2016;21:422–5.
4. Harr KE. Sample collection. Vet Clin North Am Exot Anim Pract 2018;21:579–92.
5. Neiffer DL, Hayek LAC, Conyers D, et al. Comparison of subcarapacial sinus and brachial vein phlebotomy sites for blood collection in free-ranging gopher tortoises (*Gopherus polyphemus*). J Zoo Wildl Med 2021;52(3):966–74.
6. López-Olvera JR, Montané J, Marco I, et al. Effect of venipuncture site on hematologic and serum biochemical parameters in marginated tortoise (*Testudo marginata*). J Wildl Dis 2003;39:830–6.
7. Gottdenker N, Jacobson ER. Effect of venipuncture sites on hematologic and clinical biochemical values in desert tortoises (*Gopherus agassizii*). Am J Vet Res 1995;56:19–21.
8. Hernandez-Divers SM, Hernandez-Divers SJ, Wyneken J. Angiographic, anatomic and clinical technique descriptions of a subcarapacial venipuncture site for chelonians. J Herpetol Med Surg 2002;12:32–7.
9. Wimsatt J, Johnson JD, Mangone BA. Use of a cardiac access port for repeated collection of blood samples from desert tortoises (*Gopherus agassizii*). J Am Assoc Lab Anim Sc 1998;37:81–3.
10. Quesada RJ, Aitken-Palmer C, Conley K, et al. Accidental submeningeal injection of propofol in gopher tortoises (*Gopherus polyphemus*). Vet Rec 2010;167:494–5.
11. Hernandez-Divers SJ, Cooper JE, Cooke SW. Diagnostic techniques and sample collection in reptiles. Compend Contin Educ Vet 2004;26:470–82.
12. Howerth EW. Immunopathology. In: Divers SJ, Stahl SJ, editors. Mader's reptile and Amphibian medicine and surgery. 3rd edition. St Louis (MO): WB Saunders; 2019. p. 356–60.
13. Garner MM, Homer BL, Jacobson ER, et al. Staining and morphologic features of bone marrow hematopoietic cells in desert tortoises (*Gopherus agassizii*). Am J Vet Res 1996;57:1608–15.
14. Abou-Madi N, Jacobson ER. Effects of blood processing techniques on sodium and potassium values: A comparison between Aldabra tortoises (*Geochelone gigantea*) and Burmese mountain tortoises (*Manouria emys*). Vet Clin Pathol 2003; 32:61–6.
15. Di Girolamo N, Ferlizza E, Selleri P, et al. Evaluation of point-of-care analysers for blood gas and clinical chemistry in Hermann's tortoises (*Testudo hermanni*). J Small Anim Pract 2018;59:704–13.
16. Jensen AL, Kjelgaard-Hansen M. Diagnostic test validation. In: Weiss DJ, Wardrop KJ, editors. Schalm's veterinary hematology. 6th edition. Ames: Blackwell Publishing Limited; 2010. p. 1027–33.
17. Russo EA, McEntee L, Applegate L, et al. Comparison of two methods for determination of white blood cell counts in macaws. J Am Vet Med Assoc 1986;189: 1013–6.

18. Vap LM, Harr KE, Arnold JE, et al. ASVCP quality assurance guidelines: control of preanalytical and analytical factors for hematology for mammalian and nonmammalian species, hemostasis, and crossmatching in veterinary laboratories. Vet Clin Pathol 2012;41:8–16.

19. Andreani G, Carpene E, Cannavacciuolo A, et al. Reference values for hematology and plasma biochemistry variables, and protein electrophoresis of healthy Hermann's tortoises (*Testudo hermanni* ssp.). Vet Clin Pathol 2014;43:573–83.

20. Zaias J, Norton T, Fickel A, et al. Biochemical and hematologic values for 18 clinically healthy radiated tortoises (*Geochelone radiata*) on St Catherines Island, Georgia. Vet Clin Pathol 2006;35:321–5.

21. Wilkinson R. Clinical Pathology. In: McArthur S, Wilkinson R, Meyer J, editors. Medicine and surgery of tortoises and turtles. Oxford: Blackwell Publishing; 2004. p. 141–80.

22. Raskin RE, Crosby FL, Jacobson ER. Newly recognized *Anaplasma* sp. in erythrocytes from gopher tortoises (*Gopherus polyphemus*). Vet Clin Pathol 2020;49: 17–22.

23. Broughton CA, Clark SD. What is your diagnosis? Blood smear review in a Texas tortoise (*Gopherus berlandieri*). Vet Clin Pathol 2021;50:299–301.

24. Crosby FL, Wellehan JF, Pertierra L, et al. Molecular characterization of "Candidatus Anaplasma testudinis": An emerging pathogen in the threatened Florida gopher tortoise (*Gopherus polyphemus*). Ticks Tick-borne Dis 2021;12:101672.

25. Cook CA, Lawton SP, Davies AJ, et al. Reassignment of the land tortoise haemogregarine *Haemogregarina fitzsimonsi* Dias 1953 (Adeleorina: Haemogregarinidae) to the genus *Hepatozoon* Miller 1908 (Adeleorina: Hepatozoidae) based on parasite morphology, life cycle and phylogenetic analysis of 18S rDNA sequence fragments. Parasitol 2014;141:1611–20.

26. Lainson R, Naiff RD. *Haemoproteus* (Apicomplexa: Haemoproteidae) of tortoises and turtles. Proc R Soc Lond B 1998;265:941–9.

27. Redrobe SP, Hart M, MacDonald J. Treatment of suspected Plasmodium infection in star tortoises (Geochelone elegans). IAAAM. 2000. Available at: https://www.vin.com/apputil/content/defaultadv1.aspx?pId=11125&id=3980444. Accessed January 24, 2022.

28. Jacobson ER, Schumacher J, Telford SR Jr, et al. Intranuclear coccidiosis in radiated tortoises (*Geochelone radiata*). J Zoo Wildl Med 1994;1:95–102.

29. Hellebuyck T, Simard J, Velde NV, et al. Acute ramson (*Allium ursinum*) toxicosis in captive tortoises. J Herpetol Med Surg 2019;29:34–9.

30. Christopher MM. Physical and biochemical abnormalities associated with prolonged entrapment in a desert tortoise. J Wildl Dis 1999;35:361–6.

31. Schumacher VL, Innis CJ, Garner MM, et al. Sulawesi tortoise adenovirus-1 in two impressed tortoises (*Manouria impressa*) and a Burmese star tortoise (*Geochelone platynota*). J Zoo Wildl Med 2012;43:501–10.

32. Rivera S, Wellehan JFX Jr, McManamon R, et al. Systemic adenovirus infection in Sulawesi tortoises (*Indotestudo forsteni*) caused by a novel siadenovirus. J Vet Diagn Invest 2009;21:415–26.

33. Casimire-Etzioni AL, Wellehan JF, Embury JE, et al. Synovial fluid from an African spur-thighed tortoise (*Geochelone sulcata*). Vet Clin Pathol 2004;33:43–6.

34. Sheldon JD, Stacy NI, Blake S, et al. Comparison of total leukocyte quantification methods in free-living Galapagos tortoises (*Chelonoidis* spp.). J Zoo Wildl Med 2016;47:196–205.

35. Brenn-White M, Raphael BL, Rakotoarisoa, et al. Hematology and biochemistry of critically endangered radiated tortoises (Astrochelys radiata): Reference intervals

in previously confiscated subadults and variability based on common techniques. PLoS One 2022;17:e0264111.

36. Ippen R. Ein Beitrag zu den spontantumoren bei Reptilien. Verhandlungsbericht des 1972;14:409–18.

37. Frye FL. Diagnosis and surgical treatment of reptilian neoplasms with a compilation of cases 1966–1993. In Vivo 1994;8:885–92.

38. Stacy NI, Hollinger C, Arnold JE, et al. Left shift and toxic change in heterophils and neutrophils of non-mammalian vertebrates: A comparative review, image atlas, and practical considerations. Vet Clin Pathol 2022;51:18–44.

39. Stacy NI, Hollinger C, Arnold JE, et al. Proposal for standardized classification of left shift, toxic change, and increased nuclear segmentation in heterophils and neutrophils in non-mammalian vertebrates. Vet Clin Pathol 2022;51:14–7.

40. Stacy NI, Fredholm DV, Rodriguez C, et al. Whip-like heterophil projections in consecutive blood films from an injured gopher tortoise (*Gopherus polyphemus*) with systemic inflammation. Vet Q 2017;37:162–5.

41. Stacy NI, Alleman AR, Sayler KA. Diagnostic hematology of reptiles. Clin Lab Med 2011;31:87–108.

42. Rosenberg JF, Hernandez JA, Wellehan JFX, et al. Diagnostic performance of inflammatory markers in gopher tortoises (*Gopherus polyphemus*). J Zoo Wildl Med 2018;49:765–9.

43. Neiffer DL, Lydick D, Burks K, et al. Hematologic and plasma biochemical changes associated with fenbendazole administration in Hermann's tortoises (*Testudo hermanni*). J Zoo Wildl Med 2005;36:661–72.

44. El Ridi R, Zada S, Afifi A, et al. Cyclic changes in the differentiation of lymphoid cells in reptiles. Cell Differ 1988;24:1–8.

45. Johnson AJ, Pessier AP, Wellehan JFX, et al. Ranavirus infection of free-ranging and captive box turtles and tortoises in the United States. J Wildl Dis 2008;44:851–63.

46. Christopher MM, Berry KH, Wallis IR, et al. Reference intervals and physiologic alterations in hematologic and biochemical values of free-ranging desert tortoises in the Mojave desert. J Wildl Dis 1999;35:212–38.

47. George JW, Holmberg TA, Riggs SM, et al. Circulating siderophagocytes and erythrophagocytes in a corn snake (*Elaphe guttata*) after coelomic surgery. Vet Clin Pathol 2008;37:308–11.

48. Bielli M, Nardini G, Di Girolamo N, et al. Hematological values for adult eastern Hermann's tortoise (*Testudo hermanni boettgeri*) in semi-natural conditions. J Vet Diagn Invest 2015;27:68–73.

49. Duguy R. Numbers of blood cells and their variations. In: Gans C, Parsons TC, editors. Biology of the Reptilia, vol. 3. New York: Academic Press; 1970. p. 93–109.

50. Alleman AR, Jacobson ER, Raskin RE. Morphologic and cytochemical characteristics of blood cells from the desert tortoise (*Gopherus agassizii*). Am J Vet Res 1992;53:1645–51.

51. Sypek J, Borysenko M. Reptiles. In: Rowley AF, Ratcliffe NA, editors. Vertebrate blood cells. Cambridge: Cambridge University Press; 1988. p. 211–56.

52. Keller KA, Hawkins MG, Weber EP, et al. Diagnosis and treatment of urolithiasis in client-owned chelonians: 40 cases (1987-2012). J Am Vet Med Assoc 2015;247:650–8.

53. Leineweber C, Stöhr AC, Öfner S, et al. Plasma capillary zone electrophoresis and plasma chemistry analytes in tortoises (*Testudo hermanni, Testudo graeca*)

and turtles (*Trachemys scripta elegans, Graptemys* spp.) in fall. J Zoo Wildl Med 2020;51:915–25.

54. Macrelli R, Ceccarelli MM, Fiorucci L. Determination of serum albumin concentration in healthy and diseased Hermann's tortoises (*Testudo hermanni*): a comparison using electrophoresis and the bromocresol green dye-binding method. J Herpetol Med Surg 2013;23:20–4.

55. Divers SJ. Hepatology. In: Divers SJ, Stahl SJ, editors. Mader's reptile and Amphibian medicine and surgery. 3rd edition. St Louis (MO): WB Saunders; 2019. p. 649–68.

56. Montesinos A, Martinez R, Jimenez A. Plasma bile acids concentration in tortoises: reference values and histopathologic findings of importance for interpretation. WSAVA 2002 Congress. Available at: https://www.vin.com/apputil/content/defaultadv1.aspx?pId=11147&id=3846378. Accessed January 25, 2022.

57. Dutra GH. Diagnostic value of hepatic enzymes, triglycerides and serum proteins for the detection of hepatic lipidosis in *Chelonoidis carbonaria* in captivity. J Life Sci 2014;8:633–9.

58. Redrobe SP, Scudamore CL. Ultrasonographic diagnosis of pericardial effusion and atrial dilation in a spur-thighed tortoise (*Testudo graeca*). Vet Rec 2000; 146:183–5.

59. Flanagan JP, Gibbons PM, Heard D, et al. Edema in giant tortoises. J Herpetol Med Surg 2021;31:220–38.

60. Feltrer Y, Strike T, Routh A, et al. Point-of-care cardiac troponin I in non-domestic species: a feasibility study. J Zoo Aq Res 2016;4:99–103.

61. Christopher MM, Brigmon R, Jacobson E. Seasonal alterations in plasma B-hydroxybutyrate and related biochemical parameters in the desert tortoise (*Gopherus agassizii*). Comp Biochem Physiol 1994;108A:303–10.

62. Dickinson VM, Jarchow JL, Trueblood MH. Hematology and plasma biochemistry reference range values for free-ranging desert tortoises in Arizona. J Wildl Dis 2002;38:143–53.

63. Eatwell K. Calcium and phosphorus values and their derivatives in captive tortoises (*Testudo* species). J Small Anim Pract 2010;51:472–5.

64. Selleri P, Di Girolamo N. Plasma 25-hydroxyvitamin D(3) concentrations in Hermann's tortoises (*Testudo hermanni*) exposed to natural sunlight and two artificial ultraviolet radiation sources. Am J Vet Res 2012;73:1781–6.

65. Romeijer C, Beaufrère H, Laniesse D, et al. Vomiting and gastrointestinal obstruction in a red-footed tortoise (*Chelonoidis carbonaria*). J Herpetol Med Surg 2016; 26:32–5.

66. Divers SJ, Innis CJ. Urology. In: Divers SJ, Stahl SJ, editors. Mader's reptile and Amphibian medicine and surgery. 3rd edition. St Louis (MO): WB Saunders; 2019. p. 624–48.

67. Flanagan JP. Chelonians (Turtles, Tortoises). In: Miller ER, Fowler ME, editors. Fowler's Zoo and wild animal medicine, vol. 8. St Louis (MO): WB Saunders; 2015. p. 27–38.

68. Juan-Sallés C, Garner MM, Nordhausen RW, et al. Renal flagellate infections in reptiles: 29 cases. J Zoo Wildl Med 2014;45:100–9.

69. Mans C, Foster JD. Endoscopy-guided ectopic egg removal from the urinary bladder in a leopard tortoise (*Stigmochelys pardalis*). Can Vet J 2014;55:569–72.

70. Klaphake E, Gibbons PM, Sladky KK, et al. Reptiles. In: Carpenter JW, editor. Exotic animal formulary. 5th edition. St Louis (MO): Elsevier; 2018. p. 82–166.

71. Mathes KA, Holz A, Fehr M. Blood reference values of terrestrial tortoises (*Testudo* spp.) kept in Germany. Tierarztl Prax Ausg K Klientiere Heimtiere 2006;34: 268–74.

72. Knotková Z, Doubek J, Knotek Z, et al. Blood cell morphology and plasma biochemistry in Russian tortoises (*Agrionemys horsfieldi*). Acta Vet Brno 2002; 71:191–8.

73. Lawrence K, Hawkey C. Seasonal variations in haematological data from Mediterranean tortoises (*Testudo graeca* and *Testudo hermanni*) in captivity. Res Vet Sci 1986;40:225–30.

74. Berg KJ, Schexnayder M, Grasperge BJ, et al. Single time point reference intervals for complete blood counts and select biochemistries in juvenile red-footed tortoises (*Chelonoidis carbonaria*). J Herpetol Med Surg 2021;31:124–31.

Clinical Pathology of Freshwater Turtles

Michael F. Rosser, DVM, MS, DACVP (Clinical Pathology)

KEYWORDS

- Aquatic • Biochemistry • Chelonian • Hematology • Slider

KEY POINTS

- Preanalytical factors including lymphatic contamination and anticoagulant choice may influence interpretation of chelonian hematology and plasma biochemistry.
- Baseline hematologic parameters, hemic cell morphology, and plasma biochemistry data have been reported for many freshwater chelonian species.
- Continued investigation of changes in laboratory data in response to specific disease states is needed for improved management of freshwater chelonian health in both clinical and field settings.

INTRODUCTION

Freshwater turtles are a diverse group of aquatic reptiles adapted to life on both land and a variety of freshwater habitats, including wetlands, lakes, and rivers. Studies of normal physiology are plentiful, especially in the red-eared slider (*Trachemys scripta elegans*), and reference intervals have been described for multiple species in both free-ranging and captive settings. However, clinicopathologic changes in freshwater chelonian species in response to disease processes are poorly characterized in peer-reviewed literature. Appropriate interpretation of laboratory values specific to these species is important for both conservation efforts in free-ranging populations and in captive populations, especially because these animals become increasingly popular as pets. This article will review the current knowledge of hematology, plasma biochemistry, and urinalysis in freshwater turtles, with correlates to other chelonian species when data specific to freshwater turtles are unavailable.

SAMPLE HANDLING

In a clinical setting, 10% of the total blood volume can be safely acquired from healthy turtles during venipuncture, with blood comprising 5% to 8% of total body weight.[1–3]

Department of Veterinary Clinical Medicine and Veterinary Diagnostic Laboratory, College of Veterinary Medicine, University of Illinois at Urbana-Champaign, 1008 West Hazelwood Drive, Urbana, IL 61802, USA
E-mail address: mrosser2@illinois.edu

Vet Clin Exot Anim 25 (2022) 785–804
https://doi.org/10.1016/j.cvex.2022.05.005
1094-9194/22/© 2022 Elsevier Inc. All rights reserved.

However, blood cell regeneration is relatively slow, and the safe time interval between maximal blood draws has yet to be determined for these species. Venipuncture sites in chelonians include the dorsal coccygeal vein, subcarapacial sinus, jugular veins, and ulnar or brachial venous plexuses. Detailed descriptions and diagrams of sampling techniques have been compiled elsewhere.[2,3] Cardiocentesis has also been described in a research setting but is generally not preferred in clinical practice apart from immediately before or as part of euthanasia.[2,4]

Lymphatic Contamination

Lymphatic contamination is a potential complication of venipuncture in chelonians, as venous and lymphatic vessels are closely paired. This may occur at any venipuncture site but can be minimized with appropriate jugular venipuncture technique.[2,3] Lymphatic contamination may serve as a source of preanalytical error, manifesting as a decreased red blood cell count, packed cell volume (PCV), and white blood cell counts (WBC) due to dilutional effects, along with an increased absolute lymphocyte count.[3,5–7] Effects of lymphatic dilution on plasma biochemical parameters may be variable, although significantly lower levels of total protein and potassium have been detected from blood–lymph mixtures in red eared sliders (T. scripta elegans).[7] Aspiration of clear fluid rather than blood, or an unexpected anemia and lymphocytosis should alert the clinician to potential lymphatic or extracellular fluid contamination, and resampling from a different site may be indicated.[1,3,5]

Anticoagulants

EDTA (Ethylenediaminetetraacetic acid) causes in vitro hemolysis in multiple freshwater turtle species including the spiny softshell turtle (Apalone spinifera) and the Arrau turtle (Podocnemis expansa).[8,9] However, in other species such as the yellow-blotched map turtle (Graptemys flavimaculata), EDTA does not cause hemolysis and may allow for improved cellular preservation compared with heparin.[10] Heparin is generally considered the anticoagulant of choice for chelonian plasma biochemistry and hematology unless a species-specific study suggests otherwise.[3]

Storage

Generally, blood samples should be processed as soon as possible, although this may not always be feasible in a field setting. If storage is required before biochemical analysis, the sample should be immediately centrifuged and the plasma should be separated and stored frozen, ideally at $-80°C$. Studies evaluating the effects of short-term or long-term blood sample storage in freshwater turtles are sparse; one study in Arrau turtles (P. expansa) showed that some serum analytes such as alkaline phosphatase (ALP), calcium, cholesterol, and urea are stable for up to 1 month after freezing at $-20°C$, whereas others such as creatine kinase (CK) and gamma glutamyltransferase (GGT) should be analyzed immediately.[11]

HEMATOLOGY

Complete blood count in chelonians and other reptiles is completed using manual methods because commercially available automated hematology analyzers are currently unable to produce accurate results due to the presence of nucleated erythrocytes and thrombocytes. Reference intervals for many freshwater turtle species have been described, with significant intraspecies variability depending on seasonality, sex, geographic location, venipuncture site, and other factors documented.[8,12–15] Therefore, transference of published reference intervals to varying patient or field conditions should be done with caution. Selected hematological reference values for North American freshwater turtle species are provided in **Table 1**, whereas descriptive values for other species are compiled elsewhere.[3]

Spun PCV is often used as the sole estimator of red blood cell mass in chelonians in a clinical setting. Hemoglobin concentration can be measured using the cyanmethemoglobin method, and 2 hemoglobin isoforms exist in some aquatic turtles to allow a transition from aerobic to anaerobic metabolism during winter hibernation.[16,17] Red blood cell concentrations may be obtained via hemocytometry and used to calculate mean cell volume and mean cell hemoglobin concentration (MCHC), although results should be interpreted with caution due to inherent imprecision of hemocytometric counting, even in the hands of experienced technicians. Leukocyte density may be quantified using hemocytometry and phloxine or Natt-Herrick's solution, or by manual estimation on a blood smear. Hemocytometric methods are preferred in reference laboratory settings but are relatively time consuming, require trained technicians, and are subject to significant intraassay and interassay variabilities.[18] Leukocyte estimation from a blood smear depends heavily on smear quality and is generally considered less precise than hemocytometric methods. The method of leukocyte quantification should be considered both when analyzing chelonian hematology results and when comparing to published reference intervals.[18] Thrombocytes are typically quantified subjectively, and often form clumps following exposure to lithium heparin during sample processing.[5]

Erythrocytes

The life span of reptilian erythrocytes is markedly prolonged compared with avian and mammalian species and may range from 600 to 800 days based on a study in box turtles (*Terrapene carolina carolina*).[19] Mature chelonian erythrocytes are ovoid in shape with pink-orange cytoplasm and oval-shaped, centrally located nuclei with dense nuclear chromatin (**Fig. 1**A, B). Immature erythrocytes are more rounded to spherical in shape with more blue-purple cytoplasm. Nuclear size and nuclear cytoplasmic ratio are increased in immature erythrocytes relative to mature erythrocytes (**Fig. 1**C). Approximately 1% to 2% of chelonian erythrocytes may be immature in health, although increased numbers of these cells may support active erythropoiesis. New Methylene Blue staining to enumerate reticulocytes has been described, with 2% to 3% reticulocytosis identified in healthy red-eared slider turtles (*Pseudemys scripta elegans*)[20]; however, reticulocyte counting is not typically incorporated into chelonian hematologic analysis in a clinical setting.

A relatively common finding in chelonian erythrocytes is one to multiple clear to basophilic, punctate, cytoplasmic inclusions (see **Fig. 1**B, C). These have been described in blood smears from multiple freshwater chelonian species, including painted turtles (*Chrysemys picta picta*), Asian yellow pond turtles (*Ocadia sinensis*), and yellow-bellied slider turtles (*T. scripta scripta*); these inclusions are degenerating organelles based on ultrastructural evaluation and are of no known clinical significance.[5,14,21,22] Multiple variably sized, refractile zones of cytoplasmic clearing within erythrocytes are a common artifactual finding associated with smear drying (**Fig. 1**D, E).

Anemia in chelonians is typically identified by a decreased PCV. Evidence of a regenerative response to anemia may include anisocytosis (variability in erythrocyte size), polychromasia, and increased frequency of immature red blood cells. General considerations for a regenerative anemia include causes of hemorrhage or hemolytic disease.[23] Marked regenerative anemia in response to hemorrhage has been characterized experimentally in red-eared slider turtles (*P. scripta elegans*), with removal of

Table 1
Selected hematology reference values for North American freshwater chelonians

Species:	Spotted Turtle (*Clemmys guttata*)[68]	Alligator Snapping Turtle (*Macrochelys temminckii*)[69]	Western Pond Turtle (*Emys marmorata*)[70]	Units
Sample size and characteristics:	32 captive	101–106 free ranging	20 free ranging/10 captive	
Data format:	95% CI	95% CI	10th–90th percentile	
Parameter				*Units*
PCV	20–39	22.1–24.4	20.9–31.1/23.9–31.65	%
WBC	4.8–14.7	11.2–13.4	8.95–27.3/9.46–22.5	$\times 10^3/\mu L$
Heterophils	0.1–4.4	4.076–5.355	1.13–5.1/4.1–10.85	$\times 10^3/\mu L$
Lymphocytes	0.2–6.4	2.645–3.556	0.6–8.9/0.38–7.59	$\times 10^3/\mu L$
Monocytes	0.2–2.2	n/a	0–0.12/0.48–3.23	$\times 10^3/\mu L$
Azurophils	n/a	0.560–0.760	0.29–1.02/0–0	$\times 10^3/\mu L$
Eosinophils	0–4.0	2.276–2.836	2.27–7.27/1.21–3.23	$\times 10^3/\mu L$
Basophils	0–2.9	0.813–1.733	1.16–4.39/0.63–2.43	$\times 10^3/\mu L$

20% of blood volume resulting in marked decreases in PCV, hemoglobin, and calculated MCHC with reticulocytosis and increased numbers of immature erythrocytes.[4] Anemia secondary to vehicular or other trauma has also been characterized, with PCV identified as a potential prognostic indicator.[24] Other causes of hemorrhagic anemia may include gastrointestinal ulceration, ectoparasites, coagulopathies, or neoplasia.[5] Reports of confirmed hemolytic anemias in freshwater turtles are sparse, although marked anemia with increased immature red blood cells supporting regeneration has been documented in loggerhead sea turtles exposed to crude oil.[25] Considerations for nonregenerative anemia in freshwater turtles include chronic infection, starvation or malnutrition, renal disease, neoplasia, and cold torpor or hibernation.[4,5,23,26] Conditions resulting in nonregenerative anemia often develop over a long period of time due to prolonged erythrocyte life span.[23] Hemoconcentration is the most common cause of an increased PCV in freshwater chelonians, which may occur before hibernation or secondary to dehydration.[3,27]

Intraerythrocytic hemoparasites termed hemogregarines are often observed in free-ranging freshwater chelonians, with leeches implicated as the most common vector in freshwater turtles.[28] These organisms are oblong in shape, pale basophilic in color, contain a round to ovoid, basophilic nucleus, and may cause peripheral displacement of the erythrocyte nucleus (**Fig. 1**F). Hemoparasites with this morphology may represent organisms from multiple genera within the phylum Apicomplexa, which cannot be differentiated on light microscopy but are generally considered nonpathogenic.[3,5] Heavy organism burdens and anemia have been documented in Bornean river turtles (*Orlitia borneensis*) suffering from shell necrosis, although a direct association between hemogregarine parasitemia and anemia was not firmly established.[29] Gametocytes of *Plasmodium* spp. or *Haemocystidium* spp. may seem morphologically similar to hemogregarines but may be differentiated by the presence of golden-brown hemozoin pigment granules.[5,30]

Leukocytes

The chelonian leukocyte differential generally includes heterophils, lymphocytes, monocytes/azurophils, eosinophils, and basophils (**Figs. 2** and **3**). Heterophils and

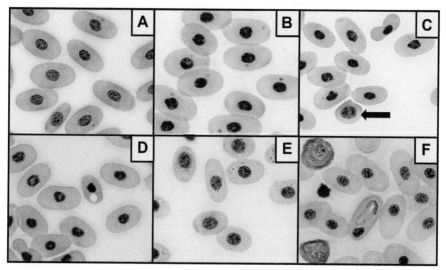

Fig. 1. Red blood cell morphology in freshwater chelonians. (*A*) Normal red blood cells in a red-eared slider turtle (*T. scripta elegans*), Wright-Giemsa, ×100 objective. (*B*) Basophilic inclusions representing degenerate organelles in a painted turtle (*C. picta*), Wright-Giemsa, ×100 objective. (*C*) Few degenerate organelles and an immature erythrocyte (*arrow*) in a painted turtle (*C. picta*), Wright-Giemsa, ×100 objective. (*D*) An irregularly round area of cytoplasmic clearing representing an artifactual change in a red-eared slider turtle (*T. scripta elegans*), Wright-Giemsa, ×100 objective. (*E*) Refractile, irregularly shaped inclusions representing water artifact in a Mississippi map turtle (*G. pseudogeographica kohni*), Wright-Giemsa, ×100 objective. (*F*) A presumed hemogregarine causing peripheral displacement of the erythrocyte nucleus in a common snapping turtle (*C. serpentina*).

lymphocytes comprise most of the leukocyte differential in many freshwater chelonian species, although some species may also display a basophil predominance. Azurophils describe a unique cell type to reptiles appearing morphologically similar to the monocyte with many fine, pink to purple cytoplasmic granules and/or few discrete, nonstaining cytoplasmic vacuoles (see **Fig. 3**C). A functional difference between chelonian monocytes and azurophils has not been elucidated, and studies vary in terms of whether azurophils are quantified separately or designated as monocytes.

Chelonian heterophils are similar to those described in other reptiles, with round to ovoid, often eccentrically located nuclei and many discrete, rod-shaped cytoplasmic granules that may range from pink-orange to red depending on the staining method used (see **Fig. 3**A). Heterophilia is often associated with causes of inflammation, which may include infectious disease, tissue injury, and necrosis (see **Fig. 2**).[5] Toxic change to heterophils provides further support for inflammatory disease, especially bacterial infections. Indicators of mild heterophilic toxic change include increased cytoplasmic basophilia and hypogranulation, whereas severe toxicity may manifest as cytoplasmic vacuolation and atypical granule morphology (**Fig. 4**).[3,5] Other potential causes of heterophilia without toxic change in chelonians include glucocorticoid-mediated stress responses or neoplasia.[31] Granulocytic leukemia in freshwater turtles has not been described. When accompanied by cytoplasmic toxic change, heteropenia supports acute or overwhelming inflammatory disease. Drug or toxin-induced heteropenia has not been reported in freshwater chelonians, although fenbendazole administration has been described as a cause of extended heteropenia in Hermann's tortoises (*Testudo hermanni*).[32]

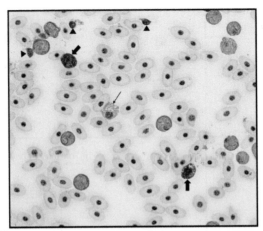

Fig. 2. Blood smear from a common snapping turtle (*C. serpentina*) with no provided clinical history. A marked leukocytosis (62,900/μL) is present, consisting primarily of heterophils with lower numbers of lymphocytes (*arrowheads*), basophils (*thick arrows*), and eosinophils (*thin arrow*). These findings support an inflammatory response. Wright-Giemsa, ×50 objective.

Lymphocytes in chelonians seem similar to other species, with a round nucleus and a high nuclear to cytoplasmic ratio. Differentiating small lymphocytes from thrombocytes may be challenging (**Fig. 5**). Conditions causing antigenic stimulation may result in the presence of plasmacytoid or reactive lymphocytes, granular lymphocytes, or lymphoblasts in circulation.[5] Lymphocytosis may be associated with wound healing, inflammation, some parasitic infections, and viral infection, whereas lymphopenia may occur with immunosuppression, cortisol-induced stress responses, and chronic malnutrition.[31] In an experimental setting, testosterone injection has also been reported as a cause of lymphopenia in Caspian turtles (*Mauremys caspica*).[33]

Chelonian monocytes are mononuclear cells with round to ovoid to reniform nuclei, a moderate-to-large amount of blue-gray cytoplasm, and occasional discrete cytoplasmic vacuoles, similar to those described in other species. Although phagocytic capacity of monocytes has been described across other reptilian species, specific reports of this finding in freshwater turtles are lacking.[5,34] Although relatively uncommon, monocytosis in turtles may suggest chronic disease states or granulomatous inflammation.[5,31]

Eosinophils in freshwater chelonians have round to ovoid to bilobed nuclei that are often eccentrically located, as well as many discrete, round, salmon-colored cytoplasmic granules (see **Fig. 3**D). Parasitic disease has been proposed as a cause of eosinophilia in reptiles, although direct correlation in freshwater turtles has not been described.[31] Basophils are commonly identified in freshwater turtles and may comprise most of the leukocyte differential in some species such as the snapping turtle (*Chelydra serpentina*), the red-bellied cooter (*P. rubriventris*), and the Pascagoula map turtle (*G. gibbonsi*).[15,35,36] Basophils are recognized morphologically by round nuclei that are often obscured by many discrete, dark purple cytoplasmic granules. Staining quality of basophil granules may vary based on species and staining method (see **Fig. 3**E, F). Basophil function in turtles is poorly understood, although evidence for immune capacity analogous to mammalian basophils or mast cells has been described.[35]

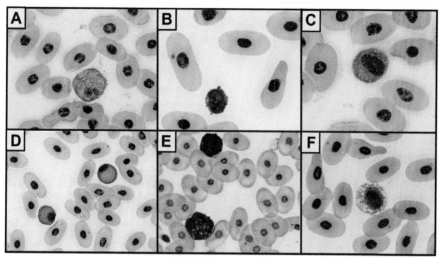

Fig. 3. White blood cell morphology in freshwater chelonians. (*A*) Heterophil from a red-eared slider turtle (*T. scripta elegans*), Wright-Giemsa, ×100 objective. (*B*) Lymphocyte from a painted turtle (*C. picta*), Wright-Giemsa, ×100 objective. (*C*) Azurophil from a red-eared slider turtle (*T. scripta elegans*), Wright-Giemsa, ×100 objective. (*D*) Eosinophils from a painted turtle (*C. picta*), Wright-Giemsa, ×100 objective. (*E*) Basophils with dark purple cytoplasmic granules from a Mata Mata turtle (*Chelus fimbriata*). Wright-Giemsa, ×100 objective. (*F*) Basophils with punctate magenta to nonstaining cytoplasmic granules from a painted turtle (*C. picta*), Wright-Giemsa, ×100 objective.

Thrombocytes

Chelonian thrombocytes range from ovoid to elliptical in shape with colorless to pale blue cytoplasm and a relatively high nuclear to cytoplasmic ratio (see **Fig. 5**). These cells can be challenging to differentiate from small lymphocytes but will often appear in clumps, which may facilitate their identification. By comparison, lymphocytes generally have a more basophilic cytoplasm and a less condensed chromatin pattern (see **Fig. 3**B). Due to the frequency of thrombocyte clumping, thrombocytes are typically subjectively quantified as increased, adequate, or decreased.[3] In a clinical

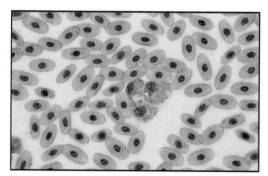

Fig. 4. Blood smear from a red-eared slider turtle presenting for ulcerative shell disease. Toxic change to heterophils is present, including hypogranulation, increased cytoplasmic basophilia, and cytoplasmic vacuolation. Wright-Giemsa, ×100 objective.

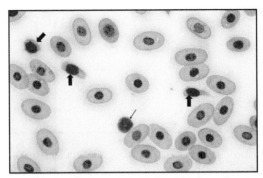

Fig. 5. Blood smear from a Mississippi map turtle (*G. pseudogeographica kohni*). Thrombocytes (*thick arrows*) can be differentiated from lymphocytes (*thin arrow*) by their relatively increased cytoplasmic volume, dense nuclear chromatin, and round to tapered shape. Identification of thrombocyte clumps may also aid in differentiation. Wright-Giemsa, ×100 objective.

setting, subjective estimations of thrombocyte mass should be correlated with clinical evidence of petechiation, ecchymosis, or disseminated intravascular coagulation.

COAGULATION/HEMOSTASIS

Documented cases of coagulopathy in freshwater turtles are very sparse, with a single case report of disseminated intravascular coagulation secondary to *Mycobacterium chelonae* sepsis in an Eastern spiny softshell turtle (*A. spinifera spinifera*) diagnosed on postmortem examination.[37] Consequently, validated methods for coagulation testing in freshwater chelonians are largely unavailable. Intrinsic pathway coagulation factors XI and XII are absent in sea turtles and partial thromboplastin time (PTT) assays in these species are of no clinical utility.[38,39] Thromboelastography (TEG) protocols have also been recently described in green sea turtles, and initial investigations support the presence of hemostatic derangements in cold-stunned turtles.[39,40] Similar investigations in freshwater turtle species have not been performed to date.

BIOCHEMISTRY

Routine biochemical parameters used for evaluation of health status in chelonians include urea, uric acid, total protein, albumin, globulins, calcium, phosphorus, electrolytes (sodium, potassium, and chloride), glucose, bile acids, and enzymatic activities including ALP, alanine aminotransferase (ALT), aspartate aminotransferase (AST), GGT, and CK.[3] Tissue activities of plasma enzymes have been described in sea turtles and eastern box turtles (*T. carolina carolina*) but have not been specifically evaluated in freshwater turtle species.[41–43] Reference intervals for many species have been published, although most of these studies do not meet the American Society for Veterinary Clinical Pathology guidelines for reference interval determination. Data from an individual patient during health may serve as more reliable baseline for comparison, especially if species-specific references are sparse.[44] Selected biochemistry reference values for North American freshwater turtle species are provided in **Table 2**; values for other species are compiled elsewhere.[3]

Table 2
Selected biochemical data for North American freshwater chelonians

Species:	Spotted Turtle (Clemmys guttata)[68]	Red-Eared Slider (T. scripta elegans)[51]	Map Turtle (Graptemys spp.)[51]	Alligator Snapping Turtle (Macrochelys temminckii)[69]	Western Pond Turtle (Emys marmorata)[70]	Units
Sample size	28–32 captive	79 captive	30 captive	102–106 free ranging	20 free ranging/10 captive	
Data format:	95% CI	10th–90th percentile	Min–Max	95% CI	10th–90th percentile	
Parameter						Units
Blood urea nitrogen		2.5–32.8	2.2–45.7	21.3–28.3	7.9–46.6/18.6–60.7	mg/dL
Creatinine				0.27–0.32		mg/dL
Uric acid	0–3.1	0.3–6.0	0.7–1.7	0.65–0.83	0.39–0.91/0.39–0.6	mg/dL
Total protein	1.9–6.6			3.9–4.4	2.96–4.53/4.4–6.45	g/dL
Albumin	0.27–1.30			0.70–0.81	0.8–1.81/1.78–2.72	g/dL
Calcium	6.6–13.8	9.6–16.0	9.6–19.2	8.9–9.7	8.79–15.2/11.11–21.87	mg/dL
Phosphorus	1.3–3.3	1.9–6.5	2.2–4.6	3.5–3.9	2.38–4.18/2.55–4.93	mg/dL
Ca: Phos	2.6–6.3					
Sodium		124.0–140.0	126.0–138.0	127.2–129.2	133.9–138.1/136.8–142.1	mmol/L
Potassium		2.8–5.7	4.1–7.1	3.6–3.8	3.09–4.43/3.07–3.82	mmol/L
Chloride					90.9–100/89.8–99.5	mmol/L
Bicarbonate				30.4–34.5	27.3–37.1/26.9–34.7	mmol/L
Glucose	36–266			43.5–52.6	32.6–97.3/38.9–72.4	mg/dL
Cholesterol				50.4–64.0	65.9–300.5/135.2–389.6	mg/dL
Total bilirubin						mg/dL
Bile acids		0.9–4.9	1.5–10.1	0.13–0.25		μmol/L
Alanine aminotransferase	3.0–6.2	8.1–35.6	5.0–50.8	20.0–25.9		U/L
Aspartate transaminase	0–145	53.1–196.7	59.5–167.5	151.2–184.2	54.8–223.3/112.4–510.5	U/L
Alkaline phosphatase		19.0–117.0	84.0–935.0		87.3–323.5/163.3–313.5	U/L
Creatine kinase	0–281	129.0–790.0	46.0–180.0	213.9–583.0	86.1–638.8/202.1–1070.8	U/L

Renal Analytes

Urea is considered the major end product of protein metabolism in many freshwater turtle species, whereas terrestrial turtles and other reptiles are typically uricotelic.[45] Urea excretion in the kidney depends on glomerular filtration, which may decrease with dehydration, renal hypoperfusion, or primary renal disease.[46] Dietary protein intake may also significantly influence plasma urea concentrations. One study in Chinese soft-shelled turtles (*Pelodiscus sinensis*) demonstrated a transient increase in plasma urea concentration following a high protein meal, reaching a maximum of a 3-fold increase from baseline 24 hours after feeding.[47] Uric acid and ammonia are minor products of protein metabolism in most freshwater chelonians but may serve as useful additional markers of glomerular filtration rate in some species.[48] Plasma ammonia analysis is currently challenging outside of a tertiary care setting due to sample handling requirements. Creatinine is not produced in significant enough quantities in reptiles to be considered useful for evaluation of renal function.[46,48]

Proteins

Total protein concentrations may be estimated via refractometry or measured using the biuret method in turtles, similar to other species. Refractometry may overestimate the total protein value and is not considered interchangeable with measured total protein concentrations.[46] Total protein is composed of albumin and globulins, with albumin being directly measured and globulins being calculated from the difference between total protein and albumin concentrations in most species. Physiologic causes of hyperproteinemia in turtles include hibernation, recent high-protein food intake, or vitellogenesis in adult females.[46,49] In clinically ill turtles, other considerations include hemoconcentration from dehydration or increased globulin concentrations from inflammation.[3,46] Hypoproteinemia is a more common finding in debilitated turtles and may result from decreased production (ie, hepatic insufficiency), decreased protein intake (ie, starvation, malabsorption), or protein loss (ie, blood loss, protein losing nephropathy, or enteropathy, and so forth).[3,46]

Fractionation of total protein into albumin and globulins provides a more comprehensive assessment of protein status but may be challenging to perform and interpret in freshwater chelonians. Commercially available benchtop reptile chemistry analyzers often use the bromocresol green dye-binding method for albumin measurement, although this method often overestimates albumin due to nonspecific protein binding and showed weak to no correlation with albumin measured via protein electrophoresis in red-eared slider turtles (*T. scripta elegans*).[50] Protein electrophoresis is considered to provide an accurate evaluation of albumin and globulin concentrations. Reference intervals for albumin and globulin fractions using capillary zone electrophoresis in red-eared slider turtles (*T. scripta elegans*) and map turtles (*Graptemys* spp.) have recently been described, although significant interspecies variation in these values has been noted in both freshwater and sea turtle species.[51] Although considered the preferred test at this time, interpretation of protein electrophoresis in freshwater chelonians is largely subjective given the paucity of available reference data. Protein electrophoresis data for selected species are provided in **Table 3**.

Minerals

Total calcium in reptiles is typically measured via the arsenazo III dye-binding method, similar to other species. In free-ranging environments, female turtles often have significantly higher total calcium concentrations compared with males, likely resulting from estrogen-induced increases in protein-bound calcium during vitellogenesis. Increased estrogen activity typically results in parallel increases in total protein and total calcium concentrations.[46,51,52] Pathologic hypercalcemia has been infrequently documented in freshwater chelonians, with hypercalcemia most commonly resulting from overzealous supplementation with calcium or vitamin D_3. Hypocalcemia is more commonly encountered in ill chelonians, often resulting from inappropriate husbandry in captive settings. Dietary vitamin D_3 or calcium deficiency or phosphorus excess may induce hypocalcemia, and adequate UV-B (Ultraviolet B) radiation is important for adequate 25-hydroxyvitamin D_3 synthesis in red-eared slider turtles (*T. scripta elegans*).[46,53] Metabolic bone disease is an important clinical consequence of hypocalcemia, although plasma total calcium concentrations in affected animals may be low-normal in advanced stages of disease due to effects of nutritional secondary hyperparathyroidism.[54] Other potential causes of total hypocalcemia include decreased protein-bound calcium secondary to hypoalbuminemia, renal secondary hyperparathyroidism associated with renal failure, and hypoparathyroidism.[46]

Phosphorus concentrations in free-ranging female freshwater chelonians are often higher than males, likely due to vitellogenesis.[3,46,52] Hyperphosphatemia in freshwater chelonians may result from excessive dietary phosphorus intake, hypervitaminosis D_3, or decreased glomerular filtration rate associated with renal disease or dehydration.[46] In patients with clinical evidence of metabolic bone disease, hyperphosphatemia is a consistent finding supportive of nutritional or renal secondary hyperparathyroidism.[54] Hypophosphatemia in turtles is typically a consequence of nutritional phosphorus deficiency or starvation.[46]

Electrolytes

Sodium is the major extracellular cation in freshwater turtles, and sodium balance is largely regulated by the kidney following gastrointestinal absorption of dietary sodium.[46] Hypernatremia is commonly based on dehydration, which may result from free water loss in some cases of renal failure or gastrointestinal disease, inadequate water intake, or excessive dietary salt intake. Species capable of estivation including the Sonoran mud turtle (*Kinosternon sonoriense*) and the Yellow mud turtle (*K. flavescens*) may maintain prolonged hypernatremia associated with water loss due to desiccation during drought conditions.[55] Hyponatremia may result from causes of hypertonic fluid loss, often secondary to diarrhea, other gastrointestinal disease, or renal disease.

Dietary potassium is absorbed via the gastrointestinal tract and regulated by renal excretion. Mechanisms of hyperkalemia are similar to other species, including decreased renal excretion (ie, renal insufficiency, urinary tract obstruction), transcellular shifting due to severe acidosis, or excessive dietary potassium intake. Hemolysis has recently been reported to cause pseudohyperkalemia in leatherback sea turtles (*Dermochelys coriacea*) presumably due to high intraerythrocytic potassium concentrations or differences in membrane transporters.[56] Similar studies have not been performed in freshwater turtle species, although visual inspection of plasma for hemolysis may be beneficial in cases of unexpected hyperkalemia. Hypokalemia may result from inadequate dietary potassium intake, excessive gastrointestinal loss, or severe alkalosis.[46]

Chloride is the major extracellular anion, and plasma concentrations are interpreted based on sodium concentrations. Proportional increases in sodium and chloride suggest free water loss or decreased water intake, whereas proportional decreases indicate hypertonic fluid loss, typically from the kidney or gastrointestinal tract. Selective hypochloremia has been anecdotally associated with gastric pathologic condition in turtles, presumably due to gastric outflow obstruction or impaired gastric motility resulting in impaired intestinal absorption, as characterized in other species.[3] Selective hyperchloremia has not been described in freshwater chelonians but is typically associated with secretory diarrhea or renal tubular acidosis in other species.

Glucose

Glucose concentrations in turtles and other species are dependent on intestinal dietary glucose absorption, gluconeogenesis, and glycogenolysis. Environmental conditions can significantly affect plasma glucose concentrations. Red-eared slider turtles (*T. scripta elegans*) display a rapid increase in blood glucose following sudden cold-shock and may maintain hyperglycemia during prolonged periods of cold torpor.[57] Diving behavior has also been associated with hyperglycemia in multiple freshwater chelonian species, likely due to increased anaerobic metabolism in anoxic conditions.[58,59] Seasonality, reproductive status, and hibernation may also affect plasma glucose concentrations, especially in free-ranging chelonians.[59]

Pathologic hyperglycemia is uncommonly described but may be identified in clinically ill turtles presenting with a variety of clinical signs, including anorexia, depression, weight loss, and lethargy.[59] Potential underlying mechanisms may include stress or concurrent disease, including neoplasia, inflammatory disease, sepsis, or endocrinopathy.[3,60] Polyuria and polydipsia are not consistent findings in hyperglycemic reptiles, and the renal glucose threshold has not been evaluated in reptilian species.[59] Spontaneous diabetes mellitus has been described in one red-eared slider turtle (*T. scripta elegans*) but is generally considered very rare in reptilian species and thoroughly characterized reports are lacking.[3,60,61] Hypoglycemia in turtles has been associated with prolonged starvation, septicemia, and severe hepatobiliary disease.[46,59] A recent study identified severe hypoglycemia (<30 mg/dL) and moderate to severe hyperglycemia (>151 mg/dL) as independent negative prognostic indicators for 7-day survival in a variety of client-owned chelonians presenting for veterinary care; however, underlying disease processes and species-specific variability were not described.[62]

Biliverdin and Bile Acids

Similar to most other reptiles, freshwater turtles lack the biliverdin reductase enzyme and are, therefore, incapable of reducing biliverdin to bilirubin during hemoglobin metabolism and bile excretion.[63] Hyperbiliverdinemia may impart a green tint to chelonian plasma, although thorough investigations of biliverdin dynamics in chelonian liver disease have not been performed.[3,63] Assays for biliverdin measurement have been developed although commercial availability of these assays is limited, and studies in loggerhead sea turtles (*Caretta caretta*) suggest that further validation and optimization are needed for clinical use in chelonians.[64,65]

Bile acids in chelonians may be measured using commercially available assays for other species but are structurally unique in that they contain a 22-hydroxyl group.[63] Studies evaluating bile acids in freshwater turtle species are limited. Serum bile acid concentrations have been described in healthy female red-eared sliders (*T. scripta elegans*) with no postprandial change detected, although some sources indicate that a prolonged fasting time of 3 days for chelonians may be needed for an accurate bile acid stimulation test.[63,66] Although serum and plasma bile acid concentrations are generally interchangeable in mammals, significant differences in serum and plasma bile acid concentrations have been documented in captive New Guinea Snapping Turtles (*Elseya novaeguineae*).[67] Although bile acid concentrations may be clinically useful in evaluating hepatic function in chelonians, studies correlating clinical or histopathologic evidence of hepatic insufficiency with bile acid concentrations have not been performed to date.[3]

Table 3
Selected protein electrophoresis data for North American freshwater chelonians

Species: (Parameter)	Spotted Turtle (Clemmys guttata)[68]	Alligator Snapping Turtle (Macrochelys temminckii)[69]	Male Red-Eared Slider (T. scripta elegans)[71]	Female Red-Eared Slider (T. scripta elegans)[71]	Male Map Turtle (Graptemys spp.)[71]	Female Map Turtle (Graptemys spp.)[71]	Units
Sample size and characteristics:	28–32 captive	105–106 free ranging	10–23 captive	10–56 captive	3–13 captive	3–22 captive	
Data format:	95% CI	95% CI	Min–Max (summer) 10th–90th percentile (fall)	Min–Max (spring) 10th–90th percentile (summer and fall)	Min–Max	Min–Max (spring and summer) 10th–90th percentile (fall)	
Parameter							*Units*
Total protein	1.9–6.6	3.9–4.4	Summer: 1.35–5.16 Fall: 3.20–6.06	Spring: 1.90–5.23 Summer: 1.57–5.67 Fall: 3.41–6.06	Spring: 2.10–2.62 Summer: 1.45–5.32 Fall: 3.19–5.15	Spring: 2.95–5.13 Summer: 3.33–5.93 Fall: 2.88–5.66	g/dL
Prealbumin	0.0–0.34						g/dL
Prealbumin %			Summer: 2.3–15.7 Fall: 2.6–7.3	Spring: 3.9–27.0 Summer: 3.8–10.3 Fall: 2.7–16.2	Spring: 3.4–5.1 Summer: 2.3–16.8 Fall: 4.5–21.8	Spring: 17.4–28.7 Summer: 5.3–15.8 Fall: 3.9–17.6	% of total protein
Albumin (Capillary zone electrophoresis)	0.27–1.30	0.70–0.81	Summer: 0.36–2.16 Fall: 0.90–1.54	Spring: 0.62–2.55 Summer: 0.44–1.44 Fall: 0.90–2.15	Spring: 0.59–0.66 Summer: 0.41–2.23 Fall: 0.83–2.33	Spring: 1.58–2.11 Summer: 1.25–2.14 Fall: 0.91–2.29	g/dL
Albumin (Bromocresol green)	n/a		Summer: 0.04–2.17 Fall: 1.12–2.44	Spring: 0.44–1.94 Summer: 0.32–2.39 Fall: 1.09–2.52	Spring: 0.97–1.09 Summer: 0.22–2.02 Fall: 1.18–2.28	Spring: 1.34–2.57 Summer: 1.35–2.90 Fall: 1.13–2.41	g/dL
α globulins %			Summer: 23.1–41.9 Fall: 28.6–38.8	Spring: 20.4–35.7 Summer: 26.4–35.8 Fall: 24.5–34.4	Spring: 33.0–49.3 Summer: 22.8–40.5 Fall: 23.3–45.8	Spring: 18.3–31.3 Summer: 20.5–35.0 Fall: 22.9–30.7	% of total protein

(continued on next page)

Table 3
(continued)

Species:	Spotted Turtle (Clemmys guttata)[68]	Alligator Snapping Turtle (Macrochelys temminckii)[69]	Male Red-Eared Slider (T. scripta elegans)[71]	Female Red-Eared Slider (T. scripta elegans)[71]	Male Map Turtle (Graptemys spp.)[71]	Female Map Turtle (Graptemys spp.)[71]	
α-1 globulins	0.23–0.65	0.12–0.15					g/dL
α-2 globulins	0.51–2.13	0.69–0.83					g/dL
β globulins %			Summer: 12.4–20.9 Fall: 13.2–21.7	Spring: 9.0–31.3 Summer: 14.6–22.9 Fall: 11.4–20.4	Spring: 14.9–20.5 Summer: 12.9–23.0 Fall: 11.0–17.1	Spring: 9.5–13.2 Summer: 14.3–15.3 Fall: 12.3–19.8	% of total protein
β-1 globulins	0.02–0.55						g/dL
β-2 globulins	0.08–0.64						g/dL
Total β globulins	0.23–1.06	1.5–1.8					g/dL
γ globulins	0.19–1.52	0.81–1.0					g/dL
γ globulins %			Summer: 16.3–27.4 Fall: 17.7–30.7	Spring: 8.5–32.2 Summer: 14.1–24.3 Fall: 15.5–28.5	Spring: 11.1–22.8 Summer: 11.5–30.0 Fall: 13.0–21.8	Spring: 15.1–15.3 Summer: 14.3–26.7 Fall: 17.9–26.4	% of total protein
A:G (Albumin: Globulin) ratio	0.18–0.39	0.21–0.23	Summer: 0.20–0.81 Fall: 0.28–0.48	Spring: 0.37–1.01 Summer: 0.29–0.60 Fall: 0.32–0.69	Spring: 0.31–0.46 Summer: 0.27–0.80 Fall: 0.34–0.83	Spring: 0.70–1.15 Summer: 0.56–0.81 Fall: 0.39–0.74	

Enzymes

Tissue specificity of routinely measured hepatobiliary enzymes has not been determined in freshwater chelonian species to date. Poor organ specificity has been described for ALT, AST, ALP, and lactate dehydrogenase across reptilian species.[46] Studies using the ASVCP (American Society for Veterinary Clinical Pathology) reference interval guidelines or linking changes in enzymatic activity to histologic evidence of hepatobiliary disease are lacking, and interpretation of these parameters in freshwater turtles should be done with caution.[44,63] CK is considered relatively muscle-specific in other reptiles, although moderate CK activity in the intestine and central nervous system has been documented in sea turtle studies.[41,43] Venipuncture, intramuscular injections, trauma, myositis, or seizure activity should be considered as causes of increased CK activity.[46]

URINALYSIS

Peer-reviewed urinalysis data is currently unavailable for chelonians, and currently published clinical observations are limited to tortoise and box turtle species. Urine specific gravity may be measured by refractometry as in other species but may be of limited diagnostic utility as chelonians are incapable of renal urine concentration.[3,48] Urinary dipsticks have been described to be of value in urine biochemistry interpretation in chelonians, although validation studies have not been performed to confirm the validity of results.[48] Wet-mount evaluation of the urine sediment may be useful in identifying crystals, cells, and infectious organisms. Some degree of bacterial contamination is expected as urine passes through the urodeum to enter the bladder, so the relative number and morphology of bacterial organisms on a sediment should be noted. A mixed bacterial population may support normal flora, whereas a monomorphic population or concurrent pyuria should alert the clinician to potential urinary tract infection.[48] Normal urinary flora has not been characterized in chelonians, which somewhat limits the utility of urine culture in many cases.

SUMMARY

Despite significant advances in recent years in the understanding of chelonian hematology and plasma biochemistry, data specific to freshwater turtles are lacking compared with terrestrial and marine chelonians. Reference intervals and baseline data are available for many species under specific conditions, although continued investigation of changes in laboratory data in response to specific disease states is needed for improved management of freshwater chelonian health in both clinical and field settings.

CLINICS CARE POINTS

- Preanalytical factors including lymphatic contamination and anticoagulant choice may significantly affect the interpretation of chelonian hematology and plasma biochemistry.

- Significant intraspecies variability due to sex, seasonality, geographic location, and other factors may limit the application of published reference intervals to all clinical or field scenarios.

- Relatively common findings on chelonian blood smear evaluation include punctate, basophilic cytoplasmic inclusions, or zones of cytoplasmic clearing within erythrocytes; these should not be misinterpreted as pathologic intraerythrocytic inclusions.

- Due to prolonged erythrocyte life span, regenerative anemia in reptilian species may manifest as large numbers of erythroid precursor cells including rubriblasts on peripheral blood smears and may mimic leukemia in extreme cases.
- Freshwater turtles diverge from terrestrial and marine chelonian species in that urea is the major end product of protein metabolism rather than uric acid.
- Commercially available benchtop analyzers commonly overestimate albumin concentrations in chelonians and other reptiles, and electrophoretic methods are preferred for accurate fractionation of albumin and globulin concentrations.
- Tissue specificity of enzymatic activity has not been firmly established in freshwater turtles, and plasma enzyme concentrations should be interpreted with caution.

Hematology, biochemistry, and protein electrophoresis reference value tables for selected North American freshwater turtle species.

DISCLOSURE

The author declares no conflicts of interest with respect to the research, authorship, or publication of this article.

REFERENCES

1. Wilkinson R. Clinical pathology. In: Mac Arthur S, Wilkinson R, Myer J, editors. Medicine and surgery of turtles and tortoises. 1st edition. Oxford, UK: Blackwell Publishing Ltd.; 2004. p. 141–86.
2. Sykes IVJM, Klaphake E. Reptile hematology. Vet Clin Exot Anim 2015;35(3): 661–80.
3. Innis C, Knotek Z. Tortoises and freshwater turtles. In: Heatley JJ, Russell K, editors. Exotic animal laboratory diagnosis. 1st edition. Hoboken, NJ: John Wiley & Sons, Inc.; 2020. p. 255–82.
4. Hirschfeld WJ, Gordon AS. The effect of bleeding and starvation on blood volumes and peripheral hemogram of the turtle, Pseudemys scripta elegans. Anat Rec 1965;153(3):317–23.
5. Stacy NI, Alleman AR, Sayler KA. Diagnostic hematology of reptiles. Clin Lab Med 2011;31(1):87–108.
6. Gottdenker NL, Jacobson ER. Effect of venipuncture sites on hematologic and clinical biochemical values in desert tortoises (Gopherus agassizii). Am J Vet Res 1995;56(1):19–21.
7. Crawshaw GJ, Holz P. Comparison of plasma biochemical values in blood and blood-lymph mixtures from red-eared sliders, Trachemys scripta elegans. Bull Assoc Reptil Amphib Vet 1996;6(2):7–9.
8. Perpiñán D, Armstrong DL, Dórea F. Effect of anticoagulant and venipuncture site on hematology and serum chemistries of the spiny softshell turtle. J Herpetol Med Surg 2010;20(2):74–8.
9. Garcia GC, Alves-Jûnior JRF, Santana AE, et al. Hematologic variables of the Arrau turtle (Podocnemis expansa) under the effects of different anticoagulants and cytologic stains. Vet Clin Path 2021;50(2):209–15.
10. Martinez-Hernandez D, Hernandez-Divers SJ, Floyd TM, et al. Comparison of the effects of dipotassium ethylenediaminetetraacetic acid and lithium heparin on hematologic values in yellow-blotched map turtles (Graptemys favimaculata). J Herpetol Med Surg 2007;17(2):36–41.

11. Camargo FC, Abrão NB, Queiroz TD, et al. Serum biochemistry of the Arrau turtle: frozen analyte stability and the effects of long-term storage. Vet Clin Path 2020; 49(1):42–7.

12. Oliveira-Junior AA, Tavares-Dias M, Marcon JL. Biochemical and hematological reference ranges for Amazon freshwater turtle, *Podocnemis expansa* (Reptilia: Pelomedusidae) with morphological assessment of blood cells. Res Vet Sci 2009;86(1):146–51.

13. Chansue N, Sailasuta A, Tantrongpiros J, et al. Hematology and clinical chemistry of adult yellow-headed temple turtles (*Hieremys annandalii*) in Thailand. Vet Clin Path 2011;40(2):174–84.

14. Chung C, Cheng C, Chin S, et al. Morphologic and cytochemical characteristics of Asian yellow pond turtle (*Ocadia sinensis*) blood cells and their hematologic and plasma biochemical reference values. J Zoo Wildl Med 2009;40(1):76–85.

15. Innis CJ, Tlusty M, Wunn D. Hematologic and plasma biochemical analysis of juvenile head-started northern red-bellied cooters (*Pseudemys rubriventris*). J Zoo Wildl Med 2007;38(3):425–32.

16. King P, Heatwole H. Seasonal comparison of hemoglobins in three species of turtles. J Herpetol 1999;33(4):691–4.

17. Damsgaard C, Storz JF, Hoffmann FG, et al. Hemoglobin isoform differentiation and allosteric regulation of oxygen binding in the turtle, *Trachemys scripta*. Am J Physiol Regul Integr Comp Physiol 2013;305(8):R961–7.

18. Winter JM, Stacy NI, Adamovicz LA, et al. Investigating the analytical variability and agreement of manual leukocyte quantification methods in eastern box turtles (*Terrapene carolina carolina*). Front Vet Sci 2019;6:398.

19. Altland PD, Brace KC. Red cell lifespan in the turtle and toad. Am J Phys 1962; 206(6):1188–90.

20. Sheeler P, Barber AA. Comparative hematology of the turtle, rabbit, and rat. Comp Biochem Physiol 1964;11:139–45.

21. Davis AK, Holcomb KL. Intraerythrocytic inclusion bodies in painted turtles (*Chrysemys picta picta*) with measurements of affected cells. Comp Clin Pathol 2008;17:51–4.

22. Hérnandez JD, Castro P, Saavedra P, et al. Morphologic and cytochemical characteristics of the blood cells of the yellow-bellied slider turtle (*Trachemys scripta scripta*). Anat Histol Embryol 2017;46:446–55.

23. Saggese MD. Clinical approach to the anemic reptile. J Exot Ped Med 2009; 18(2):98–111.

24. Savo APH, Zheng Y, Zheng Y, et al. Health status assessment of traumatic injury freshwater turtles. PLoS One 2018;13(8):e0202194.

25. Lutcavage ME, Lutz PL, Bossart GD, et al. Physiologic and clinicopathologic effects of crude oil on loggerhead sea turtles. Arch Environ Contam Toxicol 1995; 28:417–22.

26. Tavares-Dias M, Oliveira-Junior AA, Silva MG, et al. Comparative hematological and biochemical analysis of giant turtles from the Amazon farmed in poor and normal nutritional conditions. Vet Arh 2009;79(6):601–10.

27. Musacchia XJ, Grundhauser W. Seasonal and induced alterations of water content in organs of the turtle *Chrysemys picta*. Copeia 1962;3:570–5.

28. Rossow JA, Hernandez SM, Sumner SM. Haemogregarine infections of three species of aquatic freshwater turtles from two sites in Costa Rica. Int J Parasitol 2013;2:131–5.

29. Knotkova Z, Mazanek S, Hovorka M, et al. Haematology and plasma chemistry of Bornean river turtles suffering from shell necrosis and hemogregarine parasites. Vet Med Czech 2005;50(9):421–6.

30. González LP, Pacheco MA, Escalante AA, et al. *Haemocystidium* spp., a species complex infecting ancient aquatic turtles of the family Podocnemididae: First report of these parasites in *Podocnemis vogli* from the Orinoquia. Int J Parasitol 2019;10:299–309.

31. Campbell TW. Peripheral blood of reptiles. In: Exotic animal hematology and cytology. 4th edition. John Wiley & Sons; 2015. p. 67–87.

32. Neiffer DL, Lydick D, Burks K, et al. Hematologic and plasma biochemical changes associated with fenbendazole administration in Hermann's tortoises (*Testudo hermanni*). J Zoo Wildl Med 2005;36(4):661–72.

33. Saad AH, Torroba M, Varas A, et al. Testosterone induces lymphopenia in turtles. Vet Immunol Immunopathol 1991;28:173–80.

34. George JW, Holmberg TA, Riggs SM, et al. Circulating siderophagocytes and erythrophagocytes in a corn snake (*Elaphe guttata*) after coelomic surgery. Vet Clin Pathol 2009;37(3):308–11.

35. Mead KF, Borysenko M, Findlay SR. Naturally abundant basophils in the snapping turtle, *Chelydra serpentina*, possess cytophilic surface antibody with reaginic function. J Immunol 1983;130(1):334–40.

36. Perpiñán D, Hernandez-Divers SM, Latimer KS, et al. Hematology of the Pascagoula map turtle (*Graptemys gibbonsi*) and the southeast Asian box turtle (*Cuora amboinensis*). J Zoo Wildl Med 2008;39(3):460–3.

37. Murray M, Waliszewski NT, Garner MM, et al. Sepsis and disseminated intravascular coagulation in an eastern spiny softshell turtle (*Apalone spinifera spinifera*) with acute mycobacteriosis. J Zoo Wildl Med 2009;40(3):572–5.

38. Soslau G, Wallace B, Vicente C, et al. Comparison of functional aspects of the coagulation cascade in human and sea turtle populations. Comp Biochem Physiol 2004;138(4):399–406.

39. Barratclough A, Hanel R, Stacy NI, et al. Establishing a protocol for thromboelastography in sea turtles. Vet Rec Open 2018;5(1):e000240.

40. Barratclough A, Tuxbury K, Hanel R, et al. Baseline plasma thromboelastrography in Kemp's Ridley (*Lepidochelys kempii*), green (*Chelonia mydas*), and loggerhead (*Caretta caretta*) sea turtles and its use to diagnose coagulopathies in cold-stunned Kemp's Ridley and green sea turtles. J Zoo Wildl Med 2019;50(1):62–8.

41. Anderson ET, Socha VL, Gardner J, et al. Tissue enzyme activities in the loggerhead sea turtle (*Caretta caretta*). J Zoo Wildl Med 2013;44(1):62–9.

42. Adamovicz L, Griffloen J, Cerreta A, et al. Tissue enzyme activities in free-living eastern box turtles (*Terrapene carolina carolina*). J Zoo Wildl Med 2019;50(1):45–54.

43. Petrosky KY, Knoll JS, Innis C. Tissue enzyme activities in Kemp's Ridley turtles (*Lepidochelys kempii*). J Zoo Wildl Med 2015;46(3):637–40.

44. Friedrichs KR, Harr KE, Freeman KP, et al. ASVCP reference interval guidelines: determination of de novo reference intervals in veterinary species and other related topics. Vet Clin Pathol 2012;41(4):441–53.

45. Holz PH. Anatomy and physiology of the reptile renal system. Vet Clin Exot Anim 2020;23(1):103–14.

46. Campbell TW. Clinical chemistry of reptiles. In: Thrall MA, Weiser G, Allison RW, et al, editors. Veterinary hematology and clinical chemistry. 2nd edition. John Wiley & Sons, Inc; 2012. p. 599–606.

47. Postprandial increases in nitrogenous excretion and urea synthesis in the Chinese soft-shelled turtle, *Pelodiscus sinensis*. J Comp Physiol B 2007;177:19–29.
48. Divers SJ, Innis CJ. Urology. In: Divers SJ, Stahl SJ, editors. Mader's reptile and amphibian medicine and surgery. 3rd edition. St. Louis, MO: Elsevier, Inc.; 2019. p. 624–48.
49. Mumm LE, Winter JM, Andersson KE, et al. Hematology and plasma biochemistries in the Blanding's turtle (*Emydoidea blandingii*) in Lake County, Illinois. PLoS one 2019;14(11):e0225130.
50. Müller K, Brunnberg L. Determination of plasma albumin concentration in healthy and diseased turtles: a comparison of protein electrophoresis and the bromocresol green dye-binding method. Vet Clin Pathol 2010;39(1):79–82.
51. Leineweber C, Stöhr AC, Öfner S, et al. Plasma capillary zone electrophoresis and plasma chemistry analytes in tortoises (*Testudo hermanni, Testudo graeca*) and turtles (*Trachemys scripta elegans, Graptemys* spp.) in fall. J Zoo Wildl Med 2020;51(4):915–25.
52. Clark NB. Influence of estrogens upon serum calcium, phosphate, and protein concentrations of fresh-water turtles. Comp Biochem Physiol 1967;20:823–34.
53. Acierno MJ, Mitchel MA, Roundtree MK, et al. Effects of ultraviolet radiation on 25-hydroxyvitamin D_3 synthesis in red-eared slider turtles (*Trachemys scripta elegans*). Am J Vet Res 2006;67(12):2046–9.
54. Knafo SE. Musculoskeletal system. In: Divers SJ, Stahl SJ, editors. Mader's reptile and amphibian medicine and surgery. 3rd edition. St. Louis, MO: Elsevier, Inc.; 2019. p. 894–916.
55. Peterson CC, Stone PA. Physiological capacity for estivation of the Sonoran mud turtle, *Kinosternon sonoriense*. Copeia 2000;3:684–700.
56. Stacy NI, Chabot RM, Innis CJ, et al. Plasma chemistry in nesting leatherback sea turtles (*Dermochelys coriacea*) from Florida: understanding the importance of sample hemolysis effects on blood analytes. PLoS One 2019;14(9):e02222426.
57. Hutton KE. Effects of hypothermia on turtle blood glucose. Herpetologica 1964; 20(2):129–31.
58. Dessauer HC. Blood chemistry of reptiles. In: Gans C, Parsons TC, editors. Biol Reptilia3. New York: Academic Press; 1970. p. 1–72.
59. Raiti P. Endocrinology. In: Divers SJ, Stahl SJ, editors. Mader's reptile and amphibian medicine and surgery. 3rd edition. St. Louis, MO: Elsevier, Inc.; 2019. p. 835–48.
60. Juan-Sallés C, Boyer TH. Nutritional and metabolic diseases. In: Garner MM, Jacobson ER, editors. Noninfectious diseases and pathology of reptiles. Boca Raton, FL: CRC Press; 2021. p. 55–72.
61. Frye FL, Dutra FR, Carney JD, et al. Spontaneous diabetes mellitus in a turtle. Vet Med Small Anim Clin 1974;69:990–3.
62. Colon VA, Di Girolamo N. Prognostic value of packed cell volume and blood glucose concentration in 954 client-owned chelonians. J Am Vet Med Assoc 2020;257(12):1265–72.
63. Divers SJ. Hepatology. In: Divers SJ, Stahl SJ, editors. Mader's reptile and amphibian medicine and surgery. 3rd edition. St. Louis, MO: Elsevier, Inc.; 2019. p. 649–68.
64. Berlec A, Štrukelj B. A high-throughput biliverdin assay using indirect fluorescence. J Vet Diagn Invest 2014;26(4):521–6.
65. Stacy NI, Lynch JM, Arendt MD, et al. Chronic debilitation in stranded loggerhead sea turtles (*Caretta caretta*) in the southeastern United States: Morphometrics and clinicopathological findings. PLoS One 2018;13(7):e0200355.

66. Knotkova Z, Dorrestein GM, Jekl V, et al. Fasting and postprandial serum bile acid concentrations in 10 healthy female red-eared terrapins (*Trachemys scripta elegans*). Vet Rec 2008;163:510–4.

67. Anderson NL, Wack RF, Hatcher R. Hematology and clinical chemistry reference ranges for clinically normal, captive New Guinea snapping turtle (*Elseya novaeguineae*) and the effects of temperature, sex, and sample type. J Zoo Wildl Med 1997;28(4):394–403.

68. Buscaglia NA, Inham DN, Chen S, et al. Partial hematology, biochemistry, and protein electrophoresis reference intervals for captive spotted turtles (*Clemmys guttata*). J Zoo Wildl Med 2021;52(2):704–9.

69. Chaffin K, Norton TM, Gilardi K, et al. Health assessment of free-ranging alligator snapping turtles (*Macrochelys temminckii*) in Georgia and Florida. J Wildl Dis 2008;44(3):670–86.

70. Keller KA, Sanchez-Migallon Guzman D, Paul-Murphy J, et al. Hematologic and plasma biochemical values of free-ranging western pond turtles (*Emys marmorata*) with comparison to a captive population. J Herpetol Med Surg 2012;22(3–4): 99–106.

71. Leineweber C, Öfner S, Stöhr AC, et al. A comparison of thyroid hormone levels and plasma capillary zone electrophoresis in red-eared sliders (*Trachemys scripta elegans*) and map turtles (*Graptemys* spp.) depending on season and sex. Vet Clin Pathol 2020;49:78–90.

Diagnostic Clinical Pathology of Boas and Pythons

Amy N. Schnelle, DVM, MS, DACVP

KEYWORDS

- Boa • Python • Snake • Hematology • Biochemistry

KEY POINTS

- Hematologic assessment for snakes provides useful clinical information, though still relies on manual methods for assessment at this time.
- Biochemical assessment has clinical value, and clinicians should be cognizant of the limits of validation for non-domestic species in most laboratories.
- There is wide variability in the depth and quality of published information and reference ranges, necessitating diligence of clinicians in critically evaluating information used for case interpretation.
- There are large gaps in knowledge regarding all snake species, with many valuable opportunities for study for interested clinicians.

INTRODUCTION

Much is unknown about many aspects of diagnostic clinical pathology for reptiles, particularly snakes. Although we focus on boas and pythons, references assessing other snakes and taxa are included by necessity. Of note, though pythons were once considered a subfamily of Boidae, boas and pythons are now recognized as separate phylogenetic families.[1]

Clinical pathology typically includes antemortem diagnostic testing concerning the hemogram, serum biochemistry, endocrine testing, urinalysis, and cytologic evaluation of body fluids, tissues, masses, and lesions. Blood sample collection sites and techniques are discussed elsewhere.[2–4] Collection sites have been shown to influence data, at least in part due to the potential for lymph contamination.[5] For practical reasons, anticoagulated whole blood is commonly used for both erythron assessment and biochemical testing. Many biochemical analyses can be performed on lithium heparin plasma, and a few can be performed on EDTA plasma. In a comparison study

Veterinary Diagnostic Laboratory, University of Illinois, College of Veterinary Medicine, 1008 West Hazelwood Drive, MC 004, Urbana, IL 61802, USA
E-mail address: aschnel2@illinois.edu

Vet Clin Exot Anim 25 (2022) 805–821
https://doi.org/10.1016/j.cvex.2022.06.006
1094-9194/22/© 2022 Elsevier Inc. All rights reserved.

in Burmese pythons (*Python molurus bivittatus*), lithium heparin and EDTA anticoagulants were preferred over citrate anticoagulant due to PCV decreases, cell lysis, and plasma discoloration with sample storage.[6]

Absences of biochemical assay validation, experience with reptile samples, and robust reference intervals are significant hurdles for the clinician. Published reference ranges for select species are available as aggregated tables in texts, as well as in individual research articles.[7–10] The clinician should note that such ranges should be used with caution. The data may be generated from methods that differ from that performed for the patient. Additionally, the information may come from few animals and/or a population with differences from the patient: captive versus wild, healthy versus ill, sex, season, and reproductive status, among others. The practitioner should strive to identify reference ranges developed from a large, ideally healthy population with living conditions similar to the animal in question. The ASVCP guidelines recommend reference interval development from 120 animals; they also recommend not calculating reference intervals from groups of 10 to 20 animals and not reporting values from groups of 10 or fewer animals.[11] Alternatively, laboratory data collected during illness can be compared with historical wellness laboratory data from the same patient if available.

COMPLETE BLOOD COUNT (CBC)

Few research studies have worked toward some form of automated analysis of ophidian blood. Given the practical limitations of hematology analyzers at this time, the CBC commonly consists of a spun packed cell volume (PCV), manual hemocytometer counting or slide estimation of blood cells, and microscopic examination of one or more blood smears. Blood films are evaluated to determine leukocyte differential count, estimate thrombocyte mass, assess cell morphology, and evaluate for parasites and abnormal cells. Assessment of plasma color and refractometric measurement of total solids from the microhematocrit tube may also be included. Hemocytometer counting uses either Natt and Herrick stain or phloxine B stain.[12] Occasional sources indicate a preference for the Natt and Herrick method of leukocyte counting in species in which the fraction of lymphocytes is greater than heterophils, with some support in the literature.[7,12] Additional work with greater numbers of animals and more species variety for is needed more conclusive examination of this hypothesis.

Blood films may be prepared in by several methods. The goal is a blood smear with a quality monolayer and feathered edge for evaluation, with minimal cell rupture, uneven sample distribution, or excessive concentration of leukocytes in the feathered edge. Blood is typically smeared with use of two glass slides or coverslips or a combination of glass slide and coverslip.[13] Cell rupture is a significant concern, though a specific technique is not necessarily at fault.[12] The veterinary clinician should try several techniques to determine the most comfortable and successful for them. Dry slides quickly to reduce refractile artifact and to avoid cellular degeneration.[13] Quick and automated Romanowsky-type stains are typically used for blood films. Avoid exposure of blood films to formalin and formalin fumes which may result in gross and microscopic blue-green discoloration.[14] Storage times may also impact results. In a field study of anaconda health (*Eunectes murinus*), blood samples collected from anacondas within 1 day of capture had significantly higher azurophil and lower lymphocyte counts than did samples collected 2 to 10 days after capture.[15]

ERYTHROCYTES

The erythrocytes of reptiles are nucleated, larger and oval (**Fig. 1**). Cytoplasm is typically a pink-orange color when adequately stained, though may appear different with

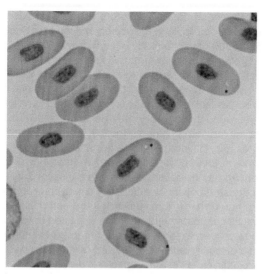

Fig. 1. Mature erythrocytes in heparinized blood of *Boa constrictor imperator*. Clinically insignificant inclusions are indicated by asterisks (Wright-Giemsa stain, original magnification 100x).

exposure to formalin or formalin fumes or with suboptimal staining.[14] Due to the increased protein content of nucleated erythrocytes, staining protocols for mammalian blood may need adjustment for adequate staining of reptile blood smears. The nuclei of snake erythrocytes may be oval or irregular in shape. Occasional non-nucleated erythrocytes (erythroplastids) may be noted and are of questionable clinical relevance.

Cutoff values of 15 or 20% packed cell volume (PCV) to suggest anemia in python species have been published (**Table 1**).[7,12] Published ranges for several python species are provided (see **Table 1**). Onset of anemia is recognized through reduced PCV, though individual laboratories may provide additional data, and the practitioner must exclude the possibility of lymph dilution of the sample. Comprehensive studies evaluating causes of anemia in snakes are not identified in review of the literature and are needed. Among a selection of 28 case reports of infectious and neoplastic diseases in boas and pythons, only five neoplastic cases included PCV information. In two reported boa cases of lymphoma with a leukemic phase, anemia was reported.[16,17] A case of pericardial mesothelioma in a tiger rat snake (*Spilotes pullatus*) documented a decrease in PCV to 25% from 30% 8 months prior to diagnosis.[18] However, in other reports, three boids with localized and systemic neoplasia lacked apparent anemia.[19–21] Thus PCV varies based on disease as in other species.

Table 1
Selection of published PCV data in pythons

Species	N	Wild/Captive	Range (%)	Mean ± SD (%)
Python molurus bivittatus[6]	10	Not specified	22–34	29 ± 3.2
Morelia spilota imbricata[8]	35	Wild	8–30	23.2, Median 24%
Python sebae[10]	19	Wild (dry season)	10–26	19.86 ± 4.22
Python regius[27]	20	Wild-caught	10.5–28	18.3 ± 5.3

Abbreviation: SD, standard deviation.

In the previously referenced cases, indicators were not provided to assess for a regenerative effort. Although reptile erythrocytes are reportedly long lived, with lifespans exceeding 500 - 800 days, no study of erythrocyte lifespan in a snake species appears extant.[22,23] Polychromatophils may be seen and have more basophilic cytoplasm and less dense chromatin, relative to mature erythrocytes (**Fig. 2**C). In health, polychromatophils typically make up less than 2.5% of circulating erythrocytes.[14] Less mature erythrocytes are more round in shape and have progressively more blue cytoplasm, larger round nuclei, and more open chromatin (**Fig. 2**B, D). Mitotic figures may also be observed in circulation (**Fig. 2**A). Increased numbers of circulating immature erythrocytes may be interpreted as evidence of active erythropoiesis.

Visible hypochromia of erythrocytes on blood film review or decreases in erythrocyte hemoglobin concentrations could suggest anemia secondary to chronic disease (presumptive iron sequestration) or iron deficiency due to chronic blood loss.[12,24] Evaluation for sources of hemorrhage, such as endo- and ectoparasites, is suggested in these snakes. Hemolysis or acute hemorrhage is expected to result in a regenerative anemia.[7] Anemia due to decreased production is an additional consideration, and inflammation, chronic disease, renal disease, and dysfunction or disease of hematopoietic tissue are possibilities, as in other species.[7] An erythrocytosis of 44% was reported in a boa constrictor with gastrointestinal T cell lymphoma; the animal was estimated to be 5% dehydrated with an unremarkable biochemistry panel.[21]

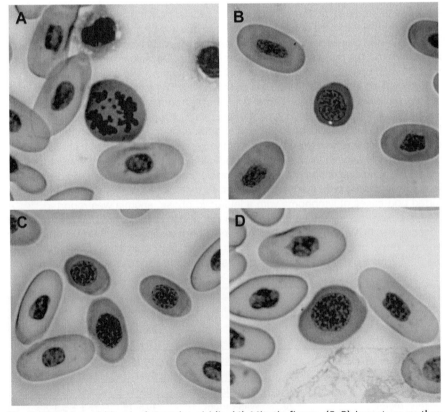

Fig. 2. Heparinized blood of *Crotalus viridis*. (*A*) Mitotic figure. (*B–D*) Immature erythrocytes. (Modified Wright stain, original magnification 100x).

THROMBOCYTES

Thrombocytes are typically small cells with rounded, oval, or somewhat spiculated borders and may be confused with small lymphocytes. They have a small or moderate amount of colorless, light gray or blue-gray cytoplasm (**Fig. 3**A–C). These cells may contain one or more discrete, colorless vacuoles or small, pink granules. The nucleus is oval or round with dense or clumped chromatin. Few to many thrombocytes may be seen in clumps. Evaluation of these groups can be useful to identify a range of thrombocyte morphology that may be observed within the sample.

LEUKOCYTES

Several types of leukocytes are expected within blood films of boas and pythons. Lymphocytes, azurophils, heterophils, and basophils are typically reported; monocytes are also commonly included.[8,10,25–27] Eosinophils are occasionally reported.[10] Using a combination of density gradient isolation, flow cytometry, and microscopic evaluation, one study confirmed the presence of heterophils, lymphocytes, azurophils, and basophils in boa constrictors, though did not report monocytes or eosinophils.[25]

Lymphocytes may range from small to large within a given sample (**Fig. 4**). Their cell and nuclear margins may be round but commonly display irregularity. Granulated lymphocytes, plasmacytoid lymphocytes, and plasma cells may also be seen. Lymphocytes outnumbered heterophils and were similar in number to azurophils in a group

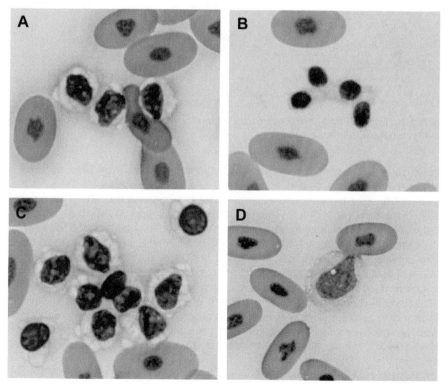

Fig. 3. Heparinized blood of *Boa constrictor imperator*. (*A–C*) Thrombocytes. (*D*) Monocyte. (Wright-Giemsa stain, original magnification 100x).

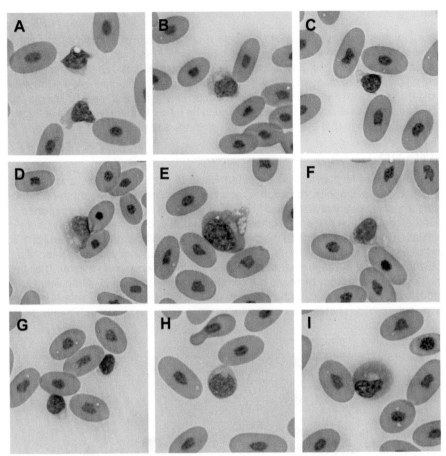

Fig. 4. Heparinized blood of *Boa constrictor imperator*. (*A–I*) Lymphocytes. (Wright-Giemsa stain, original magnification 100x).

of wild caught *Boa constrictor amarali*.[27] Lymphoid leukemia has been reported in several species.[16,17,24]

Azurophils are a large mononuclear cell type unique to reptiles. They have basophilic cytoplasm with pink to magenta granular material within the cytoplasm (**Fig. 5**). Monocytes lack pink cytoplasmic material and may be included with azurophils or reported as a separate fraction (**Fig. 3**D). Azurophils were more than 25 times more prevalent than monocytes in a group of 20 ball pythons, *Python regius*.[26] A pattern of positive staining with Periodic Acid Schiff (PAS), Sudan Black B, and benzidine peroxidase has been described in azurophils from several snake species.[28–30] This azurophil staining pattern is reminiscent of mammalian neutrophils.[28] Staining for benzidine peroxidase activity in snake azurophils is dissimilar to heterophils and azurophil staining in other reptiles, apart from some lizards.[31] In light of cytochemical staining results, it has been recommended that azurophils be reported separately from monocytes in snakes.[24]

Heterophils have abundant colorless or pale blue cytoplasm that is typically filled with pink-orange granules (**Fig. 6**). Where visible, the granules commonly are rounded, oval, and/or rod-shaped. The nucleus is rounded, frequently eccentric, and may not

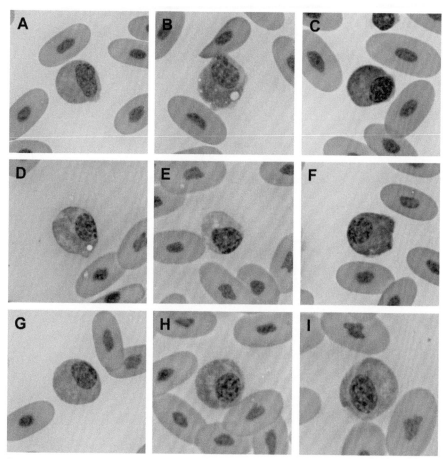

Fig. 5. Heparinized blood of *Boa constrictor imperator*. (*A–I*) Azurophils. (Wright-Giemsa stain, original magnification 100x).

completely stain, and the chromatin is clumped. Cytoplasmic extensions have been observed and may represent a response akin to Neutrophil Extracellular Traps described in mammals.[32] Heterophils were more numerous than lymphocytes and azurophils/monocytes in small groups of southwest carpet pythons (*Morelia spilota imbricata*), African rock pythons (*Python sebae*), and ball pythons (*Python regius*).[8,10,26]

Basophils have a low to moderate nuclear to cytoplasmic ratio, and the cytoplasm is typically filled with dark purple (metachromatic) rounded granules or may appear vacuolated (**Fig. 7**). The nucleus is round, often central, and typically has dense chromatin.

Some sources indicate the absence of eosinophils in snakes or in certain species.[28,33] However, eosinophils have been described in certain snake species, though granule colors vary from basophilic to homogenous eosinophilic.[30,34] While eosinophils have not been listed within the differential counts from several boa and python species, presumptive eosinophils from *Boa constrictor imperator* are pictured (**Fig. 8**).[6,8,25–27]

LEUKOCYTE RESPONSES IN DISEASE

Heterophilia is a possible finding in animals with inflammatory disease. A marked leukocytosis of 86 × 10⁹ leukocytes/L with a majority heterophils has been reported in a

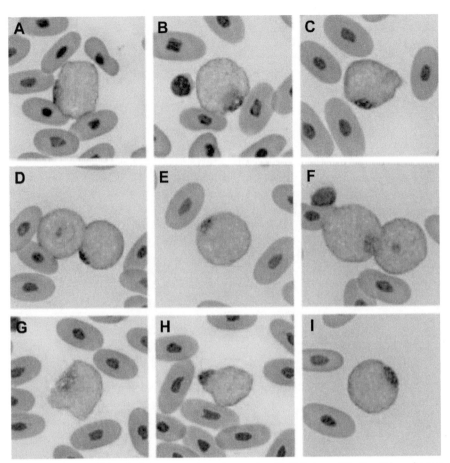

Fig. 6. Heparinized blood of *Boa constrictor imperator*. (*A–I*) Heterophils. Small lymphocyte also pictured in B & F. (Wright-Giemsa stain, original magnification 100x).

diamond python (*Morelia spilota spilota*) with inflammatory disease related to a chronic respiratory tract infection.[35] In a field study of anaconda health *(E murinus),* injured anacondas had significantly higher heterophil counts and lower potassium and uric acid levels than did uninjured snakes.[15] Relative to males, females were more likely to have been injured and had significantly higher heterophil counts with lower lymphocyte counts and packed cell volumes; they were also significantly heavier and longer.[15] A case report of an anaconda with systemic cryptococcosis found no significant alterations on blood work.[36] Azurophils may also play a role in acute inflammation.[37] Another case report of an injured wild-caught anaconda with a severe *Hepatozoon* spp. infection identified a mild to moderate leukocytosis that consisted primarily of lymphocytes.[38] Post-mortem blood smear evaluation in an Indian python (*Python molurus*) revealed a severe lymphocytosis, with a mix of smaller and large cells; the snake was diagnosed with lymphoma of multiple tissues on histopathology.[39]

EFFECTS OF SEASON

In 2 free-living species (*Boa constrictor amarali*, African rock pythons), statistical or clinically relevant differences in PCV based on season were not observed.[10,27] In

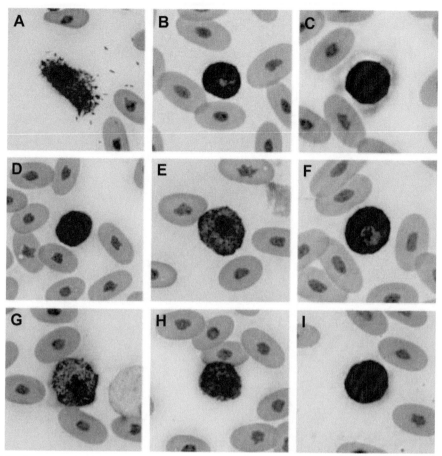

Fig. 7. Heparinized blood of *Boa constrictor imperator*. (*A–I*) Basophils. (Wright-Giemsa stain, original magnification 100x).

wild caught African rock pythons, statistically and clinically significant increases in leukocytes and heterophils occur in the dry season, relative to wet season. A clinically significant increase in lymphocytes was occurred that approached but did not achieve statistical significance.[10] In *Boa constrictor amarali*, total leukocyte counts were clinically and statistically significantly higher in the summer, relative to winter. Significant differences in lymphocyte and monocyte counts were reported, but included data proved difficult to interpret.[27]

CELLULAR INCLUSIONS

Hemogregarines, intracellular erythrocyte parasites, have been reported in wild caught boas and pythons.[40,41] Therefore, animals ending up in the pet trade may show evidence of infection. These organisms consist of the genera *Hemogregarina*, *Hemolivia*, *Hepatozoon*, and *Karyolysus*, and members of the genus *Hepatozoon*.[42] The inclusions are basophilic, nonpigmented, sausage-shaped or oblong structures within erythrocytes. They may curve around or displace the nucleus, and smaller oval or rounded forms may also be identified.

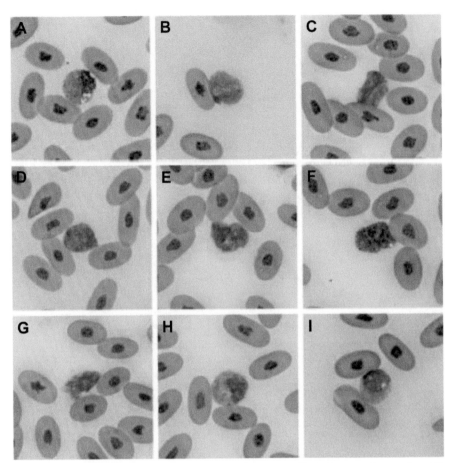

Fig. 8. Heparinized blood of *Boa constrictor imperator*. (*A–I*) Presumptive eosinophils. (Wright-Giemsa stain, original magnification 100x).

Round to oval pale blue cytoplasmic inclusions within the cytoplasm of boa and python erythrocytes may represent viral inclusions, particularly those of the contagious Inclusion Body Disease (IBD) Arenavirus in boas and pythons (**Fig. 9**B, D). In addition to erythrocyte inclusions, identification of larger structures within lymphocytes and other leukocytes is helpful to differentiate viral inclusions from artifact in erythrocytes (**Fig. 9**A, C).

Prevalence of IBD within captive populations of boas and pythons varies widely.[43–45] A 19% prevalence was found in 131 animals of mixed boa and python species from 28 collections.[43] Most infected animals were among the 53 boa constrictors *(Boa constrictor)* sampled, with a prevalence of 42%. None of 22 tested ball pythons (*Python regius*) were positive.[43] In a study from Belgium, 292 boas and pythons from 40 collections were tested, yielding an overall disease prevalence of 16.5%. Among Boidae, only boa constrictors were positive, with a disease prevalence of 35.4%; among Pythonidae, prevalence was 5.3%.[45] An evaluation of 36 snakes from an Australian zoo collection found an overall prevalence of 22.2% by PCR; inclusions were not observed in any of ten blood films examined.[44] Overall, agreement between blood film examination and PCR in these studies was good, but not

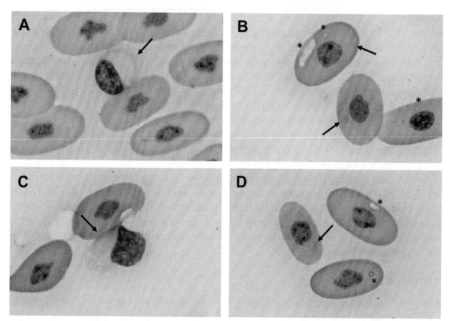

Fig. 9. Heparinized blood of *Boa constrictor imperator*. (*A–D*) Light blue, glassy inclusions of Inclusion Body Disease are indicated by arrows. Asterisks in B & D indicate clinically insignificant inclusions or artifact. (Wright-Giemsa stain, original magnification 100x).

perfect.[43,44,46] Therefore, this author recommends PCR testing for the causative arenavirus for confirmatory diagnosis of inclusions found on blood smears. Screening of breeding animals may be useful, due to reported evidence of vertical transmission.[45]

BIOCHEMISTRY

Published information about biochemical assessment of reptiles is limited and validation status of the analyses is typically unknown. Preanalytical factors, such as hemolysis and lipemia, have the potential to alter biochemical analyte results and should be minimized. Specific testing of interfering substances using boa or python serum or plasma is not identified in the literature. In a field study of anaconda health *(E murinus)*, blood samples processed within 12 hours of collection had significantly higher glucose, total CO_2, total bilirubin, and iron values and lower lactate dehydrogenase values than samples processed after storage on ice in a cooler or refrigerated for 1 to 2 days before processing.[15]

TOTAL PROTEIN AND ALBUMIN

Total protein of serum or plasma is measured in automated analyzers via the biuret reaction. Total solids may be determined via refractometry, but this method is affected by other factors, including hemolysis, hyperbilirubinemia, lipemia, and hyperglycemia, among others.[47]

Automated analyzers in veterinary laboratories typically utilize bromocresol green (BCG) dye binding to measure albumin. In reptiles, however, this method has weak to moderate correlation with albumin determined via protein electrophoresis and commonly overestimates serum or plasma albumin concentration relative to protein electrophoresis.[48] This is likely due to nonspecific binding of the dye to fibrinogen in plasma.[49–51] In the author's experience with a group of *Boa constrictor imperators*, overestimations of albumin via BCG relative to albumin determined via agarose gel electrophoresis ranged from clinically relevant to irrelevant in heparinized plasma without lipemia, hemolysis, hyperbilirubinemia, or hyperbiliverdinemia. Müller and colleagues concluded that the difference between methods could lead to clinical misinterpretation of results. Consequently, protein electrophoresis of serum or plasma is the preferred method for determination of albumin and globulin concentrations.[48,52] Total protein by the biuret method is used for calculations of electrophoretic fractions.[53,54] Agarose gel electrophoresis (AGE) and capillary zone electrophoresis (CZE) results are both reported in the reptile literature.[53,54]

Comparison of protein electrophoretic profiles of healthy controls to boa constrictors that were PCR positive for Inclusion Body Disease (Arenavirus), revealed virus positive snakes with clinical signs had lower albumin, lower A:G ratios, lower alpha globulins and higher gamma globulins.[54] Compared with virus negative healthy snakes, subclinical virus positive snakes had similar albumin but lower alpha globulins and higher gamma globulins.

CREATININE AND URIC ACID

At this time, sensitive and specific testing for renal disease in boas and pythons is not available. Creatinine is not a useful analyte in these species.[55] In a small study, urate excretions of members of Boidae (*Sanzinia madagascariensis*) and Pythonidae (*Python regius*) consisted mainly of uric acid, differing from colubrids and viper excretions that consisted primarily of ammonium urate.[56] Measurement of serum or plasma uric acid is commonly used for clinical assessment of renal health. Unfortunately, uric acid alterations have been shown to be affected by factors other than glomerular filtration rate. Uric acid significantly increases by feeding a high protein meal in reptiles and may last for 1 to 5 days in snakes[57,58]; however, these increases, and the window of time have not been confirmed for boas or pythons. Given this information, serial measurements of uric acid may be more helpful to the clinician to accumulate evidence of renal dysfunction overtime. More work is needed to identify biomarkers that may be of use in diagnosis of renal disease early in the process.

ENZYMES

Most studies of snake tissue enzymes are of colubrids and therefore are summarized elsewhere.[59] In a field study of anaconda health, male anacondas had significantly higher alkaline phosphatase, creatinine, and amylase plasma activities.[15] A single study determined gastrointestinal and pancreatic tissue enzyme activities in pre- and post-prandial Burmese pythons.[60] Postprandial activities of pancreatic (amylase and trypsin) tissue enzymes were obtained from tissues of pythons fasted and at 0.25 - 15 days post rodent consumption. Feeding triggered a 5.7- and 20-fold increase in peak activities of pancreatic trypsin and amylase, respectively; peak enzyme activities occurred from 2 - 4 days postprandially and values returned to fasting levels by day 10.[60] However, no plasma enzyme activities were determined in this study and the results are of uncertain relevance to clinical practice at this time. A transient postprandial increase in alanine aminotransferase was also reported in Burmese pythons in another study.[61]

Snake plasma contains bilirubin in addition to biliverdin; however, metabolic processing of bilirubin is slower in snakes than in mammals.[55] Information on snake bilirubin and biliverdin is scarce in the literature. Visibly green plasma consistent with hyperbiliverdinemia was reported in a diamond python with septic pneumonia.[62] Reported bilirubin values in snakes are commonly 0.2 mg/dL or less.[63,64]

BILE ACIDS

Cholic acid has been detected in many species and is likely the chief bile acid of snakes. Pythocholic acid, however, has not been found other than in pythons, and its nature was investigated based on the absence of a hydroxyl group at C-7.[65] The python liver makes cholic acid from cholesterol and conjugates this with taurine. Intestinal micro-organisms then remove the C-7 hydroxyl group and deoxycholic (3a, I za-dihydroxycholanic) acid or its taurine conjugate returns to the liver via enterohepatic circulation. The liver then inserts a new hydroxyl group at C-16a to give pythocholic acid, the taurine conjugate which functions as the chief bile salt in these species. Pythons appear unique in their possession of liver enzymes capable of C-16a hydroxylation of deoxycholic acid. The gall-bladder bile of pythons contains also some cholic acid that presumably has escaped microbial action.[65] The validity, sensitivity, and specificity of bile acids assays as a diagnostic for liver disease in some pythons and boids remains suspect as demonstrated by a recent case report of hepatic encephalopathy in a red-tailed boa (Boa constrictor imperator) with a plasma bile acids concentration of less than 35 Umol/L.[66]

GLUCOSE

In the viperid Bothrops jararaca, fasting glucose concentrations ranged from 47 to 64 mg % [mg/dL].[67] Intracoelomic injection of dextrose resulted in blood glucose elevations for 36 hrs, which were greater than in sham animals. Animals that were force fed meat did not demonstrate significant blood glucose elevations for days following feeding.[67] Total pancreatectomy of 84 colubrid Xenodon merremii yielded a decrease in blood glucose from an average of 44 mg/dL prior to surgery to an average of 26 mg/dL for 3 to 4 days. After this point, blood glucose gradually rose for approximately 60 days, with a peak of 295 mg/dL. In animals in which approximately 85% of the pancreas was removed, variations in blood glucose were not appreciated.[68] Significant increases in glucose were not identified post-prandially in Burmese pythons.[62]

LIPIDS

A study of Burmese pythons (Python molurus bivittatus) measured and reported pre- and post-prandial concentrations of total triglycerides, low density lipoprotein (LDL) triglycerides, total cholesterol, very low density lipoprotein (VLDL) cholesterol, LDL cholesterol, and high density lipoprotein cholesterol.[68] Post-prandial VLDL/chylomicron triglycerides were measured but pre-prandial values were not available for comparison. The total triglyceride and LDL triglyceride concentrations increased substantially, with an 88-fold increase in total triglycerides observed on day three post-feeding; significant decreases were identified on day ten post-feeding. Cholesterol values did not change substantially in response to feeding.[61]

SUMMARY

Clinicopathologic work up of boas and pythons has the potential to provide valuable clinical information for veterinarians overseeing individual cases and managing populations. However, a substantial amount of methodical research following ASVCP guidelines is needed to maximize the depth, reliability, and value of such testing.

Practitioners are encouraged to reach out to institutions about unique or unusual cases to broaden investigational opportunities and build material for case series publications.

CLINICS CARE POINTS

- Clinicians should critically evaluate the source populations of published reference ranges before utilizing values for patient assessment.
- At this time, there is no anticoagulant preference (lithium heparin vs EDTA) for CBCs in pythons and boas.
- Protein electrophoresis should be utilized for accurate measurement of albumin concentrations in boas and pythons.

REFERENCES

1. Alethinophidia N. Integrated Taxonomic Information System – Report. 1923. Available at: https://www.itis.gov/servlet/SingleRpt/SingleRpt?search_topic=TSN&search_value=634390#null. Accessed November 11, 2021.
2. Lloyd M, Morris PJ. Phlebotomy techniques in snakes. Bull Assoc Rept Amph Vet 1999;9(4):30–2.
3. Saggese MD. Clinical approach to the anemic reptile. J Exot Pet Med 2009;18(2): 98–111.
4. Sykes JM, Klaphake E. Reptile hematology. Clin Lab Med 2015;35:661–80.
5. Bonnet X, El Hassani MS, Lecq S, et al. Blood mixtures: impact of puncture site on blood parameters. J Comp Physiol B 2016;186:787–800.
6. Harr KE, Raskin RE, Heard DJ. Temporal effects of 3 commonly used anticoagulants on hematologic and biochemical variables in blood samples from macaws and Burmese pythons. Vet Clin Pathol 2005;34(4):383–8.
7. Campbell TW. Ch 20: Hematology of Reptiles. In: Thrall MA, Weiser G, Allison RW, et al, editors. Veterinary hematology and clinical Chemistry. 2nd edition. Ames (IA): John Wiley & Sons, Inc; 2012. p. 277–97.
8. Bryant GL, Fleming PA, Twomey L, et al. Factors affecting hematology and plasma biochemistry in the southwest carpet python (*Morelia spilota imbricata*). J Wildl Dis 2012;48(2):282–94.
9. Chiodini RJ, Sundberg JP. Blood chemical values of the common boa constrictor (*Boa constrictor constrictor*). Am J Vet Res 1982;43(9):1701–2.
10. Jegede HO, Omobowale TO, Okediran BS, et al. Hematological and plasma chemistry values for the African rock python (*Python sebae*). Int J Vet Sci Med 2017;5:181–6.
11. Friedrichs KR, Harr KE, Freeman KP, et al. ASVCP reference interval guidelines: determination of de novo reference intervals in veterinary species and other related topics. Vet Clin Pathol 2012;41(4):441–53.
12. Campbell TW. Exotic animal hematology and cytology. 4th edition. Ames (IA): John Wiley & Sons, Inc; 2015.
13. Harvey JW. Atlas of Veterinary Hematology: blood and bone marrow of domestic animals. Philadelphia: Saunders; 2001. p. 9–11.
14. Heatley JJ, Russell KE. Ch 33: Hematology. In: Divers SJ, Stahl SJ, editors. Mader's reptile and Amphibian medicine and surgery. 3rd edition. Saint Louis (MO): Elsevier Inc; 2019. p. 301–18.

15. Calle PP, Rivas J, Munoz M, et al. Health assessment of free-ranging anacondas (Eunectes murinus) in Venezuela. J Zoo Wildl Med 1994;25(1):53–62.

16. Schilliger L, Selleri P, Frye FL. Lymphoblastic lymphoma and leukemic blood profile in a red-tail boa (*Boa constrictor constrictor*) with concurrent inclusion body disease. J Vet Diagn Invest 2011;23:159–62.

17. Schilliger L, Rossfelder A, Bonwitt J, et al. Antemortem diagnosis of multicentric lymphoblastic lymphoma, lymphoid leukemia, and inclusion body disease in a boa constrictor (*Boa constrictor imperator*). J Herp Med Surg 2014;24(1–2):11–9.

18. Yan J, Margiocco ML, Strobel M, et al. Pericardial mesothelioma and associated pericardial effusion in a tiger rat snake (*Spilotes pullatus*) treated with pericardiocentesis. J Zoo Wildl Med 2020;51(4):1077–81.

19. Simpson M. Hepatic lipidosis in a black-headed python (*Aspidites melanocephalus*). Vet Clin Exot Anim 2006;9:589–98.

20. Steeil JC, Schumacher J, Hecht S, et al. Diagnosis and treatment of a pharyngeal squamous cell carcinoma in a Madagascar ground boa (*Boa madagascariensis*). J Zoo Wildl Med 2013;44(1):144–51.

21. Summa NM, Sanchez-Migallon Guzman D, Hawkins MG, et al. Tracheal and colonic resection and anastomosis in a boa constrictor (*Boa constrictor*) with T-cell lymphoma. J Herp Med Surg 2015;25(3–4):87–99.

22. Rodnan GP, Ebaugh FG Jr, Spivey Fox MR. The life span of the red blood cell and the red blood cell volume in the chicken, pigeon, and duck as estimated by the use of $Na_2Cr^{51}O_4$, with observations on red cell turnover rate in the mammal, bird, and reptile. Blood 1957;12(4):355–66.

23. Sypek J, Borysenko M. Ch 4: Reptiles. In: Rowley AF, Ratcliffe NA, editors. Vertebrate blood cells. Cambridge: Cambridge University Press; 1988. p. 211–56.

24. Stacy NI, Alleman AR, Sayler KA. Diagnostic hematology of reptiles. Clin Lab Med 2011;31:87–108.

25. Carvalho MPN, Queiroz-Hazarbassanov NGT, Massoco CO, et al. Flow cytometric characterization of peripheral blood leukocyte populations of 3 neotropical snake species: *Boa constrictor, Bothrops jararaca, Crotalus durissus*. Vet Clin Pathol 2016;45(2):271–80.

26. Johnson JH, Benson PA. Laboratory reference values for a group of captive ball pythons (*Python regius*). Am J Vet Res 1996;57:1304–7.

27. Machado CC, Silva LFN, Ramos PRR, et al. Seasonal influence on hematologic values and hemoglobin electrophoresis in Brazilian *Boa contrictor amarali*. J Zoo Wildl Med 2006;37(4):487–91.

28. Alleman AR, Jacobson ER, Raskin RE. Morphologic, cytochemical staining, and ultrastructural characteristics of blood cells from eastern diamondback rattlesnakes (*Crotalus adamanteus*). Am J Vet Res 1999;60(4):507–14.

29. Egami M, Sasso WS. Cytochemical observations of blood cells of *Bothrops jararaca* (Reptilia, Squamata). Revista Brasilieira de biologia. Rev Bras Biol 1998; 48(1):155–9.

30. Salakij C, Salakij J, Apibal S, et al. Hematology, morphology, cytochemical staining, and ultrastructural characteristics of blood cells in king cobras (*Ophiophagus hannah*). Vet Clin Pathol 2002;31:116–26.

31. Stacy N, Heard D, Wellehan J. Ch 8: Diagnostic sampling and laboratory tests. In: Girling S, Raiti P, editors. BSAVA manual of reptiles. 3rd edition. Quedgeley (England): British Small Animal Veterinary Association; 2019. p. 115–33.

32. Stacy NI, Harvey JW. Whip-like heterophils projections: Best in show. Vet Clin Pathol 2021;50:176–7.

33. Montali RJ. Comparative pathology of inflammation in the higher vertebrates (reptiles, birds and mammals). J Comp Pathol 1988;99:1–26.

34. Troiano JC, Vidal JC, Gould J, et al. Haematological reference intervals of the South American rattlesnake (*Crotalus durissus terrificus*, Laurenti, 1768) in captivity. Comp Haem Int 1997;1:109–12.

35. Stock GJ, Feltrer Y, Flach EJ, et al. Pathology in Practice: Blood smear from a diamond python (*Morelia spilota spilota*). J Am Vet Med Assoc 2013;243(9):1265–7.

36. McNamara TS, Cook TA, Behler JL, et al. Cryptococcosis in a common anaconda (*Eunectes murinus*). J Zoo Wildl Med 1994;25(1):128–32.

37. Jacobson ER, Adams HP, Geisbert TW, et al. Pulmonary lesions in experimental ophidian paramyxovirus pneumonia of Aruba Island rattlesnakes, *Crotalus unicolor*. Vet Pathol 1997;34:450–9.

38. Ortunho VV, de Oliveira e Souza L, Lobo RR, et al. [Hemoparasite in Sucuri of the species *Eunestes* [sic] *murinus*, at the Centro de Conservação da wild fauna of Ilha Solteira]. Spanish. Braz J Anim Hyg Health 2014;8(3):72–8.

39. Finnie EP. Lymphoid leucosis in an Indian python (Python molurus). J Path 1972; 107:295–7.

40. Sloboda M, Kamler M, Bulantova J, et al. A new species of *Hepatozoon* (Apicomplexa: Adeleorina) from *Python regius* (Serpentes: Pythonidae) and its experimental transmission by a mosquito vector. J Parasitol 2007;93(5):1189–98.

41. Allen KE, Yabsley MJ, Johnson EM, et al. Novel *Hepatozoon* in vertebrates from the southern United States. J Parasitol 2011;97(4):648–53.

42. Strik NI, Alleman AR, Harr KE. Ch 3. Circulating inflammatory cells. In: Jacobsen ER, editor. Infectious diseases and pathology of reptiles. Boca Raton (FL): Taylor & Francis Group, LLC; 2007. p. 167–218.

43. Chang L-W, Fu A, Wozniak E, et al. Immunohistochemical detection of a unique protein within cells of snakes having inclusion body disease, a world-wide disease seen in members of the families Boidae and Pythonidae. PLoS One 2013; 8(12):e82916.

44. Hyndman TH, Marschang RE, Bruce M, et al. Reptarenaviruses in apparently healthy snakes in an Australian zoological collection. Aust Vet J 2019;97:93–102.

45. Keller S, Hetzel U, Sironen T, et al. Co-infecting reptarenaviruses can be vertically transmitted in *Boa constrictor*. PLoS Pathog 2017;13(1):e1006179.

46. Simard J, Marschang RE, Leineweber C, et al. Prevalence of inclusion body disease and associated comorbidity in captive collections of boid and pythonid snakes in Belgium. PLoS ONE 2020;15(3):e0229667.

47. Melillo A. Applications of serum protein electrophoresis in exotic pet medicine. Vet Clin Exot Anim 2013;16:211–25.

48. Müller K, Brunnberg L. Determination of plasma albumin concentration in healthy and diseased turtles: a comparison of protein electrophoresis and the bromocresol green dye-binding method. Vet Clin Pathol 2010;39(1):79–82.

49. Andreasen CB, Latimer KS, Kircher IM, et al. Determination of chicken and turkey plasma and serum protein concentrations by refractometry and the biuret method. Avian Dis 1989;33:93–6.

50. Tsai I-T, Chi C-H, Yu P-H. Hematologic, plasma biochemical, protein electrophoretic, and total solid values of captive oriental turtle doves (*Streptopelia orientalis*). Zool Stud 2018;57:e11.

51. Katsoulos PD, Athanasiou LV, Karatzia MA, et al. Comparison of biuret and refractometry methods for the serum total proteins measurement in ruminants. Vet Clin Pathol 2017;46(4):620–4.

52. Proverbio D, Bagnagatti de Giorgi G, Della Peppa A, et al. Preliminary evaluation of total protein concentration and electrophoretic protein fractions in fresh and frozen serum from wild Horned Vipers (Vipera ammodytes ammodytes). Vet Clin Pathol 2012;41(4):582–6.

53. Leineweber C, Stohr AC, Ofner S, et al. Reference intervals for plasma capillary zone electrophoresis in Hermann's tortoises (*Testudo hermanni*) depending on season and sex. J Zoo Wildl Med 2019;50(3):611–8.

54. Leineweber C, Simard J, Kolesnik E, et al. Protein electrophoresis of plasma samples from boa constrictors with and without reptarenavirus infection. J Zoo Wildl Med 2020;51(2):350–6.

55. Divers SJ, Innis CJ. Ch 66: Urology. In: Divers SJ, Stahl SJ, editors. Mader's Reptile and Amphibian Medicine and Surgery. 3rd edition. Saint Louis (MO): Elsevier; 2019. p. 624–48.

56. Thornton AM, Schuett GW, Swift JA. Urates of colubroid snakes are different from those of boids and pythons. Biol J Linn Soc 2021;133:910–9.

57. Smeller JM, Slickers K, Bush M. Effect of feeding on plasma uric acid levels in snakes. Am J Vet Res 1978;39(9):1556–7.

58. Maixner JM, Ramsay EC, Arp LH. Effects of feeding on serum uric acid in captive reptiles. J Zoo Anim Med 1987;18(2–3):62–5.

59. Mason AK, Perry SM, Mitchell MA. Plasma and tissue enzyme activities of banded water snakes (*Nerodia fasciata*) and diamondback water snakes (*Nerodia rhombifer*). Am J Vet Res 2022;83(1):1–10.

60. Cox CL, Secor SM. Matched regulation of gastrointestinal performance in the Burmese python, *Python molurus*. J Exp Biol 2008;211:1131–40.

61. Magida JA, Tan Y, Wall CE, et al. Burmese pythons exhibit a transient adaptation to nutrient overload that prevents liver damage. J Gen Physiol 2022;154(4): e202113008.

62. Divers SJ. Ch 67: Hepatology. In: Divers SJ, Stahl SJ, editors. Mader's Reptile and Amphibian Medicine and Surgery. 3rd edition. Saint Louis (MO): Elsevier; 2019. p. 640–68.

63. Noonan NE, Olsen GA, Cornelius CE. A new animal model with hyperbilirubinemia: the indigo snake. Dig Dis Sci 1979;24(7):521–4.

64. Lamirande EW, Bratthauer AD, Fischer DC, et al. Reference hematologic and plasma chemistry values of brown tree snakes (*Boiga irregularis*). J Zoo Wildl Med 1999;30(4):516–20.

65. Bergstrom S, Danielsson H, Kazuno T. The metabolism of bile acids in python and constrictor snakes. J Biol Chem 1960;235(4):983–8.

66. Di Giuseppe M, Oliveri M, Morici M, et al. Hepatic encephalopathy in a red-tailed boa (*Boa constrictor imperator*). Abstract. J Exot Pet Med 2017;26(2):96–100.

67. Prado JL. Glucose tolerance test in Ophidia and the effect of feeding on their glycemia. Rev Can Biol 1946;5(5):564–9.

68. Houssay BA, Penhos JC, Lujan MA. Blood glucose changes in reptiles after total pancreatectomy. Acta Endocrinol 1960;35:313–23.